In the Name of Science

In the Name of Science

Issues in Responsible Animal Experimentation

F. BARBARA ORLANS

New York   Oxford
OXFORD UNIVERSITY PRESS
1993

Oxford University Press

Oxford   New York   Toronto
Delhi   Bombay   Calcutta   Madras   Karachi
Kuala Lumpur   Singapore   Hong Kong   Tokyo
Nairobi   Dar es Salaam   Cape Town
Melbourne   Auckland   Madrid

and associated companies in
Berlin   Ibadan

Copyright © 1993 by Oxford University Press, Inc.

Published by Oxford University Press, Inc.,
200 Madison Avenue, New York, New York 10016

Oxford is a registered trademark of Oxford University Press

Library of Congress Cataloging-in-Publication Data
Orlans, F. Barbara.
In the name of science : issues in responsible animal experimentation /
F. Barbara Orlans.
p.   cm.
Includes bibliographical references and index.
ISBN 0-19-507043-7
1. Animal experimentation—Moral and ethical aspects—Public policy.
I. Title.   HV4915.O75   1993
179'.4—dc20   92-39344

Parts of this book have been previously published by F. B. Orlans as follows:
Fig. 2.1 In: *Lab Animal* 1993:April issue. Fig. 3.1 In: Policy Issues in the Use of Animals in Research, Testing, and Education.
The Hastings Center Report Special Supplement, 1990:May/June:25–30. Chapter 6. In: Research Protocol Review for Animal
Welfare. *Investigative Radiology* 1987:22(3):253–258. Also, the section on prolonged water deprivation. In: Prolonged Water
Deprivation: A Case Study in Decision Making by an IACUC. *ILAR News* 1991:33(3):48–52. National Academy of Sciences,
Washington, D.C. Chapter 9. In: Animal Pain Scales in Public Policy. *ATLA* 1990:18:41–50. FRAME, Nottingham, U.K. Chapter
14 — various parts. In: Use of Animals in Education: Policies and Practices in the United States. *Journal of Biological Education*
1991:25(1):27–32. In: Debating Dissection: Pros, Cons, and Alternatives. *The Science Teacher* 1988:November:36–40. National
Science Teachers Association, Washington, D.C. Also in: Editorial Responsibilities. *CBE Views* 1993:16(1):3–7. Council of
Biology Editors, Chicago, IL.

9 8 7 6 5 4 3 2 1

Printed in the United States of America
on acid-free paper

To
Herb:

I can no other answer make but thanks,
And thanks, and ever thanks.

Twelfth Night

Preface

Some thirty years ago, I was drawn into the examination of animal welfare issues by a deeply troubling experience. In the late 1950s, I was working as an animal researcher at the National Institutes of Health on developing new drugs for heart disease. I was interested in biology education, and so visited a local science fair where I saw exhibits of teenage student projects. Among some laudable projects, I also saw a number that involved substantial animal pain and lingering death and that had been performed in students' bedrooms or basements. Typical was a project in which a thirteen-year-old student had put a guinea pig into a shoe box and then had blown in cigarette smoke until the animal suffocated and died. This was supposed to be educational in demonstrating the deleterious effects of nicotine. On further investigation, I found that such projects were common nationwide. Some were even more inhumane. What I was seeing was mainstream biology "education" of that day. I could not walk away from this situation, and so began my involvement with humane issues of animal experimentation.

At first, I thought it would be a simple matter to establish policies and enforcement procedures that would prohibit such projects. It was not that I was against the study of living organisms in the classroom, nor was I against animal experimentation when conducted by well-trained, professional scientists to discover new knowledge that had a social purpose. But I thought that reasonable limits should be set. After all, rules had been established over a hundred years ago for student projects involving animals, yet these rules, still valid today, were being blatantly ignored.

To my surprise, when I proposed changes, I encountered a harsh environment. I found that some members of the medical research and teaching community could see nothing wrong with what was going on (indeed they were directly involved since they were the judges and awarded the prizes), and often those who saw something wrong were not prepared to do anything about it. This resistance served to reinforce my resolve.

Slowly, and with a great deal of effort, some improvements were finally made. It took thirty years and many further episodes of improper animal use before a professional biology teachers' association established a policy to deal effectively with these issues. The policies have yet to be enforced nationwide, so the problems are not yet solved.

I learned much along the way. Reforms do not come easily; setting limits — a worthy objective — is hard to achieve. Each step of the way is a struggle against a weight of resistance to any change in the status quo. The case for change must be argued convincingly; examples of current problems have to be repeatedly brought forward even though there are costs in so doing; reasonable, achievable alternatives to accomplish the same purpose but which avoid the objectionable aspects have to be suggested and demonstrated to be effective, the climate of opinion has to be congenial, and the benefits of change must be recognized within the biomedical and teaching professions. All this takes a long time.

A major obstacle to any reform in this field is the polarization of viewpoints — the issues are usually argued in terms of total approval or total disapproval of animal experimentation: there is no middle ground, for myself, I find both ends of the spectrum equally implausible — that all animal experimentation is evil or that all animal experimentation is good. Cannot some ground of mutual trust and respect be established by the polarized groups? I would like to think so. This text seeks to stake out an area between the extremes of banning all animal experimentation and the other extreme of obstructing every reform that is suggested. This book does not claim to be the last word on the issue; it seeks only to promote a more reasonable dialogue.

Over the years, I have become increasingly involved not just in the use of animals in education, but in the use of animals in all scientific endeavors, especially in research and testing, as well as in the historical, moral, and policy-making aspects of the treatment of animals by human beings. As a scientist who participated in research in which animals were used, I am fully aware of the usefulness of animal subjects, if not of their current indispensability in some situations. I have also become aware of the abuses that have sometimes been carried out in the name of science. But the legitimacy of animal experimentation is not at issue in this book. My focus is on such questions as: How much societal voice should there be in what goes on in a laboratory? By what mechanism should this input be made? What policies can best serve the current state of the art of animal experimentation and what practices should be curbed or encouraged without harming the scientific enterprise? And what are the ethical aspects of animal experimentation in which the voice of society at large — or its many voices — should be taken into account?

This book, the result of years of thinking about the issues and trying to become sensitive to many points of view, is about setting limits. One of its main purposes is to make recommendations for policy changes that are achievable within the foreseeable future and that would improve the lot of animals used for experimentation without hampering the scientific process. The normative standards presented fit an animal welfare perspective with a moral conviction that alternatives to harming and killing animals should be vigorously pursued. I recognize that current social standards are such that animals are quite often killed or harmed for human purposes, but public acceptance does not necessarily make it right. For me, a reasonable way of looking at these issues is to ask the question. "Can the harms be reduced?"

In 1976, the late W. Lane Petter of Cambridge Unversity and an influential figure in establishing standards for animal experiments wrote: "If man is motivated to discover new knowledge, subscribing to the severe intellectual discipline of the scientist, but at the same time ignores the existence of moral principles that may moderate his pursuit, he may run the risk of vitiating his originally altruistic motivation. The question is, therefore, not whether experimentation should recognize restraints, but what restraints should be recognized."[1] This book seeks to identify and explore what restraints should be recognized.

Washington D.C.   F. B. O.
March 22, 1993

---

[1]Lane Petter, W., 1976. The ethics of animal experimentation. *J. Med. Ethics* 2:118–26.

Acknowledgments

Many people made significant contributions to this book by discussing issues with me and by critically commenting on the manuscript. Their suggestions and perspectives have been invaluable. My sincere thanks go to the following:

Michael Balls, Tom L. Beauchamp, John E. Cooper, Richard L. Crawford, Anthony J. DeLucia, Peter A. Doris, R. G. Frey, Stephen D. Gettings, Michael A. Giannelli, Rosalina V. Hairston, Frederic L. Holmes, Edward J. Huth, B. Julie Johnson, Hugh LaFollette, Susan E. Lederer, Timothy D. Mandrell, John McArdle, David B. Morton, John Miller, David G. Porter, Tom Regan, Jenny Remfry, Harriet Ritvo, Harry C. Rowsell, Christine Stevens, Joyce Tischler, Farol N. Tomson, and Manfred Zimmermann.

Also, I wish to thank the many people too numerous to mention individually — government officials and persons who serve on national policy-making bodies — who have kept me informed about national policies on animal experimentation in other countries, Canada, UK, Australia, the Netherlands, Denmark, Sweden, New Zealand, and elsewhere.

My gratitude goes to Jeremy Stone who sparked the events that allowed me to devote full-time to animal welfare issues. He has provided unswerving support.

Especial thanks go to my husband, Herbert C. Morton. He has provided expert advice, constant encouragement, and keen insightful analysis. The innumerable discussions we have enjoyed on animal topics over the years have helped to sharpen and clarify my own thinking and his reading of the manuscript has been a major contribution.

I started writing this book during residence as a scholar at the Rockefeller Foundation's Study Center in Bellagio, Italy. I wish to thank the Foundation for this support. Also, I am indebted to the Kinnoull Foundation for their continued encouragement and financial help.

Contents

In the Name of Science

1

The Beginnings of Institutionalized Animal Experimentation: Nineteenth-Century Highlights

Animal experimentation has been an issue of intense public controversy for the past two centuries. In the early nineteenth century, animal experiments emerged as an important method of science and marked the birth of experimental physiology and neuroscience as we know it today; they also marked the birth of the antivivisection movement. By the end of the century, vivisection, which Claude Bernard defined as "the art of carrying observation to the deep-seated organs of animals," had become institutionalized—it is now an established approach. The ethical and political issues raised in the nineteenth century remain alive today.

Before the nineteenth century, there had been some animal experimentation, but it was not widespread. The first recorded use of live animals was the study of body humors by Erasistratus in Alexandria in the third century B.C. Later, the physician Galen (A.D. 129–200) used live pigs to investigate the effects of severance of various nerves and also to demonstrate the position of the ureter. His influence in the history of medicine persisted until the thirteenth century. The Renaissance sparked a new interest in scholarship. Andreas Vesalius (1514–1564) conducted a number of experiments on monkeys, swine, and goats, from which he made remarkably accurate anatomical drawings, and challenged some of Galen's by now outworn concepts. Among other scholars who conducted animal experiments were Francis Bacon (1561–1626), William Harvey (1578–1657) (whose studies on live deer and many other species of animals contributed to his important discovery of blood circulation), René Descartes (1596–1650), Anthony van Leeuwenhoek (1632–1723), and Stephen Hales (1677–1761).

From the late seventeenth century through the eighteenth century, a strong tradition emerged in England and in France of animal experimentation based on the notion that animals are incapable of feeling pain. The way had been paved for this view by the influential French philosopher Descartes, whose ideas have persisted into the twentieth century. He said. "The greatest of all the prejudices we have retained from our infancy is that of believing that the beasts think" (Descartes, 1989). He likened animals to machines; according to this thinking, the cries of animals are like the ticking of a clock, no more.

Not everyone went along with this exclusion of animals from the universe of suffering creatures. Jeremy Bentham (1748–1832), the English Utilitarian philosopher, published a contrary view in his *Introduction to the Principles of Morals and Legislation* in 1789. In his most widely quoted passage on animals' rationality and capacity to feel pain, he argued that:

"a full grown horse or dog is beyond comparison a more rational, as well as a more conversable animal, than an infant of a day, or a week or even a month old. But suppose the cause were otherwise, what would it avail? The question is not, can they *reason?* Nor, can they *talk?* but can they suffer?" (Bentham, 1962).

The Utilitarians under Bentham formalized this concern by making pain and pleasure the main criteria of morality. Bentham's words and ideas about the evil of pain captured the imagination of people of his time; they continue to be influential to this day among philosophers and others who oppose Descartes' views.

However, it was not until the nineteenth century that these issues matured into major political concerns. Two French physiologists, François Magendie (1783–1855) and his pupil Claude Bernard (1813–1878), revolutionized methods of scientific discovery by establishing live animal experimentation as common practice. The experiments of both Magendie and Bernard attracted adverse public comment. It was in their wake that the antivivisection movement became formally organized on a national basis. Although the experiments were conducted in France, the protests occurred mainly in England, and it was here that the antivivisection movement first set its roots.

Nineteenth-century England saw the rise of humane and civilizing charity concerning many issues. The slave trade was abolished in Britain in 1807 and throughout the Empire in 1833. There was a movement to humanize the penal code and capital punishment was drastically reduced. The industrial revolution brought with it inhumane conditions in factories, but the Factory Acts brought some relief, at least with regard to the exploitation of children. A humanitarian concern was fostered by the peaceful times (broken only by the Crimean War), a moneyed class of increasing affluence, and the mistaken belief that pain could be easily banished with the advent of anesthesia. There were few external threats to distract the upper classes from considering the sufferings of others.

The antivivisectionists gained support because they could document the infliction of animal pain that was beyond the limits of public tolerance. Experimental
scientists also won public support by showing that animal experiments were
justified because of their scientific value. An endless bitter conflict arose, with
both sides taking an all-or-nothing approach.

What follows are some highlights of this early conflict. The period covered is
from the early nineteenth century up to the enactment of the landmark 1876
Cruelty to Animals Act in England, the first legislation in the world to regulate
the use of animals in research. The events of this period illustrate some enduring
attitudes encountered among scientists and the public concerning animal
experimentation.

Magendie's experiments and philosophy

François Magendie, (Figure 1.1), the pioneer nineteenth-century experimentalist,
was known as an impetuous, hard-working man. His contributions left a mark on
almost every branch of physiology.

In 1811, Magendie qualified in medicine at the University of Paris and worked
there for two subsequent years teaching surgery and physiology. After a falling
out with a powerful professor at the school, he was forced to find a means to
support himself. Magendie established a private laboratory where he conducted
research and ran a series of courses in experimental physiology for medical
students and others who paid to observe his animal experiments. It was not until
1830 that Magendie managed to reenter academia when he took up the chair of
experimental medicine at the College of France in Paris.

Magendie's animal experiments raised storms of controversy because of several intertwining issues. One was his emphasis on the revolutionary new scientific method of deduction from physiological experimentation which was in
direct conflict with the previous approach of deductive inference from anatomy.
The old methods of anatomical deduction, defended by prestigious establishment
scientists, proved hard to dislodge. This was a period beset with medicine men
and quackery; cures for ailments were based on anecdotal evidence. So the early
physiologists' emphasis on evidence by experimentation was a radical departure
from the past. After many decades the approach of Magendie and his followers
prevailed, and physiological experimentation became the prime method of biomedical science.

The morality of animal experiments was a major issue. In the vast majority of
Magendie's experiments, there was no limit to the amount of animal pain inflicted since most were conducted before the discovery of anesthetics in 1846. He
was 63 when the pain-killing effects of ether were first demonstrated at the
Massachusetts General Hospital in Boston. During the remaining nine years

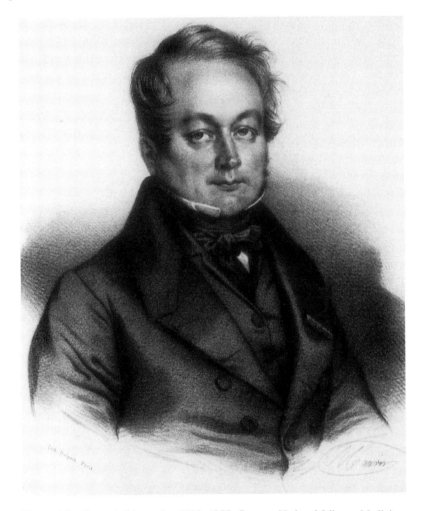

Figure 1.1   François Magendie, 1783–1855. Source: National Library Medicine.

before his death in 1855, he probably did start using anesthetics since Claude Bernard, who worked in the same laboratory, did.

Magendie and the spinal roots

The Cartesian disregard for animal suffering was evident in Magendie's work. A typical experiment was that of 1809 when Magendie investigated the absorption of poisons through various tissues of the body. According to Frederic L. Holmes, a historian of the period, Magendie isolated a section of the dog intestine so that it was attached to the rest of the body only by a single artery and vein (Holmes, 1974). This of course was done without anesthesia. Magendie injected various powerful poisons including prussic acid into the intestinal segment and found that the animal was poisoned just as if the normal connections had been intact. Holmes continues, "He obtained a similar result by injecting a leg detached except for its crural artery and vein. In 1820 he showed that a poison can be absorbed directly through the walls of a vein." The animals' deaths must have been excruciating.

In 1822, Magendie published a major discovery. In this paper (reprinted in Fulton, 1966), he described how he had experimented on a litter of eight puppies and then repeated the experiment on other species. The highly invasive procedures involved cutting through the skin and surrounding tissue to expose the spinal column, and then severing either separately or together the dorsal and ventral roots (bundles of nerves) as they enter and leave the spinal cord. Over the next few days Magendie observed the animals for the effects of loss in sensation and paralysis in affected limbs. He tested the animals by administering "nux vomica" (a dried seed extract comprised mainly of strychnine) to see if the well-known convulsions it causes would still occur. In this manner he established that the dorsal root carries sensory nerves into the spine and the ventral root carries motor nerves out of the spine. This finding was of great significance in helping to establish how the nervous system works.

The cost in animal suffering was high. The animals experienced convulsions and intense and protracted pain. In a publication of 1966, John Fulton, Sterling Professor of Physiology at Yale, judged Magendie's work to be "fearless, and at times unnecessarily cruel."

Not only were these experiments conducted in order to make the original discovery, but they were repeated many times in public demonstrations (see Figure 1.2). Such demonstrations were a feature of the times and brought monetary reward and prestige for the demonstrator. In 1824, Magendie visited London to give such a demonstration. He was greeted with an angry public outcry, and efforts were even made in the British Houses of Parliament to deport him for the cruelties witnessed (Olmsted, 1944a). The ensuing uproar also led to the first Parliamentary efforts to enact legislation in England to control animal experiments. Some fifty years later, when legislation finally did come, the 1876 Royal Commission report stated, "It is not to be doubted that inhumanity may be found in persons of very high position as physiologists. We have seen that it was so in Magendie" (quoted in French, 1975a).

Controversy within the scientific community

It was not only the public but also members of the scientific community who expressed hostility to Magendie's work. For instance, Sir Charles Bell, the

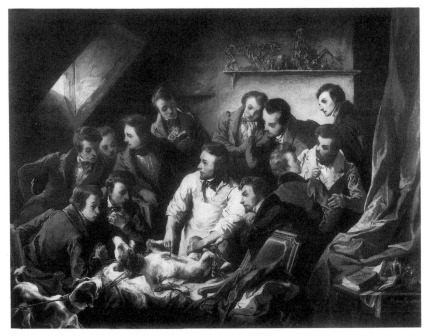

Figure 1.2   This depiction of an animal experiment is from an 1832 oil painting by Emile Edouard Mouchy. Wellcome Institute Library, London.

eminent English anatomist, openly declared his opposition, describing Magendie's work as "experiments without number or mercy" and "prosecuted with cruelty and indifference" (Gordon-Taylor and Walls, 1958).

Bell himself conducted only one animal experiment. He stated at that time, "I was deterred from repeating the experiment by the protracted cruelty of the dissection" (Bell, 1824). In a letter dated July 1, 1822, Bell stated, "I cannot perfectly convince myself that I am authorized in nature, or religion, to do these cruelties—for what?—for anything else than a little egotism or self-aggrandisement . . . " (quoted by Olmsted, 1944b).

Debate on the morality of animal experimentation appeared in the scientific literature of the day. For instance, the London Medical Gazette carried an editorial written by a physician who defended the general principle of animal experimentation "*under certain restrictions*" (emphasis in original) but criticized Magendie for his "profligacy and cruelty" (Anonymous, 1839). This physician judged Magendie's frequent repetition of experiments involving animal pain, the results of which were already well-known facts, as "odious."

This same author expressed an increasingly popular view that animal experiments are not only justified but laudable "if they lead to the good of mankind, by suggesting remedies for disease and pain." He anticipated the modern concept of alternatives by stating that the experimenter should never conduct animal experiments "till it is sufficiently clear that the fact pursued neither is, nor can be, proved by any other evidence which is within reach, nor by any more gentle mode of inquiry." Further, the experiment must be performed with the "least possible pain" and the animal "should be deprived of sensation." At that time, a common method for depriving an animal of sensation was stunning.

Additional criticism came from scientists who had personally visited Magendie's laboratory. French, who has written the definitive account of the vivisection controversy in nineteenth-century England, tells of an English physician, James Macaulay, who attended Magendie's classes in 1837 and described them as "revolting" (French, 1975b).

There is also an account of Magendie's classes by an American physician who, writing in The Medical Times, said, "At [Magendie's] first lecture, a basketful of live rabbits, a glass receiver full of frogs, two pigeons, an owl, several tortoises and a pup were victims ready to lay down their lives for the good of science! His discourse was to explain the function of the fifth pair of nerves. The facility was very striking with which the professor could cut the nerve at its origin, by introducing a sharp instrument through the cranium, immediately behind and below the eye. M. Magendie drew attention of the class to several rabbits in which the fifth pair of nerves had been divided several days before. They were all blind of one eye, a deposition of lymph having taken place in the cornea, from inflammation of the eye always following the operation. . . . M. Magendie had not lost all feeling for the victims he tortures, but he really likes his business. When the animal squeaks a little, the operator grins; when loud screams are uttered, he sometimes laughs outright" (Anonymous, 1840).

J.M.D. Olmsted, professor of physiology at the University of California and author of a biography of Magendie, rose to Magendie's defense. He stated that the American's "implied charge of sadism" should not go unchallenged (Olmsted, 1944c). Olmsted asserted that the "grins" and "laughs" were "automatic reactions caused by a desire to reassure spectators, whose discomfiture at evidences of pain or fright displayed by an experimental animal Magendie understood only too well." These forgiving remarks may help refute charges of sadism, but they leave unanswered Magendie's indifference to the suffering of experimental subjects.

Jeri Sechzer (1983), a psychologist at Cornell University, says that if Magendie had waited until anesthesia was discovered, "the delay in the critical discovery of the function of the spinal roots and the use of this finding may have been more costly to humans in the end." But she provides no amplification of this claim. The urgency of a scientific quest for knowledge has on occasion been invoked by scientists as an overriding factor that takes precedence over humane standards, but this is highly questionable. A contrary view is voiced by Hans Jonas (1969), a bioethicist: "Progress is an optional goal, not an unconditional commitment . . . and its tempo has nothing sacred about it . . . a slower progress in the conquest of disease would not threaten society . . . but would indeed be threatened by erosion of those moral values whose loss, possibly caused by the too ruthless a pursuit of scientific progress, would make its most dazzling triumphs not worth having." Although these words were used in the context of unethical human experimentation, they apply also, in my opinion, to unacceptable animal experimentation.

Bernard's animal experiments

What Magendie had started was brought to fruition by his pupil and successor Claude Bernard. Bernard was a brilliant scientist and his discoveries illuminated wide-ranging aspects of physiology. For instance, Bernard demonstrated that digestion is not completed in the stomach, as had been believed, but is continued in the intestine, and he investigated the function of various digestive juices. He described the "internal environment" or *milieu intérieur* of the body and paved the way for the discovery of hormones. In addition, he demonstrated that sympathetic nerves constrict blood vessels, thus laying down the fundamentals of vasomotor physiology.

At the height of his career in 1865, Bernard published his *Introduction to the Study of Experimental Medicine,* which brought him many accolades. "Never," wrote Louis Pasteur shortly after this book was issued, "has anything clearer, more complete, more profound been written about the true principles of the difficult art of experiment." By the end of his life, he had attained the highest honors attainable by a French man of letters.

The son of a winegrower, Bernard (Figures 1.3 and 1.4) was born in 1813 in St. Julien near Lyon. He achieved some success in his early years as a playwright before moving to Paris and turning to medicine. In 1841, while still a medical student, he became Magendie's assistant. After graduation, Bernard continued to work at the College of France and on Magendie's death in 1858 succeeded him in the chair of medicine.

At times, Bernard's animal research attracted unfavorable attention. Around 1844, a dog escaped from Bernard's laboratory and was found in the streets with a cannula protruding from its belly wall. Bernard was prosecuted and it was discovered that this dog belonged to the commissary of police from whom it had been stolen! Bernard recounts this episode, revealing that it was not he who had stolen the dog, but "persons who sold dogs to physiologists who said that they were employed by the police to collect stray animals" (Bernard, 1867, as quoted in Olmsted, 1938). Bernard had unwittingly experimented upon this pet animal, which he restored to full health and returned to its owner. Bernard was given a fair hearing at the trial and he managed to convince the commissary of police of the importance of his physiological experiments. He was lucky in this outcome. This episode illustrates that the public outrage about the use of people's pets for

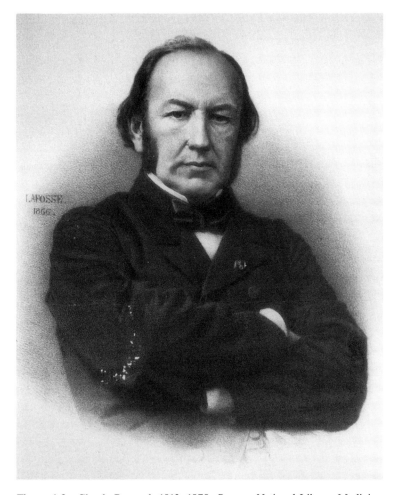

Figure 1.3   Claude Bernard, 1813–1878. Source: National Library Medicine.

experimental purposes—still a thorny issue today—goes back a long way and
that scientists may be held accountable for the animals they use.

At that time, laboratory conditions were poor. The experimental animals were
kept in a damp, gloomy basement. The apparatus Bernard used was constructed
by himself amid great difficulties. Dr. George Hoggan, who served four months
as a research assistant to Bernard, provided a scaring account of the conditions:
"[We] sacrificed daily from one to three dogs, besides rabbits and other animals. . . . I have witnessed many harsh sights, but I think the saddest sight I ever
witnessed was when the dogs were brought up from the cellar to the laboratory
for sacrifice. Instead of appearing pleased with the change from darkness to
light, they seemed seized with horror as soon as they smelt the air of the
place. . . . One of the most revolting features of the laboratory was the custom of

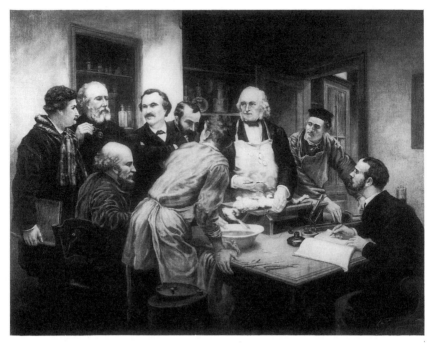

Figure 1.4 Claude Bernard in his laboratory. This 1889 anonymous oil painting, after Léon Augustin Lhermitte, is held by the National Academy of Medicine, Paris. Wellcome Institute Library, London.

giving an animal, on which the professor had completed the experiment, and which had still some life left, to the assistants to practice the finding of arteries, nerves, etc." (quoted in French, 1975c). For these training purposes, the more humane practice of using dead animals could have been substituted. It is not clear from the account in exactly what year the above events had happened, but Hoggan's remarks appeared in the *Morning Post* (an English newspaper) just one year before the enactment of the British legislation of 1876, and they helped fuel the fire for regulation.

Bernard's troubles regarding his animal experiments spilled over to his domestic life. Funding for some of his research had been provided by his wife, who was the daughter of a rich man. But his wife came to disapprove of his experiments because of the condition of the animals and the marriage subsequently fell apart. Vyvyan reports that one night in 1849 Bernard brought home a dog on which he had experimented that day, which had "pus running from its nostrils and an open wound in its side through which fluids were drawn off from time to time" (Vyvyan, 1988). Bernard's wife and two daughters joined the newly formed antivivisection movement and actively campaigned on the issue.

Curare experiments

Perhaps the most often cited example of Bernard's questionable use of experimental animals is the research he started in 1844 involving the deadly poison curare. At this period he was still with Magendie. A colleague and chemist, Theophile Jules Pelouze, gave Bernard several Indian hunting arrows tipped with curare. With no method of pain relief, Bernard administered this drug to conscious frogs, rabbits, and dogs, and then dissected out their nerve and muscle systems. Since curare causes paralysis of the whole body, surgery can be conducted with little trouble to the operator because no pain responses are manifest. But curare does not deaden pain perception, so these animals perceived full measure of pain. Finally, when the nerve-controlled respiratory muscles also became paralyzed, the animals died of asphyxiation.

From repeated experimentation, Bernard uncovered the mechanism of action of curare, which is to block transmission of nerve impulses to muscles. This finding was of fundamental significance. From Bernard's work emerged an understanding of how nerve impulses are transmitted and how they can be blocked.

These experiments would be impermissible by today's standards. Curare causes "the most atrocious suffering which the imagination can conceive," states Olmsted (1939). But one could argue that until Bernard uncovered the drug's action, he did not know how inhumane it is to administer curare to a conscious being. He could have mistaken the animals' quietness as a sign that they were not suffering. Judgments about the humaneness of the work have to be considered within the context of the state of knowledge at the time.

Some time after Bernard's experiments, it became generally recognized that curare should never be used alone, that it can only be humanely administered if the subject is under general anesthesia. Many of the early national policies on humane practices singled out curare for special mention and established strict rules for its use. This is true of policies of the United Kingdom, United States, Canada, and New Zealand, among other countries. Unusually strong language is found. For instance, Canada's current national policy speaks of the "excruciating pain" and "terrifying" effects of curare when used alone without an anesthetic (CCAC, 1980).

Experiments after the advent of anesthesia

Bernard did not suffer the intensity of criticism from the public and scientific community that Magendie had experienced. This was due in part to his attitude (which was not insensitive to the moral issues), but also to improved experimental techniques that reduced at least to some extent the amount of animal suffering.

Technical advances began to revolutionize the humaneness of surgery. According to Holmes, within months of the discovery of the anesthetic effects of ether, Bernard tested these effects on animals in January 1847 (Frederic L. Holmes, personal communication, February 26, 1990), but he did not immediately begin to use ether regularly. Probably there was a gradual increase in his use of it over the years. Also, based on the new discoveries of Pasteur in the 1860s, Bernard like others began to pay attention to antisepsis during surgery, which further contributed to the reduction of the pain associated with surgery.

The science of anesthesia was only in its infancy during Bernard's life, and using anesthesia did not necessarily mean that the experiments were devoid of pain. The practice was that volatile anesthetics (ether or chloroform) were applied by means of a sponge soaked in the liquid. These anesthetics are relatively short-acting. They might have been administered at the start of animal surgery but the effects could easily have worn off before completion of the procedure.

Bernard's attitude toward animal experimentation

In his classic work *An Introduction to the Study of Experimental Medicine,* Bernard (1865) addressed the issues of both human and animal experimentation. "Morals," he wrote, "do not forbid making experiments on one's neighbors or on one's self. . . . So, among the experiments that may be tried on man, those that can only harm are forbidden, those that are innocent are permissible, and those that may do good are obligatory."

Animal experimentation he addressed at some length. A chapter on vivisection contained these remarks: "Have we the right to make experiments on animals and vivisect them? As for me, I think we have that right, wholly and absolutely. It would be strange indeed if we recognize man's right to make use of animals in every walk of life, for domestic service, for food, and then forbade him to make use of them for his own instruction in one of the sciences most useful to humanity. No hesitation is possible: the science of life can be established only through experiment, and we can save living beings from death only after sacrificing others. Experiments must be made on man or on animals. Now I think that physicians already make too many dangerous experiments on man, before carefully studying them on animals. I do not admit that it is moral to try more or less dangerous or active remedies on patients in hospitals, without first experimenting with them on dogs; for I shall prove, further on, that results obtained on animals may all be conclusive for man when we know how to experiment properly . . . it is essentially moral to make experiments on an animal, even though painful and dangerous to him, if they may be useful to man" (Bernard, 1865). The "use to man" at that time was largely physiological knowledge. As Richards (1987b) points out, Bernard, writing toward the end of his life's work, "could apparently cite few examples of clinical application in concrete support of experimental medicine."

In this period of history, the continuity of biological function between humans and other animals was gaining acceptance. Charles Darwin's influence served to heighten this sense of continuity. With such words as *The Descent of Man* (1871) and *The Expression of the Emotions in Man and Animals* (1872), Darwin helped establish the close relationship of man to other animals. In this light, it is notable that Bernard set certain limits on his animal experimentation—he would not experiment on monkeys because of their resemblance to human beings. Yet he also said: "The physiologist is not an ordinary man: he is a scientist, possessed and absorbed by the scientific idea he pursues. He does not hear the cries of animals, he does not see their flowing blood, he sees nothing but his idea, and is aware of nothing but an organism that conceals from him the problem he is seeking to resolve" (Bernard, op. cit., chapter 2).

Some people find the Cartesian ring of these words chilling. Others would accept these remarks uncritically as merely descriptive of the passion of discovery. In any case, their truth reveals the all-too-real problems that investigators face in remaining always sensitive to what should be overriding humane demands.

What is clear is that Bernard was sensitive to the moral issues raised by animal experimentation, that he cannot be blamed for not using anesthetics for his curare work because no one knew the action of curare at that time, and that he did use anesthetics within months of the first demonstration of the pain-killing effects of ether. The limitations of humaneness in his animal experiments (such as using pet animals) must be judged within the limitations of his time.

Student handbook of physiology

Considerable public protest greeted the first English language manual for the physiological laboratory, which appeared in 1873. It was a two-volume work entitled *Handbook for the Physiologists,* edited by John Scott Burdon Sanderson, FRS, and authored by leading scientists. Sanderson was professor of physiology at University College, London, and he had at one time worked under Bernard. This book provides the "closest approximation available of what it was actually like to do physiology at the time" (Richards, 1987c). The book was taken to presage widespread animal experimentation for educational purposes. Its appearance was ominous to those concerned about the use of animals in research, who feared that unacceptable standards of animal experimentation were being fostered.

French (1975d) has written of the book that "Failing to specify the use of anesthetics, as it largely did, it gave no assurance as to the painless nature of such vivisection. Prefaced for 'Beginners,' as it was, it seemed to set no limits to callow youth being indoctrinated in animal experiments."

Many of the experiments included in this Handbook were in violation of recommended humane policy that had been issued by the British Association for the Advancement of Science in 1871. There were many infractions of the policy's first recommendation that "No experiment which can be performed under the influence of an anesthetic ought to be done without it." Not only was this policy not followed, it was not even referred to. Since Sanderson had actively participated in the development of this policy only two years before the Handbook's publication, its omission is revealing. (The policy's full text is given below in the section headed "Early Policies on Animal Experimentation.")

In analyzing the vertebrate experiments included in the Handbook, Richards (1987d), who is a physiologist, found a total of 120 experiments, of which 66 were calculated to give pain, in the section authored by Sanderson. Of these 66, 20 used anesthetics (for at least part of the time), 19 were performed under curare, and in 27 no mention was made of anesthetic use. In a section written by Emmanuel Klein, 179 experiments were described; 32 were calculated to give pain, none used anesthetics, and 6 were performed under curare. These are maximum figures based on the authors' failure to specify anesthesia; if, as the authors claimed, anesthetics were nevertheless often applied, the figures may exaggerate the number of painful experiments. Richards's study was funded by the Royal Society, and it forms part of an authoritative historical study of the rise of the antivivisection movement in the nineteenth century published by the *Wellcome Institute series in the History of Medicine.*

As a witness before the 1876 Royal Commission on animal experimentation, Sanderson defended the casualness of mention of anesthetics on the ground that it was "taken for granted" among physiologists that anesthetics would be used. (This unconvincing defense persists to this day. For instance, at an Upjohn conference in Kalamazoo, Michigan in 1985, A. Clifford Barger, MD, a Harvard professor of physiology and historian of nineteenth-century science, publicly stated that the authors of this 1873 work "forgot" to mention that anesthetics should be used).

Even more revealing than Sanderson's 1876 testimony was that of Klein. According to Richards, Klein testified that he never used anesthetics except for teaching purposes or for his own convenience—to prevent being bitten or scratched. Asked about his attitude to the suffering of animals, Klein answered at once, "No regard at all."

Surgical practice at Alfort Veterinary School

Sanderson's 1876 contention that anesthetics would be used whenever necessary can be challenged. Earlier reports had come from France that in the veterinary school at Alfort, near Paris, students practiced surgery skills on conscious, aged horses. Reports of these mutilated horses reached the RSPCA in England in the 1840s and protests appeared in the French and British press and in several British scientific journals. In *The Lancet* in 1860, the English physician Alfred Perry recounted what he had personally witnessed when he visited the Alfort veterinary school in order to make some anatomical drawings. "Every week old and worn out horses and mules are provided, and the students of the two senior classes commenced, soon after nine in the morning with slighter operations of bleeding from the neck and feet, nicking the tail . . . etc. At midday . . . [they] proceeded to perform the more serious operations of firing, lithotomy, neurotomy [respectively, burning with a hot iron, removal of stones, and dissection or cutting of a nerve] . . . and other operations equally painful. This lasted till near five in the afternoon when the classes were dismissed, and the animals, if not already dead from pain and loss of blood were dragged into the yard and destroyed." Perry tells how he remonstrated with the professor in charge who "admitted the cruelty" but defended the practices because it "accustomed the students to the shrinking of the animal when touched by the instruments; and it made them cool at operating."

In condemning these student experiments, Perry made the important distinction between experiments whose goal is to elucidate new physiological phenomena (which he believed were "perhaps excusable") and those that were student exercises, or drill, to render the students expert in the use of operating instruments. Perry called for abolition of these student exercises. He said they demoralized and brutalized the students.

The protests about Alfort veterinary school had a sympathetic reception from scientists and the public in England. The Society for the Protection of Animals, a London-based organization, petitioned the French government to take some action to rectify the situation. The government turned to the French Academy of Medicine, which formed a committee to address the matter.

The fact that the complaints had come from England exacerbated the situation. According to an anonymous 1863 editorial in the *British Medical Journal* (*BMJ*), the French Academy "was evidently much annoyed at the language of *perfide Albion,* and annoyed that complaints should have come from this side of the water." Out of all the committee members, only one, M. Dubois, an eminent pathologist, spoke up for reforms. M. Dubois had himself witnessed what he described as "atrocities" at Alfort. "[S]o pungent were [M. Dubois'] censures," said the *BMJ* writer, "that some of the academicians left the hall without waiting the end of his discourse. The veterinary part of his audience heard him to the end; and it is to be hoped profited by the picture he drew."

M. Dubois recommended that the Academy of Medicine make a statement that henceforth veterinary students practice their skills on "dead bodies, and no more on living horses." This recommendation was roundly defeated. Instead, the Academy passed a resolution stating:

The Academy declares that the complaints brought forward by the Society for the Protection of Animals are without foundation; that no notice need be taken of them; and that the performance of vivisections and of surgical operations, as practiced in the veterinary schools, should be left to the discretion (*sagesse*) of men of science.

The *BMJ* editorial scathingly remarked that the French Academy's action "is entirely opposed to the facts." The view expressed by the French Academy, that scientists should be left alone to determine their own affairs, finds its corollaries in today's attitudes. It is significant that this exclusion from public accountability, so evident in the Academy's remarks, was made in the face of complaints coming from members of their own community, from other scientists. M. Dubois, who spoke his conscience, was rebuffed by other Academicians.

Early policies on animal experimentation

The good that did come out of these sorry affairs was that the British scientific community responded with some sound policy recommendations. The British Association for the Advancement of Science issued a report in 1871 that sought to establish a code for physiological experiments involving animals. It was drawn up by eminent scientists of the day (including Sanderson, as previously mentioned). The recommendations were:

  i. No experiment which can be performed under the influence of an anesthetic ought to be done without it.
 ii. No painful experiment is justifiable for the mere purpose of illustrating a law or fact already demonstrated; in other words, experimentation without the employment of anesthetics is not a fitting exhibition for teaching purposes.
iii. Whenever, for the investigation of new truth, it is necessary to make a painful experiment, every effort should be made to ensure success, in order that the suffering inflicted may not be wasted. For this reason, no painful experiment ought to be performed by an unskilled person with insufficient instruments and assistance, or in places not suitable to the purpose, that is to say, anywhere except in physiological and pathological laboratories, under proper regulations.
 iv. In the scientific preparation for veterinary practice, operations ought not to be performed upon living animals for the mere purpose of obtaining greater operative dexterity   (French, 1975e).

These are important concepts, still valid today. Over a hundred years later, the enforcement of such a sensible code is still at issue. For a discussion of modern-day violations of this code, prevalent in some American secondary school science fair competitions, see chapter 12.

Provisions of the 1876 law and its aftermath

In the United Kingdom, decades of protests by the antivivisectionists, along with support coming from the scientific community for reasonable policies, set the stage for passage of legislation. It was the combined public and scientific support for control of animal experimentation that made legislation a reality. Many eminent Victorians, including Queen Victoria herself, the Roman Catholic leader Cardinal Newman, John Ruskin, and Charles Dodgson, author of *Alice's Adventures in Wonderland,* were among those who spoke out for strong legislation. They helped exert pressure on Benjamin Disraeli's conservative government.

The 1876 Cruelty to Animals Act embodied a compromise that sanctioned animal experiments but set limits on the amount of animal pain—it required that animal pain be kept to a minimum. The Act required the registration of places where animal experiments are conducted, thus limiting animal experimentation to designated places and effectively outlawing such private laboratories as that of Magendie. It also required the licensing of investigators and that all experiments had to be carried out under terminal anesthesia. However, exemptions were made through granting certificates. For instance, those experiments in which no anesthetics were to be given had one sort of certificate, those in which the animal would recover from anesthesia another sort, and so on. Record-keeping and reporting was required of licensees. The law remained unchanged for 110 years. By contrast, it was not until 1963 that the first French legislation controlling animal experiments was passed.

Disenchanted with the compromise, the nineteenth-century antivivisectionists immediately withdrew their support for the law. Frances Power Cobb, the leading antivivisectionist, said that the effect of the 1876 law would be to anesthetize the public, not the animals! This pattern of antivivisectionists' withdrawal of support of reform legislation has been repeated over and over again since then.

The next chapter will recount some controversies surrounding animal experimentation in the United States that led to the passage of the first American law on this issue.

2

Current Attitudes and Ethical Arguments

During the past century, animal experimentation has become an accepted method of scientific inquiry. Both the number of animals used and the number of people who conduct animal experiments have increased greatly—indeed, worldwide thousands of scientists are committed to helping human patients by means of experimental work involving animals. The humanitarian purpose is commanding. The uses of laboratory animals are more complex and the effect on human life greater than ever before. The human benefits from animal experimentation are more impressive. Also, an industry has been developed that helps to promote and sustain animal experimentation.

At the same time, public sympathy for animals and concerns about interference with their lives have increased. Many common human practices have been questioned—not only animal experimentation but also meat-eating, hunting, and the wearing of luxury furs. There has been mounting pressure to impose more stringent limits on human exploitation of animals. The battle over animal experimentation is now more intense because much more is at stake.

To lay the foundations for understanding the current situation, this chapter will address the range of current attitudes toward animals and the moral underpinnings of some human beliefs.

Attitudes

Human attitudes about animals range from love and reverence to indifference and hatred. Love does not necessarily translate into humane behavior. People who participate in bull or cock fighting may say that they love and admire the animals that they are responsible for brutally killing. People who exploit animals for their own purposes may claim that they really care about the animals they are harming. For instance, trophy hunters may claim that they care about the deer or antelope that they kill for sport. Those who seem indifferent do not necessarily condone suffering or cruelty. People's views about animals are often strongly held and are not usually subject to much modification, and strong views can engender antagonism against others who hold different beliefs.

How is it that views on animals have become so polarized? What are the fundamental attitudes that clash so violently that the various factions seem unable to live together without mistrust, denial of freedom to express views, and inability to appreciate the other person's point of view? Are our attitudes to animals so basic to our view of the world that they profoundly color our relationships with each other? Is it possible that with a greater understanding of these attitudes we could arrive at some diminution of the polarization of viewpoints?

Perhaps these questions are unanswerable, but at least some understanding of the range in viewpoints can be achieved. Figure 2.1 sketches five major points of view that are encountered in Western society. The categories overlap since such attitudes are a continuum. At one end of Figure 2.1 are the animal exploiters who believe that animals are our property and we can use them as we wish. At the other end are animal liberationists who hold that illegal and even violent actions are justified to prevent or stop animal suffering. At each end of this spectrum people are willing to break the law (item 5). The other groups identified—animal use, animal welfare, and animal rights—hold various attitudes toward the law— they either want less or more regulation and legislation.

The polarization of views that has occurred presents a false black-and-white view of available alternatives. Instead of five or more major viewpoints, the major protagonists commonly recognize only two. Thus, the animal users and animal exploiters and abusers are treated by their critics as a single group while all those who espouse animal welfare, animal rights, and animal liberation are forced into another group. The rhetoric of the antagonists often becomes extreme in its anger and unfairness. Among the resulting distortions are (1) that animal experimenters are all portrayed as insensitive persons who use animals as tools, and (2) that animal advocates are all portrayed as anti-science and anti-intellectual terrorists.

Both (1) and (2) are false. Common sense tells us that there are many compassionate and responsible animal experimenters and many sensible and responsible animal advocates. In fact, the major humane societies and leaders of the animal rights movement have made public statements deploring the violence that has emerged in some of the laboratory raids. Many researchers have sought to minimize and reduce unnecessary use of animals. Obviously, there are many people in the middle who agree with some, but not all, animal experimentation,

Attitudes to Animals: An Overview of Animal-Related Organizations
A Preliminary Classification

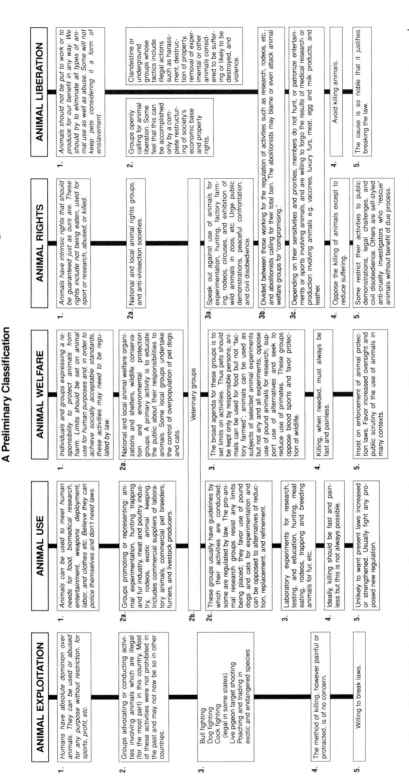

	ANIMAL EXPLOITATION	ANIMAL USE	ANIMAL WELFARE	ANIMAL RIGHTS	ANIMAL LIBERATION
1.	Humans have absolute dominion over animals. They can be used or abused for any purpose without restriction, for sports, profit, etc.	Animals can be used to meet human needs for food, biomedical research, entertainment, weapons deployment, labor, and clothes etc. Believe they can police themselves and don't need laws.	Individuals and groups expressing a responsibility to protect animals from harm. Limits should be set on animal use for human purposes and, in order to achieve socially acceptable standards, these activities may need to be regulated by law.	Animals have intrinsic rights that should be guaranteed just as ours are. These rights include not being eaten, used for sport or research, abused, or killed.	Animals should not be put to work or to produce for our benefit in any way. We should try to eliminate all types of animal use as well as abuse. Some will not keep pets considering it a form of enslavement.
2.	**2a.** Groups advocating or conducting activities involving animals which are illegal (for the most part) in this country. Most of these activities were not prohibited in the past and may not now be so in other countries.	**2a.** Groups promoting or representing: animal experimentation, hunting trapping and fur industry, meat and poultry industry, rodeos, exotic animal keeping. Includes commercial suppliers of laboratory animals, commercial pet breeders, furriers, and livestock producers. **2b.**	**2a.** National and local animal welfare organizations and shelters, wildlife conservation and environmental protection groups. A primary activity is to educate the public about their responsibilities to animals. Some local groups undertake the control of overpopulation of pet dogs and cats. **2b.** Veterinary groups	**2a.** National and local animal rights groups, and anti-vivisection societies.	Groups openly calling for animal liberation. Some feel that this can be accomplished only by a complete restructuring of society's economic base and property rights.
3.	Bull fighting Dog fighting Cock fighting (legal in some states) Live pigeon target shooting Poaching and trading in exotic and endangered species	**2c.** These groups usually have guidelines by which their activities are conducted; some are regulated by law. The pro-animal research groups resist any limits being placed; they favor use of pound dogs and cats for experimentation and can be opposed to alternatives of reduction, replacement, and refinement. **3.** Laboratory experiments for research, testing, and education, hunting, meat eating, rodeos, trapping and breeding animals for fur, etc.	The broad agenda for these groups is to set limits on activities. Thus pets should be kept only by responsible persons; animals can be used for food but not "factory farmed"; animals can be used as subjects of selected animal experiments but not any and all experiments; oppose use of pound animals for research; support use of alternatives and seek to reduce use of primates. These groups oppose blood sports and favor protection of wildlife.	**3a.** Speak out against use of animals for experimentation, hunting, factory farming, rodeos, circuses, and exhibition of wild animals in zoos, etc. Urge public demonstrations, peaceful confrontation, and civil disobedience. **3b.** Divided between those working for the regulation of activities such as research, rodeos, etc. and abolitionists calling for their total ban. The abolitionists may blame or even attack animal welfare groups for "compromising." **3c.** Depending on their sensitivities and priorities, members do not hunt, or patronize entertainments or sports involving animals, and are willing to forgo the results of medical research or production involving animals e.g. vaccines, luxury furs, meat, egg and milk products, and leather.	Clandestine or underground groups whose tactics include illegal actions such as harassment, destruction of property, removal of experimental or other animals considered to be suffering or likely to be destroyed, and violence.
4.	The method of killing, however painful or protracted, is of no concern.	Ideally, killing should be fast and painless but this is not always possible.	Killing, when needed, must always be fast and painless.	Oppose the killing of animals except to reduce suffering.	Avoid killing animals.
5.	Willing to break laws.	Unlikely to want present laws increased or strengthened. Usually fight any proposed new regulation.	Insist on enforcement of animal protection laws. Favor increased oversight and public scrutiny of the use of animals in many contexts.	Some restrict their activities to public demonstrations, legal challenges, and civil disobedience. Others are self-styled anti-cruelty investigators who "rescue" animals without benefit of due process.	The cause is so noble that it justifies breaking the law.

Figure 2.1 This classification is a first approximation to highlight the differences among major points of view. The categories overlap. In reality, the value judgments are a continuum, so this chart, with its sharp lines of demarcation, is an oversimplification. The box numbers refer to (1) statement of belief, (2) groups represented, (3) activities, (4) attitude to killing, and (5) attitude to the law. This classification is based on a ... of Katherine D. Mason, a former editor and publisher, and with her permission has been substantially revised.

who believe that laws are reasonable, and who favor public accountability for what goes on inside labs.

Rancor is not limited to the extremists. One might have thought that adjacent groups in Figure 2.1 would share a closer perspective than those more distant and would therefore be more friendly, but this is not necessarily so. For instance, a great political divide separates the animal users from the animal welfarists. Scientists who espouse the animal welfare perspective can suffer rejection from the scientific community—they are perceived as having "gone over to the other side." Also, with varying degrees of intensity, the animal rights activists and animal liberationists attack not only the animal exploiters and animal users but also the animal welfarists for their more moderate stand on issues. These tensions will be explored further in subsequent chapters.

What is clear is that over the last couple of decades there has been a considerable swing of public opinion toward the animal welfare and animal rights perspectives though the support for animal experimentation has continued to be strong. Public opinion surveys in recent years have tended to show that about 60 to 80 percent of the population favors some animal experimentation. For instance, a survey conducted in 1985 by Medic General Research Survey asked 1,421 adults questions concerning the uses of animals in different areas of research. When the respondents were asked if animals are necessary for studying health problems, including research on cancer, heart disease, and diabetes, 81 percent agreed that animals could be used for these studies, 12 percent said that animals should not be used, and 7 percent did not know. However, when asked about using animals to study less threatening ailments, such as allergies, only 61 percent believed animals should be used.

In a 1989 survey conducted by the Gallup Organization and commissioned by the AMA, some 77 percent of the 1,500 adults surveyed agreed with the statement that the use of animals in biomedical research is necessary for progress in medicine, 17 percent disagreed, and 6 percent were unsure. A somewhat smaller group, 64 percent said they actually support the use of animals in biomedical research, 29 percent opposed it, and 6 percent were unsure.

Over time, surveys in general have indicated an upswing in public sympathy toward animals. For instance, a recent poll found that 80 percent of the American public agrees with the statement that animals have rights that should limit how humans use them. (*Parents Magazine* commissioned a random poll of American adults which it published in May, 1990.) The majority of those polled believed that certain activities were not only wrong but should be made illegal: 63 percent said that killing animals to make fur coats should be prohibited by law and 58 percent said using animals for cosmetics research should be illegal. On the other hand, 85 percent of respondents said it is acceptable to kill animals for food, and 58 percent approved using animals for medical research. When people were asked if they would favor using animals for research if that were the only way to find a cure for AIDS, the approval rating went up to 78 percent.

Beliefs: moral views about animal experimentation

Over recent decades, moral views about animal experimentation have been much debated and a number of new theories have been put forward. But this field is in its infancy; a consensus is yet to be reached on who or what has moral standing and what is the nature of the moral relationship between humans and animals. Can ethical principles of animal experimentation be worked out that would gain widespread public acceptance? If some basic generalizable ethical principles could be established that set limits on animal experiments, then public policy could be built around them.

By contrast, on some other bioethical issues, after much deliberation, philosophers, ethicists, and physicians have reached a rough consensus that meets with general acceptance. They have agreed, for example, that a human subject of scientific experimentation must provide informed consent before the experiment starts, must be allowed to withdraw from the experiment at any time without penalty, and must be accorded certain other important protections. Ethical debate has also helped establish a consensus that competent adult human patients have a right to refuse medical treatment.

The following section provides a brief summary of some contending and often incompatible ethical theories that could be used for defining ethical principles for animal experimentation. The views presented are those of two philosophers who oppose animal experimentation (Peter Singer and Tom Regan), two who uphold it (Carl Cohen and R. G. Frey), and the kinship views of Mary Midgley.

The recent rise of the animal rights movement dates back to Peter Singer's publication in 1975 of his revolutionary book *Animal Liberation*. This important book changed the way many of us look at animals; it inspired a worldwide movement. By 1989, over 300,000 copies of Singer's book had been sold and it had been translated into five languages; in 1990 a second edition was published. Other philosophers soon followed with significant challenges to long-held views about the moral relationship between people and animals.

Singer's book found a receptive audience. It appeared on the heels of the civil rights movement of the 1960s and the women's liberation movement. There had also been a rise in concern over medical experimentation on vulnerable groups starting with the shocking revelations of the Nazi experiments on prisoners and later concerning American experiments on syphilitic patients, those terminally ill with cancer, and the mentally disabled. A new field of bioethics had emerged, mainly led by philosophers and ethicists who developed arguments and guidelines to protect the rights of humans used as subjects of experiments. Now Singer's book extended the compass of concern to animals as well.

Ethical views opposing animal experimentation

Singer challenged many current views about animals. He rejected Descartes's view that we can treat animals as we like because they are without sensations. Singer argued that animals have feelings, desires, and preferences and that their moral status should be based on their capacity to suffer or experience pleasure. He observed that stimuli that cause pain to humans (such as hitting, burning, and so on) cause pain to animals. However, the capacity to experience pain and to suffer varies—animals higher on the phylogenetic scale (above mollusks, he thought) are capable of perceiving pain. He argued that these higher animals, like humans, share an interest in not being subjected to pain.

His position is not, as is often mistakenly supposed, that animals are equal in moral status to humans; it is that equal harms should be counted equally and not downgraded for animals. Nor is he arguing that equal stimuli cause the same amount of pain in each species. "If I give a horse a hard slap across its rump with my open hand, the horse may start, but it presumably feels little pain. Its skin is thick enough to protect it against a mere slap. If I slap a baby in the same way, however, the baby will cry and presumably does feel pain, for its skin is more sensitive. So it is worse to slap a baby than a horse, if both slaps are administered with equal force. But there must be some kind of blow—I don't know exactly what it would be, but perhaps a blow with a heavy stick—that would cause the horse as much pain as we cause a baby by slapping it with our hand. This is what I mean by 'the same amount of pain' and if we consider it wrong to inflict that much pain on a baby for no good reason then we must, unless we are speciesists, consider it equally wrong to inflict the same about of pain on a horse for no good reason" (Singer, 1975, page 17). "The animal liberation movement is NOT saying that all lives are of equal value," Singer says, but that equal interests (such as not being hurt) count equally. "A simple point, no doubt, but nevertheless part of a far-reaching ethical revolution."

The word *speciesism,* first coined by Richard Ryder of the Royal Society for the Prevention of Cruelty to Animals, is like racism and sexism, says Singer. Species membership—considered solely as such—is as morally irrelevant as race or gender. Racism and sexism fail to accord equal consideration to equally significant interests and are morally wrong. By similar reasoning, human undervaluation or disregard of the central interests of other species is also morally wrong. "To discriminate on the basis of species is really fundamentally just the same moral mistake as discrimination on the basis of race or sex," he says.

The bulk of Singer's book documents the abusive treatment of animals in "factory" farms, and in medical, psychological, and commercial research. His views supporting vegetarianism are also explained. (One review of his book noted that it is perhaps the only philosophical work that includes recipes.)

Animals have rights

Another type of ethical argument against animal experimentation is made by Tom Regan, professor of philosophy at North Carolina State University. He is the leading proponent of the position that animals have "rights"—the right to be treated in a certain way, an assertion that implies a great claim (Regan, 1982, 1983, and 1987). To assert that some entity has a "right" is powerful language. It immediately sets strict boundaries on what can be done to that entity. Animal advocates have in general adopted this language to make claims and demands.

Animals have a basic moral right to respectful treatment, says Regan. Animals have preferences, goals, and desires; they have mental states that enter into the explanation of their behavior. In Regan's words, animals are "subjects of a life" just as human beings are, and a subject of a life has "inherent value." They are, in Kant's sense, ends in themselves. This inherent value is not respected when animals are reduced to being mere tools in a scientific experiment. To conduct any animal experiment is morally wrong no matter how much humans may benefit from the results because the animal's basic right has been infringed. "Risks [such as being given a toxic substance] are not morally transferable to those who do not choose to take them" says Regan. He thinks the morally sound way to proceed is to develop alternative ways of testing toxic substances that will not infringe animal rights, perhaps using cell and tissue cultures.

Regan establishes a strong set of boundaries to protect weak and vulnerable subjects. He holds that special protections should be accorded to vulnerable groups of human beings (such as the mentally disabled, the insane, prisoners, children, and fetuses). If retarded and insane human beings have moral rights— as Regan thinks they do—to live their lives without being used as tools of science, then so do mammals. He argues that higher mammals are at least as sophisticated mentally as cognitively deficient human beings who are accorded both moral and legal rights. These "marginal cases" provide a view that mammals should be accorded rights just as are mentally handicapped human beings.

Singer's and Regan's views in support of the animal rights movement have met with some public acceptance. People have been drawn to Singer's appeal against domination and exploitation of any kind and to Regan's ideas that animals have inherent value and that vulnerable subjects deserve protection. By now, many other philosophers have contributed arguments that oppose animal experimentation on ethical grounds; among these are Bernard E. Rollin, Stephen R. L. Clarke, Steven F. Sapontzis, and co-authors Harlan B. Miller and William H. Williams, to mention just a few. An extensive literature exists that is beyond the scope of this chapter to summarize. Some suggested readings are provided in Additional Reading, page 271.

Denial of ethical issues

The mainstream view in the Western world is that animal experimentation is morally justified. This view is supported in a number of ways. One way is to deny that any ethical issues are raised by experimenting on animals. A nineteenth-century proponent of this view, mentioned in the last chapter, is Klein, who said that he had no regard at all for the suffering of experimental animals. Such views persist and fit the Animal Exploitation column of Figure 2.1.

David Baltimore, a microbiologist who later received the Nobel prize, appeared on public television in 1974 to discuss Frederick Wiseman's controversial documentary movie on the use of primates in scientific experiments at Yerkes Primate Research Center. Other scientists and moral philosopher Robert Nozick also participated in the program. Nozick asked the scientists whether the fact than an experiment would kill hundreds of animals is ever regarded by them as a reason for not performing it. One of the scientists answered: "Not that I know of." Nozick pressed his question: "Don't animals count at all?" A scientist countered: "Why should they?" Baltimore then interjected that he did not think that experimenting on animals raises a moral issue at all (*The Price of Knowledge,* 1974).

Another proponent of this view is Robert J. White, M.D., Professor of Surgery at Case Western Reserve University in Cleveland. In 1990, White sharply criticized a report on the ethical issues of animal experimentation that appeared in a highly respected journal of biomedical ethics, the *Hastings Center Report*. This 32-page report summarized the project undertaken by the Hastings Center to explore the "middle ground" which holds that some, but not all, animal experimentation is justified (Donnelley and Nolan, 1990). The journal later printed a letter of complaint from White, who expressed his "extreme disappointment" at this series of articles which "quite frankly, has no right to be published. . . . Animal usage is not a moral or ethical issue and elevating the problem of animal rights to such a plane is a disservice to medical research and the farm and dairy industry."

White's view is long held; in a 1971 article, he argued that "antivivisection theory and practice have no moral or ethical basis." White (1988) also opposes review of animal experiments for compliance with national standards by Institutional Animal Care and Use Committees which, he says, "shackles" the experiments.

White is not alone in not wanting ethical concerns aired. Scientists who acknowledge that moral issues are involved may try to avoid their discussion in relation to animal experimentation because they are uncomfortable with such debates. Scientific journals generally reject publication of manuscripts such as those by Singer, Regan, and Rollin and ethical arguments about animal experiments are rarely addressed in their pages. What does appear in the scientific literature about animal experimentation (apart from the description and results of the experiments) tends to be politically motivated—why and how various reform measures should be resisted. There is scant discussion of what limits a scientist's "right" to experiment on animals or of the conflicts involved in conducting science within the general standards of the public. In current public policy governing animal experimentation in the United States, the issues are not directly cast as ethical issues. (This contrasts with public policy in countries such as Canada and Australia, where ethical dilemmas are openly addressed.) So, even though this viewpoint does not involve outright denial of the existence of ethical issues in animal experimentation, it is an indication of substantial resistance to their analysis.

Pro-research mainstream views

The mainstream views favoring animal experimentation rest primarily on important distinctions that separate humans from other animals. The argument goes that these distinguishing features are morally significant so that humans are justified in killing and harming animals for human purposes.

Support of this view is based on a widespread assumption of human superiority over other creatures. A typical position among scientists is that once you accept that a "line" distinguishes man from other animals, there is no reason to debate the justification for using animals for human purposes any further. As one scientist put it to me, "Further discussion is needless." Not only is no discussion necessary, but philosophical views that present the case for moral concern over animals should not be countenanced. It is as if, once having demonstrated that human benefits are derived from some animal experimentation, there is no need to provide any ethical argument that justifies harming millions of animals each year. It is typically argued that since animals are used for many human purposes including food, transport, sports, and entertainment, then animal experimentation is just another example of how animals can be used for human benefit. In the scientific literature, very little new gets said to defend animal experimentation other than documentation of the many human benefits that derive from them. During recent years, the biomedical community has been active in documenting these benefits.

A few philosophers have come to the defense of animal experimentation. Among them is Carl Cohen from the University of Michigan. In an article, much heralded by the biomedical community, that appeared in the *New England Journal of Medicine* in 1986, he argued that animals have no rights. He defended speciesism ("essential for right conduct") and maintained that more, not less, animal experimentation should be done. Cohen's view is that animal experimentation is justified virtually without restriction.

Rights involve claims, or potential claims, that one party may exercise against another, says Cohen. But to exert rights claims, "we must know who holds the right, against whom it is held, and to what is it a right." Animals lack certain capacities and therefore have no rights, he claims. The essential ingredients that are lacking in animals are the ability to respond to moral claims, the capacity to comprehend rules of duty, and the capacity to recognize certain conflicts between what is in their own interest and what is just. "Membership in a community of moral agents . . . remains impossible" for animals.

Cohen, who acknowledges that he is a speciesist, uses a utilitarian argument of weighing benefits and harms. He concludes that the sum total of benefits from animal experimentation (which are so great for humans as to be "beyond calculation") easily outweighs the animal suffering.

As an aside, in the context of utilitarian weighing of benefit and harm, bioethicist Arthur L. Caplan establishes a boundary. What is put on the scale for human benefit should not include human selfishness. In a discussion that was later published in *Harpers* magazine, Caplan took the example of cures for baldness. He said that when you depart from important benefits to human health and get to baldness cures and "people say, 'I don't care about animals. My interests are a hell of a lot more important than the animals' interests. So if keeping hair on my head means sacrificing those animals, painlessly or not, I want it.' It's not utilitarian—it's selfish" (Caplan, 1988).

Cohen believes we should load the scale of weighing benefits against harms with the "terrible" human pains that would have resulted had animals not been used. His defense of increasing animal experimentation is based on the premise that we should "avoid when feasible the use of humans as experimental subjects." He does not address the possibility that non-harmful human experimentation could replace some injurious animal experiments (as in substitution of human clinical research).

In concert with Cohen's view, many scientists who have commented on the matter reject the idea that animals have moral standing or a "right" to anything. The argument goes that the generous treatment of animals is a matter of charity and compassion. It stems from human benevolence, not from the animal's moral claim.

Quality-of-life arguments

A different defense of animal experimentation is made by Raymond G. Frey. This philosopher from Bowling Green State University, who is frequently called upon to defend the use of animals in research in campus debates, rejects the views of both Singer and Regan (Frey, 1980, 1989, and 1991). He has devoted a book to refuting Singer's arguments on vegetarianism and he rejects "rights" talk about animals completely. Furthermore, he believes it is unnecessary to argue in terms of "speciesism" in order to establish that some lives are more valuable than others.

Frey identifies himself with the "middle position" that some but not all animal experiments are justified. In holding this position he says, "Many experiments will have to go but many will survive." He believes that human life is more valuable than animal life, but cedes some value to animal lives. He has publicly stated that he objects to AIDS research on any primates (not only chimps), reasoning that primates are integrative creatures with a quality of life that should exclude them from this experimentation. He favors greater restrictions on the use of primates in research in the United States.

Frey appeals to "quality-of-life" considerations. He points out that many decisions that have now become serious ethical issues regarding sustaining human life draw on "quality-of-that-life" assessments. As an example, the problem of choosing whether to perform a fourteenth operation on a three-month-old baby in order to sustain life for another few days can be judged on quality-of-life considerations. He argues too that not all human lives are of equal value—there are rich, valuable lives, and there are diminished lives such as those of persons in a permanent vegetative state. With similar reasoning, he argues that all animal lives are not equal. In Frey's words, animal life is inferior in "richness" to the life of a normal adult human. On Frey's account, life becomes progressively less valuable as the riches are stripped away. From this, he concludes that we can use those less valuable lives for experiments. Richness, he says, is measured not simply as a product of addition of experiences but essentially involves the integration of experience and the creation of a personality.

Frey straightforwardly acknowledges that this theory is not fully developed—a "safety net" is needed to protect vulnerable subjects. He is at pains to point out that he is not saying that in situations where the quality of life of a nonhuman primate exceeds that of a human being with a diminished quality of life there is justification for experimenting on the human being. Obviously such a judgment would be repugnant.

In my opinion, quality-of-life judgments could be used as a substitute for sentience level, but only within certain confines. Quality-of-life judgments could be used in determining the justification for experimenting on a non-human animal only. They do not hold for judgments of experimenting on human beings with different qualities of life, nor can they be used for judgments of "marginal cases."

I believe there are many persons who oppose the absolutist view that no animal experimentation is ever justified, and who also oppose the view that unlimited animal experimentation is justified. What is not yet fully developed at this stage is a workable ethical theory and ethical principles that allow some, but not all, animal experimentation to proceed—a theory that satisfies the "middle position" point of view that I believe many people espouse. It has proved difficult. Some suggestions based on a utilitarian approach of how to proceed in making ethical judgments are presented in the following chapter.

Kinship views

Another philosopher, Mary Midgley (1983), makes the case that many species of animals fall within the compass of human concern because of our feeling of kinship with them. The extent of our concern over living creatures is related to our sense of kinship, says Midgley. She explains that a sense of kinship can be likened to a series of concentric circles around a human being, each further and further afield. First there is the individual's family, then personal friends, followed by colleagues, tribe or race, non-human primates, other warm-blooded vertebrates, cold-blooded vertebrates, invertebrates, and other living things. In general, the more distant the circle, the less the sense of kinship.

Kinship views can help define the limits of what is justified because there is an ethical pull that coincides with kinship. Kinship is related to the degree of permissible harming of other creatures—indeed, it is what makes tribal wars possible and could conceivably be used to justify speciesism. The kinship view asserts that we have stronger obligations to our own children and other family members than to strangers; that we have stronger obligations to our own community as a whole than to other communities. We tend to favor our own kin and our own species over the lives of other animals.

Certain relationships may in and of themselves generate specific personal duties, both positive and negative. Close kinship requires certain actions, such as altruism and self-sacrifice, and prohibits killing. With more distant kin, killing may not be prohibited, but there is a moral duty to minimize suffering. With even more distant kin, (for instance, beyond the boundaries of sentient life) there is a duty to respect life.

Altruism and self-sacrifice are not limited to human beings; there are a number of documented accounts of these qualities occurring in other species. For instance, in a laboratory setting, Masserman and his colleagues (1964) set up an experiment in which macaques, also known as rhesus monkeys, were fed only if they were willing to pull a chain and electrically shock an unrelated macaque whose agony was plainly seen through a one-way mirror. Otherwise they starved. The monkeys frequently refused to pull the chain; in one experiment only 13 percent would do so—87 percent preferred to go hungry. One macaque went without food for nearly two weeks rather than hurt its kin. As another example, in this case of altruism extending beyond the circle of conspecifics, there are many documented accounts of dolphins helping to rescue drowning humans. By repeated nudging, dolphins can manage to keep distressed persons at the water's surface and lead them to dry land.

Recently, the attitude of many people has shifted to include circles further away from the center. This new concern is shown not only for dogs, cats, and other pets, but for chimpanzees, gorillas, other non-human primates, whales, frogs, snail darters, spotted owls, squid, butterflies, trees, and some other plants, to mention a few.

The kinship that exists among all animals has not always been acknowledged. But over time, especially during the last century, the understanding of similarities between humans and other animals has gained ground. The idea of a continuum of life forms was thrust into public attention by Charles Darwin in the nineteenth century. In *The Descent of Man* Darwin wrote that "there is no fundamental difference between man and the higher mammals in their mental facilities," only a difference in degree (Darwin, 1871). Nowadays, this concept of kinship finds wider acceptance. (When faced with the boiling controversy in the 1870s over animal experimentation, Darwin's humanitarian view collided with his desire to see science advance, and he was uncomfortably caught in the middle. When pressed to choose, he chose science.)

Discussion of kinship and the similarities between humans and other animals can be emotionally laden. In Darwin's day and ever since, some people have been disturbed when others focus on close and relevant similarities. Some people believe that the more love, respect, or recognition of abilities is given to animals then the less is given to human beings—humans are diminished. If appreciation of animals is upgraded then humans are downgraded. It is as if there is a limited, fixed amount of human bountiful concern or compassion to be divided rather than the reality that, at least for some people, there is an extensive appreciation and compassion for a wide universe.

Distinctions between humans and other animals

The significant distinctions between humans and other animals are central to ascribing a right to humans to use animals for human benefit—Cohen argues that animals lack moral agency, and Frey argues that some animals have a different grade of quality of life. Human interests can override animal interests because of these distinguishing features. Mainstream scientific perspectives rely heavily on these distinctions—humans are "special."

This search for distinctions is centuries old. In the seventeenth century, philosophers and scientists debated whether or not animals could feel pain or suffer. In the twentieth century, some distinctions that were once believed to be true distinctions have been shown to be false. Scientific research has played an important role in shaping our understanding of the many similarities between humans and animals. Thorpe (1974) pointed out that it used to be said that animals cannot learn, cannot plan ahead, cannot conceptualize, cannot use, much less make, tools, have no language, cannot count, etc. All these assertions have been shown to be untrue for some species, and Thorpe provides evidence for this. In recent years, the linkages between humans and other animals have become even further strengthened and the list of "special" human characteristics smaller and smaller. It has been established, for instance, that chimpanzees and human beings share 98 percent of their genetic material. Another example is that the electroencephalograms (EEGs) of animals are analogous to those of humans, in fact the EEGs of gorillas and other primates are nearly indistinguishable from those of humans. Carl Sagan and Ann Druyan's 1992 book *Shadows of Forgotten Ancestors: A Search for Who We Are* includes an interesting discussion of the similarities and differences between humans and other primates.

In a book on animal consciousness, the Radners (1989) have this to say about the time-honored precept of human uniqueness:

Only humans have or do *x*. The value of *x* has to be changed from time to time as more evidence comes in, but there must be an *x* because humans are unique. . . . Darwin remarks that he once made a collection of such aphorisms and came up with over twenty, "but they are almost worthless, as their wide difference and number prove the difficulty, if not the impossibility, of the attempt". . . .

Obviously there are differences between humans and other species. Every species is different from every other species: this much is plain biology. The ideology lies not in the search for differences, but in the unwavering belief that humanity is defined by attributes that have absolutely no precedent in the rest of the biological world

(Radner and Radner, 1989).

In some respects, some animals have innate capacities that far exceed those of humans. To mention but a few, dogs and several other species have a better sense of smell and range of hearing than humans, hawks and other birds can see better, mice can see ultraviolet light, bats have an innate ability to use radar and to orient themselves by the sun's rays, bees with their waggle dance can convey information about the direction, distance, and desirability of a food source, and whales have ability to communicate with each other over hundreds of miles. It is difficult to know just where to draw lines of what is "special."

Beauchamp (1992) has assembled a current list of cognitive conditions considered essential to distinguish between humans and other animals. These conditions are (1) self-consciousness (consciousness of oneself as existing over time, with a past and future), (2) freedom to act and to engage in purposive sequences of actions, (3) having reasons for actions and the ability to appreciate reasons for acting, (4) capacity to communicate with other persons using a language, (5) capacity to make moral judgments, and (6) rationality. According to Beauchamp's view, one or more of these capacities are essential to moral standing. (It should be noted that Beauchamp has argued that it is permissible to inflict some harms on animals in research but that there is an upper limit to this which must not be exceeded.)

However, even if we could reach consensus about exactly which attributes are uniquely human, we still would be left wondering why this list of cognitive conditions, or any other list, provides a moral basis for animal experimentation, says Beauchamp. "How intelligent does a chimpanzee have to be before killing him constitutes murder?" asks Carl Sagan. Why is it that there is nothing wrong with killing or placing at risk a creature lacking certain attributes asks Beauchamp.

Agreement on ethical principles to guide animal experimentation is still a long way off. Philosophers and ethicists at least have succeeded in opening up the debate.

3

Major Issues

Ethical theories get you only so far. Then comes the problem of translating moral concerns into practical judgments about real day-to-day issues. Given the current state of affairs, this chapter introduces some of the major issues about animal experimentation that must be considered when deciding whether to approve or disapprove a particular experiment.

There are many complications in moral decisions about animal experiments. In order to delineate some of the major issues, a schematic representation is offered in Figure 3.1.

Infringements of animal interests

When an animal becomes a subject of an experiment, some or many of its interests are compromised or obliterated. The first three bars in Figure 3.1 represent questions that should be asked about whether or not the animal is harmed in any way, and if so how much. The first two bars are (1) pain and suffering and (2) all other infringements of interests (or harms). Also relevant is the place of the species on the phylogenetic scale (third bar) since the sentience level of an animal is intimately related to its ability to perceive pain and to experience suffering. Furthermore, the third bar includes mention of endangered species, since it is a group interest of those species to continue to exist and not to become extinct.

What is meant by "infringement of an animal's interest"? Animal interests

Animal Pain or Suffering [1]

- none
- invertebrate animal pain
- some short-lasting vertebrate animal pain or suffering
- significant but unavoidable animal pain or suffering

Degree of Infringement of Other Animal Interests [2]

- none
- minimal
- great

Classification of Sentience Level

- non-biological systems (computer simulation)
- little or no sentience (protozoa, plants)
- less sentient invertebrates (worms, insects)
- highly sentient invertebrates (octopi)
- cold-blooded vertebrates (fish, amphibians, reptiles)
- warm-blooded vertebrates (birds, mammals)
- non-endangered primates and marine mammals
- endangered primates and marine mammals

Purpose of Experiment

- to gain original knowledge (high social worth)
- for product safety and drug testing
- for professional training
- for other educational purposes [3]

36

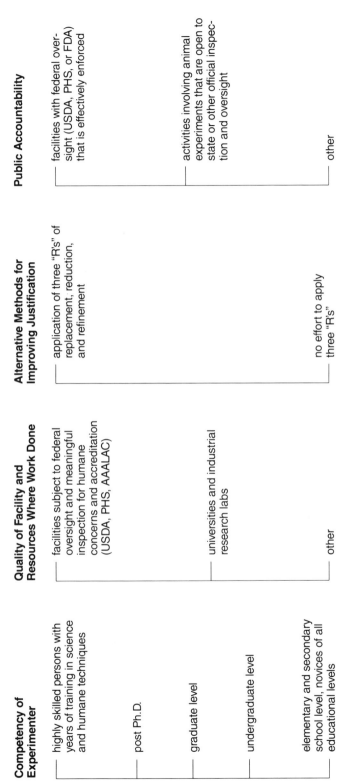

Figure 3.1 The bars represent some major issues to be considered in assessing potential approval or disapproval of an animal experiment. Items placed at the top of the bar indicate situations where there is the greatest or most readily conceded justification. Those at the bottom of the bar carry the least justification or alternatively are those situations most vulnerable to improper use of animals.

1. Also see another version of pain scale in Table 6.1.

2. "Other" refers to other than animal pain and suffering and includes death, confinement, and other harms; see text for discussion.

3. Distinction must be made between educational projects involving animals that carry *no* ethical costs of which there are many (i.e., do not involve harming or destroying a sentient animal), and those that *do* carry an ethical cost (that do involve harming or destroying a sentient animal). Those that do carry an ethical cost are depicted here.

The content of the figure is as follows:

Competency of Experimenter
- highly skilled persons with years of training in science and humane techniques
- post Ph.D.
- graduate level
- undergraduate level
- elementary and secondary school level, novices of all educational levels

Quality of Facility and Resources Where Work Done
- facilities subject to federal oversight and meaningful inspection for humane concerns and accreditation (USDA, PHS, AAALAC)
- universities and industrial research labs
- other

Alternative Methods for Improving Justification
- application of three "R's" of replacement, reduction, and refinement
- no effort to apply three "R's"

Public Accountability
- facilities with federal oversight (USDA, PHS, or FDA) that is effectively enforced
- activities involving animal experiments that are open to state or other official inspection and oversight
- other

include some negatives (things to be avoided), and some positives (desirable things that should be present). Among the negatives are the following: not to be afflicted with physical pain or mental suffering; not to be killed; not to be harmed by fear, held captive, confined, or immobilized; and not to be captured from the wild and separated from family and social group (as many monkeys are). The positive interests of animals include freedom to choose where to live, and ability to establish territorial rights; freedom to express the natural range of behavioral repertoire common to that species such as social interaction with their own and other species; freedom to select preferred food; enough space to be able to express all forms of natural movement such as stretching, walking, running, rolling, and swinging; and freedom to be able to escape harms and to make other self-determining choices.

It must already be obvious that this schematic representation only begins to suggest the nature of possible animal harm. Determining the infringement of interests to an animal is very complicated. Deciding how much an animal's interests have been compromised cannot be represented by straight lines—it is not that simple. Take the example of death, which is included in the second bar in this schema. Untimely death is the ultimate deprivation, the ultimate loss of opportunity to find satisfaction, the ultimate infringement of an animal's interest. Yet the quality of the animal's life may be such that death might be a better option than continued life. Indeed, in most laboratory animal legislation killing is mandatory to prevent or stop unrelievable severe pain, so in that sense a dead animal is regarded as less of a moral problem than an animal in pain.

Furthermore, it is not only the time of death that matters, but the manner of death. If the animal's death is protracted and painful, such as from terminal cancer or from poisoning, then the harm is greater than if the death is quick and painless. Also the number of animal deaths resulting from a particular experiment must surely be a factor. This is not significant to the individual animal, but it should be taken into account by people who have to decide whether or not to approve a particular experiment.

Another example of the limitations of this schema concerns the source of the animals, whether they are wild-caught, purpose-bred, or previous pets (as are some dogs and cats). Human levels of responsibility are different for each of these groups—the ethical pull is greater the closer the relationship of that animal with human beings. To put it another way, there are increasing degrees of kinship going from wild, to domesticated, to pet animals.

But again, this is not a simple matter. There is deep concern about taking primates from the wild. These sensitive creatures can be seriously traumatized by captivity, and many may die because of inhumane trapping and transportation methods for each one that arrives at the laboratory. Even if they live, some wild-caught animals may never really adjust to captivity, especially if they are maintained in barren environments. So, does it lessen the ethical cost if these animals are purpose-bred, thus avoiding the trauma of transition in life-style but not changing the harms that befall them as a result of experimentation? It would seem that taking an animal from the wild into captivity is a more serious infringement of an animal's interest than using animals that are purpose-bred and thereby captive from the moment of birth. Should previous life histories of the animal before the animal arrives at the laboratory door be taken into account? Should pound animals be used? What if all laboratory animals were purpose-bred? Would this make experimentation more acceptable?

So, this schema must be taken for what it is—a rough chart for illustrating some of the major issues.

Purpose of the experiment

The fourth bar, the purpose of an experiment, needs to be considered in the broad context of the social merit or promise of the work. There are three major reasons for animal experiments: (1) research to obtain original knowledge, (2) testing of products for safety or efficacy, and (3) pedagogic purposes as in veterinary or biology education. These uses are distinct.

Research

Much original research is for biomedical purposes—indeed, this is the most commonly thought of reason for animal experimentation. Biomedical research is conducted for two broad purposes: (1) to add to scientific understanding of basic biological functions, processes, and behavior (basic research); and (2) to improve human or animal health by studying the natural history of disease, its pathophysiology and prevention, and by developing diagnostic and therapeutic methods (applied research).

But there are other types of animal use in experiments, such as in weapons development and deployment. In the United States, dolphins have in the past been used as carriers of lethal weapons; the animals are killed when the weapon reaches its target. (Under the German law of 1986, it is prohibited to use animals to develop or test weapons.) Other areas include space research, agricultural research to improve food animal yield and therefore commercial profit, veterinary research aimed at improving animal health, zoological research to study wildlife in free-living states, and behavioral research to probe the mental state of animals, which may or may not have application to human ailments. Not all these uses of animals in research are equally justified.

Testing

Testing is conducted to assess the potency, effectiveness, or toxicity of substances that have established or potential usefulness for medical, scientific, or commercial purposes. For instance, new drugs are tested for efficacy and safety before clinical trials are conducted on humans. In addition, tests on animals are conducted to establish safety levels for humans of known toxic substances (for instance, those that occur as human hazards in the chemical production industry or as environmental pollutants from toxic waste deposits). Justification for these tests is based on the reasonable assumptions that adverse effects caused by chemical substances in animals are usually the same as those encountered in humans, and that the dose causing toxicity in animals permits risk assessment for exposed humans.

Education

Animals are used to teach humane concepts at all levels of education, to instruct students of the biological sciences in biology, physiology, pharmacology, and to teach certain skills, such as surgery. The purpose of advanced educational projects involving animals is to train the next generation of scientists. The actual experimental results obtained have little significance, in contrast to research and testing where the results are all-important.

Obviously, not all purposes are equally justified. Some purposes carry significant public benefit, others are trivial or nonexistent. For some purposes suitable alternatives are available, for others they are not. To some extent, public sanction varies according to the significance and dignity of the goal of the work. Approval rate depends on the experiment's purpose—high for cancer or heart disease research and lower for less threatening human diseases such as allergy. Approval rate tends to fall again if the experiment's purpose is product safety testing. My guess would be that public approval of the use of dolphins to carry lethal military weapons or of primates in car crashes to test car safety would be relatively low. The non-biomedical uses of animals as experimental subjects are frequently challenged by animal advocates, but any argued defense of such use is rare. To the extent that the procedures cause harm to sentient animals, that they are nonessential, and that alternatives exist, they may be judged of trivial social worth and fail to gain public support.

Alternative methods

Many of the other bars are self-explanatory, but a definition is needed for the term *alternatives* (bar 7). This bar has three components: *replacement* using experimental subjects that are phylogenetically lower or using non-animal systems; *reduction* in the number of animals used; and *refinement* of experimental design and methods to reduce ethical costs. These are often referred to as the three Rs of Russell and Burch (1959), the English scientists who first described them. In using the word alternatives, it is important to include all three components, not just one or two as is sometimes done.

The state of the art is such that the availability of alternatives for immediate application varies with different situations. In research, refinements are the most readily available and are therefore those most commonly used. Certainly in research there is place for reduction alternatives, and these are also currently being applied, although to a lesser extent than refinements. In research, replacement alternatives are not well developed, indeed some would say they will never be developed. In testing and in education, all three alternatives of refinement, reduction, and replacement are currently available and are increasingly being applied.

"Threshold" and "on-balance" questions

This schematic outline of issues is further complicated by other assessments. To begin with, certain "threshold" questions must be addressed, and only when these have been raised and answered affirmatively do "on balance" questions arise.

An important threshold question involves infringement of an animal's interests. People with different perspectives will answer this question in different ways. For instance, to total antivivisectionists no animal experimentation is ever justified; the threshold would never be passed to permit a single experiment on any animal. No matter how noble the purpose, how qualified the experimenter, how fine the facility, or how slight the animal harm, no animal should be experimented on.

Others would argue that some infringements of animal interests are permissible but that there is an upper limit of what harms can be inflicted. Some infringements go beyond what is morally justified. Jane Goodall takes this view and, I would imagine, so do many scientists and members of the public. The question might be posed, is it ever justified to put animals into condition x that will result in harm y irrespective of any benefits that might be anticipated from research or other uses? Thus, to take an extreme example, is it ever justified to blow-torch pigs irrespective of how much we stand to learn about burns? If the answer is no, then assessment goes no further. This view incorporates an upper limit of permissible harm. In human experimentation, there is similarly a sense of an upper limit of what can ever be permitted.

There are also other threshold questions, such as: Is the purpose of the experiment trivial, for mere curiosity, or for repetition of well-known facts? What are the qualifications of the experimenter—novice, incompetent? Where will the experiment be done—in a high school student's bedroom or garage or other unsuitable facility? It might seem to those unfamiliar with the recent battles for reform that such questions would so automatically be checked and unqualified experiments rejected that even to mention these issues is unnecessary. But events in the United States and other countries indicate that exclusions are not always rigorously made on these counts.

Thresholds are not fixed points, but move with time. Thus, as alternatives are developed to reduce or eliminate the infliction of animal harms while maintaining scientific progress, thresholds become more restrictive.

A third view holds that there are no thresholds—there is no situation in which animal pain or suffering or other animal interests should override scientific inquiry. Proponents of these views would place minimal or no restrictions on animal experiments, arguing that restrictions infringe an experimenter's academic freedom.

For those who agree with some animal experimentation (at least for the time being because alternatives are not yet available), the final set of questions are the "on-balance" ones—that is, on balance with the value of the research, is infliction of this animal harm justified? At this level, all the issues depicted in Figure 3.1 come into play. These decisions are influenced by many crosscurrents. Each decision must take into account the weight to be given to each issue and how the many intertwining and often conflicting factors are to be resolved. Considering the complexities, it is no wonder how controversial these issues are and how many conflicting views are encountered.

Timetable for reduction of animal experimentation

Is there a timetable that should be applied to animal experimentation? Should efforts be made to reduce reliance on animal experimentation as far as possible? Some people would reject outright the idea that eliminating painful animal experimentation is an achievable or even desirable goal, but this attitude may represent only a short view of history and may not be defensible on moral grounds.

Philosopher T. L. S. Sprigge of the University of Edinburgh and other scholars such as Arthur L. Caplan argue that the burden of proof is on those who support animal experimentation and not on those who criticize it: the burden "must always be on those who seek to justify an act which is, in the first place, one of hurting, injuring, frustrating, or killing" (Sprigge, 1985). As Caplan (1990) says, the animals have to prove nothing: "[T]he animal simply has its abilities and capacities, it runs around in the field, it moves around in its cage, it does what it wants to do. I think the basic assumption should be, it should be allowed to do that. There's no reason to assume that anyone has the right to interfere with it."

Sprigge presents a rational case for espousing a "temporary event" view of animal experimentation. He reasons that when confronted with a practice that has obvious victims and that is justified as necessary, we should consider whether another way of proceeding, with no such victims, and not worse for sentient beings all round, is not available for exploration. Surely we do not have to look forward to a world in which humans have set up a pattern for themselves indefinitely in which a reasonably good life for humans is grounded on the suffering of non-humans. It is unacceptable to Sprigge that humans should be content that this is how it will always be, and he cannot believe that it is best for the total happiness of sentient life upon this globe in general. "We should have learned from plenty of past episodes of human history," he says, "that subjection or exploitation of some group, can usually be changed without people in general finding themselves much the worse for the change when things have worked their way through."

This perception that animal experimentation at current levels is an *interim measure* is also conveyed in a passage from a 1991 report of a Working Party from the Institute of Medical Ethics in Britain, which stands as the most thoughtful analysis of ethical issues of animal experimentation to date (Smith and Boyd, 1991). The report examines moral claims in terms of asking what benefits might serve a sufficiently serious purpose to be weighed against the cost to the animals used. The Working Party notes that an argument still vigorously used in defense of the use of animals in biomedical research is that their use is "necessary." The report states:

The defense of necessity can be seen in terms of the Common Law doctrine that an act which is normally unlawful may be lawful if it is done as the only way of achieving a greater and lawful benefit. One example of this might be when a highjacker is killed in order to save other passengers. . . .

In ethics, as in law, the defense of necessity requires to be examined carefully and the necessity proved. It has to be shown:

(1) that the evil prevented is greater than that done; and
(2) that there is no less drastic method of achieving the stated aim.

Thus, if a scientist claims it is necessary to use animals in a particular project in order to achieve some goal, he is required morally to demonstrate at least four things:

(1) that the goal is worthwhile;
(2) that it has a high moral claim to be achieved;
(3) that there is no less drastic method of achieving it; and
(4) that there actually is some reasonable possibility of the project achieving the goal. . . .

As these conditions suggest, justification by necessity often relies on crucial judgements of a scientific rather than a moral nature. This means, importantly, that any judgement that the use of animals is necessary, is normally an interim judgement. That is, it may change over time and with scientific advance, so that the necessity of animal use may diminish.

The diminution of reliance on animal experimentation is a goal worthy of pursuit, and ways must be sought to achieve it.

4

Legislation and the Growth of Protagonist Organizations

Legislative battles sharply reveal the profound differences in outlook between defenders of animal research and animal welfare reformers. This chapter gives a brief history of legislative events in the United States, not in strict chronological order. First, the procurement of laboratory dogs and cats from pounds is addressed; conflicts started in the 1940s and continue up to the present. Then the legislation on laboratory animal husbandry and experimental procedures starting in the 1960s is discussed. The chapter ends with a discussion of legislative issues that are still being debated. Additional discussion of legislative confrontations are found in the chapters on testing, education, and raids.

Battles over dog and cat procurement

The first confrontation between the biomedical community and humane societies concerned where the labs should get their dogs and cats. In 1945 the American Association of Medical Colleges formed an organization called the National Society for Medical Research (NSMR), a primary purpose of which was to work for passage of laws to permit researchers to have access to unwanted and unclaimed animals in pounds. The American Medical Association supported NSMR financially, and AMA representatives served on its committees, on its board, and as its senior officers. Many of the meetings were held in the AMA building. NSMR was the focal point for other scientific organizations that were interested in this matter. Their first success came in 1948 with a state law in

Minnesota, followed in 1949 by Wisconsin, and then in 1950 by city ordinances in Los Angeles and Baltimore. The Wisconsin law was particularly severe in that it required any stray animal to be made available on request to a scientific institution. Thus, shelters operated wholly by charitable funds as well as publicly funded shelters were compelled to supply animals for experiments. During the next few years, similar laws were passed in several other states. These procurement laws reflect the virtually unchallenged support the biomedical community commanded at that time.

The animal protection societies were at first dormant and the biomedical community met little resistance to these legislative initiatives. Indeed, in the 1940s and the early 1950s, the issues of animal experimentation were beyond the interests of many traditional humane societies, and antivivisection societies were not a major force.

But increasingly, some segments of the humane movement realized that this acquisition of dogs and cats was a violation of the purpose of an animal shelter, which is to be a sanctuary for animals. They believed that shelters should operate only in ways that are beneficial to animals. Thus, the early success of NSMR sparked the formation of several new humane organizations.

One of the most enduringly effective organizations, the Animal Welfare Institute (AWI), was formed in 1952. Its formation was unusual because it was formed on the initiative of Robert Gesell, M.D., professor and chair of the department of physiology at the University of Michigan. Although he had supported NSMR's formation initially, Gesell became disenchanted because "NSMR has had but one idea since its organization, namely, to provide an inexhaustible number of animals to an ever growing crowd of career scientists" (remarks of Gesell made at the business meeting of the American Physiological Society, April 15, 1952, quoted in Fox et al., 1984). Gesell continued by saying, "With the aid of the halo supplied by the faith of the American people in medical science, the NSMR converts sanctuaries of mercy into animal pounds at the beck and call of experimental laboratories regardless of how the animals are to be used." Professor Gesell and his daughter, Christine Stevens, formed both the AWI and its sister organization the Society for Animal Protective Legislation. These have been among the most politically successful of all animal welfare organizations; they have helped establish legislation or regulations on a wide range of issues including humane slaughter of livestock, protection of endangered species, ocean mammal protection, and air shipment standards, to mention but a few.

Later in the 1950s, other new organizations were formed that shared a common concern for the welfare of animals. In 1954, The Humane Society of the United States broke off as a splinter group from what was then the largest member society, the American Humane Association. In the late 1950s, the United Action for Animals and Friends of Animals were formed. During the 1950s and 1960s,

these and other organizations combined efforts toward passage of federal legislation controlling the care and use of laboratory animals, which culminated in the
passage of the 1966 Animal Welfare Act, discussed later in this chapter.

The care and use issues consumed the efforts of the humane movement, so
there was something of a lull in the state legislative battles on pound animals
until 1972 when a law was passed in Rhode Island that favored the humane
societies' viewpoint, prohibiting the requisitioning of pound animals by researchers. Similar laws soon followed in other states (Giannelli, 1986). An
intense battle occurred between the warring sides in New York State, ending in
1979 with a partial victory for the humane societies. The Metcalf-Hatch Act was
repealed and partial protection was afforded to unwanted animals (only strays are
protected, not owner-relinquished animals).

By the 1980s use of pound animals came to dominate state legislative battles
on animals. Where state and local laws mandated the release of pound animals to
research institutions, humane societies made efforts to repeal them. Where opposite laws existed, the biomedical community sought to undo them. Fair game for
either side to extend their territory were the many states where no laws existed or
where the state law left this matter up to local option. Today animal welfarists
and biomedical researchers confront each other in many of these states.

Each side allocates considerable resources to this battle. During the 1980s
major new organizations that lobby on this issue emerged. Maps of "won" states
were regularly published by the opposing organizations. As the confrontations
intensified, media coverage increased, and the battle became more emotional.

Revitalization of pro-research efforts

In 1979 a new organization was formed that became the dominating force for the
biomedical community. Initially called the Association for Biomedical Research,
its name was changed to the National Association for Biomedical Research
(NABR) when it amalgamated with what was left of NSMR. For several years
the NSMR had been foundering because its tactics did not win favor within the
biomedical community. A severe blow was given when J. Russell Lindsey, a
well-known and influential laboratory animal veterinarian from the University of
Alabama, openly criticized NSMR. In a widely circulated 1979 statement (later
published in 1980) he said that NSMR had pursued ineffective strategies of
rigidly maintaining a defensive posture of "claiming that all practices of animal
use and care within the biomedical community have been 'lily white,'" and of
relentlessly following the erroneous concept that all who speak out for the humane interests of animals are "arch enemies of medical progress." Although
overtones of these postures are still seen within NABR's ranks, NABR has been
successful in unifying the biomedical community in its political action.

NABR is the brainchild of the biggest supplier of laboratory animals in the world, Charles River, Inc. Henry Foster, the veterinarian who built up Charles River from a two-room rat breeding business into a multimillion dollar international corporation, and his son, an attorney, wrote the necessary legal papers. At least up until 1984, Frankie L. Trull, the president, described the new group as a "trade association." But as universities joined in, this description was dropped. The Charles River company was recently sold to Bausch & Lomb, the industrial conglomerate, reportedly for 38 million dollars. Since its inception, NABR has been intensely opposed to regulatory legislation that affects the laboratory animal industry or its clients.

NABR emerged as a major force to resist change. Among other issues, it continued NSMR's fight to retain and expand the use of pound animals for research. It is funded by its constituent groups which, by 1990, included 325 member institutions and companies (not individuals). Of these 325, about 70 percent are non-profit organizations—mostly academic institutions or associations; pharmaceutical, cosmetic, and chemical companies make up the rest. NABR and its offshoot, the Foundation for Biomedical Research, have a combined annual budget of approximately 1.2 million dollars. In 1990, 60 to 70 percent of funding came from industry and animal dealers and 30 to 40 percent from academe. This constituency has a commonality in their interest in the continuance of animal experimentation.

In the 1980s new state organizations that work with NABR were formed with a major focus on lobbying for use of pound animals and public education about the benefits of animal research. By 1991 a total of 12 state affiliates had been established including Michigan, Massachusetts, California, and Texas—important states for biomedical research.

Old established professional organizations of scientists have joined forces to lobby with NABR. Highly influential groups such as the AMA, the American Association of Medical Colleges, the American Physiological Society, the American Veterinary Medical Association, and the Society for Neuroscience, add to their strength.

Strategies of pro-research groups

With financial backing from the AMA, the association of the "incurably ill for Animal Research" (iiFAR) was formed in 1985 and soon joined in on the legislative battles about pound animals. This group uses a new and effective strategy— it makes heart-rending emotional appeals to the public from people who say that they would not be alive today were it not for health benefits derived from animal experiments. As an example, among iiFAR members is a mother whose four-year-old child has a heart pacemaker. The pretty child appears on television to advocate animal experiments, saying that she would willingly give up her pet rabbit to be used for research purposes.

This strategy of using patients to argue the case for animal experimentation had its beginning in 1984 at a conference organized by the National Institutes of Health—the first public conference of this federal agency to discuss animal experimentation. At this conference, several patients who had experienced life-threatening illnesses gave testimonials to describe their ailments, treatment, and recovery, always paying tribute to the role that animal experimentation had played in the development of that therapy. Typical of these presentations was a man who had survived a heart/lung transplant who said, "Human heart/lung transplantation first became possible as a result of experimental work in primates. . . . [Stanford University] has now performed 18 [human] operations and 12 of these patients remain alive today. . . . All of them would have been dead if it had not been for the discovery of these techniques and new drugs using animal research" (Jamieson, 1985).

The strategy of using patient testimonies was controversial at the time, and there was much discussion in the corridors among the scientists who attended the NIH conference. Some said it was stooping to the level of the antivivisectionists in being too emotional. The journal *Nature* published an unsigned opinion piece entitled "Double-Talk on Animals; NIH seems more ready to risk its reputation than to meet serious critics on animal care" (Anonymous, 1984). This article, commenting on the use of patients at this NIH-sponsored conference states, "While the sincerity of what these patients had to say is indisputable, one has to feel uncomfortable at the exploitation of their misfortune inevitably at play when the federal government stands them up to say how much they love their husbands and how grateful they are that medical research has kept their children's daddies alive."

Others countered that as long as animal welfarists use pathetic pictures of dogs and cats behind bars, then the scientific community is justified in trying to counter this with equally emotional appeals. The defenders of patient testimonials seem to have prevailed. In 1989, the AMA announced it would "[c]ombat emotion with emotion" in its official action plan for dealing with animal activists. AMA's stated strategy is to contrast "fuzzy" animals (that they say are the propaganda of animal activists) with "'healing' children" (AMA, 1989). Figure 4.1 provides an example of a poster, widely distributed by lobbyists for the biomedical community, of just such an approach.

iiFAR helps provide patients who are willing to testify at legislative sessions and in media events. On the pound dog issue for instance, in 1989 a paralyzed boy in a wheelchair pleaded dramatically with Virginia state legislators not to interfere with research that could bring cures. A University of Virginia medical school doctor commented that after that effective testimony "it was like shooting fish in a barrel" to persuade the legislators to severely water down a proposed law to ban the use of pound animals, (quoted in Blumenstyk, 1989). The law that was eventually passed provided that all animals, except those having a tag, license, or tattoo identification, may be provided to any research institution in Virginia.

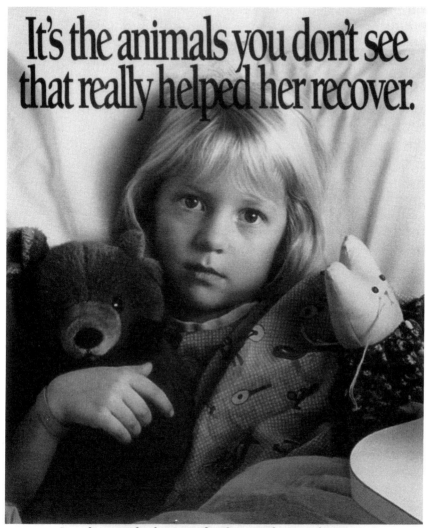

It's the animals you don't see that really helped her recover.

Recently, a surgical technique perfected on animals was used to remove a malignant tumor from a little girl's brain. We lost some lab animals. But look what we saved.

Figure 4.1 This poster illustrates the once controversial but now accepted approach of the pro-animal research organizations of focusing on "fuzzy animals" and "healed children," as recommended in the 1989 action plan of the American Medical Association. The poster was prepared and distributed by the Foundation for Biomedical Research.

But of course these new initiatives did not go unchallenged. Almost immediately the humane front formed retaliatory groups. They are called "Incurably Ill Because of Animal Research," and "Disabled and Incurably Ill for Alternatives to Animal Research." Their members would like to see the money currently used to finance animal experiments related to their disease redirected to provide services for patients suffering these disabilities and to finance clinical research on naturally occurring human cases.

The battles over dog and cat procurement are still ongoing, and an update on the status of current legislation is provided in the chapter on the source of laboratory dogs.

Inside the labs: standards of husbandry and experimentation

Although there had been brief flurries of activity previously, it was not until the 1960s that successful efforts to legislate what happened within research facilities began. The 1960s were a period of political activism for causes involving compassion and extension of concern. There was a mood of special concern for minorities, for the civil rights movement, for the disabled, for the poor. Various "Pride" and "Liberation" movements took hold. Part of this mood was reflected in the emergence of environmental issues and a new concern for animals.

As a result of an initiative by Christine Stevens, president of the Animal Welfare Institute, federal legislation was proposed in 1960 to establish legislation similar to the British law requiring licensing of individual investigators. Despite support from thirteen senators, the proposals languished for six years in Senator Lister Hill's committee without a hearing. Strong opposition to protective legislation was lead by the NSMR and its president Maurice Visscher.

Then suddenly the issue flared with the February 4, 1966, publication in *Life Magazine* of a photo-article that exposed the shocking abuse of dogs at the hands of animal dealers, many of whom sold the dogs to laboratories (Wayman, 1966). Photographs of the animal dealers' facilities showed malnourished, severely mistreated animals and filthy conditions. The article recounted how a Dalmatian dog was stolen from its owner and found some days later in a research facility awaiting experimentation.

Public outrage was intense. A bill to prevent dog theft, introduced by freshman Congressman Joseph Resnick, which required licensing of animal dealers and research facilities, quickly gathered momentum. In one week more mail was received by Congress on these issues than on civil rights or Vietnam. At that time, the Humane Society of the United States (HSUS) estimated that 50 percent of all missing pets were stolen by "dognappers" who then sold them to research laboratories. Opponents of regulatory legislation for laboratory animals, who thought the issue had been buried in that Senate Committee, now modified their position by attempting to have laboratories exempted instead; however, they failed and the Laboratory Animal Welfare Act was signed into law on August 24, 1966. (For a blow-by-blow account of these political battles—typical of Capitol Hill—see Stevens, 1990.)

The 1966 law included provisions to protect the public from having dogs and cats stolen for experimental purposes and required registration of research facilities and dog dealers with the U.S. Department of Agriculture. Research facilities were required to buy their dogs and cats only from licensed dealers. In addition, the law sought to ensure that six groups of animals intended for research—dogs, cats, non-human primates, rabbits, hamsters, and guinea pigs—are provided humane care and treatment. Numerous other animals were left unprotected. Thus federal legislation began.

Subsequent strengthening amendments, in 1970, 1976, and 1985, broadened the scope of the act. Among the new requirements were a qualified provision on use of pain-relieving drugs, the establishment of Institutional Animal Care and Use Committees, and a change in name to the Animal Welfare Act.

Another mechanism of control that emerged around that time related to grantees of the National Institutes of Health, which is part of the Public Health Service. NIH had provided federal grants for animal experiments since 1946. In 1963, in an effort to forestall the increasing efforts to establish federal legislation, the NIH published for the first time voluntary guidelines called the Guide to the Care and Use of Laboratory Animals (commonly called the NIH Guide, now the PHS Guide, 1985, and its accompanying PHS Policy on Humane Care and Use of Laboratory Animals, 1986, see references under Public Health Service). Initially these guidelines dealt with husbandry standards—minimal caging size, sanitation, nutrition, and the like. Over time, as a result of many revisions, the scope has broadened to include provisions on experimental procedures as well. At first the NIH recommendations were non-binding, but since 1985 they have been federal law.

Thus became established the two primary mechanisms for maintaining standards that continue to this day—the Animal Welfare Act and its amendments administered by the Animal and Plant Health Inspection Service (APHIS) of USDA, and the policy of NIH/PHS administered by the Office for the Protection from Research Risks (OPRR) of NIH. These two mechanisms have authority over different constituencies although there is overlap in their purview. Many revisions in these policies have occurred over time, and recently significant efforts have been expended to make the provisions of each compatible with the other.

Also, a voluntary mechanism for control of standards emerged with the American Association for Accreditation of Laboratory Animal Care. Alongside this beneficial accreditation approach, a new branch of veterinary medicine developed—the specialty of laboratory animal medicine, including technical training in husbandry of laboratory animals and in humane techniques of experimentation. A large measure of the improvements in humane animal experimentation has come from these highly trained veterinarians who have been in the forefront in improving anesthetic methods and in introducing alternatives.

Emergence of the animal rights movement

In the 1970s the environmental movement expanded to include specific animal issues. Public concern was expressed about pollution of the earth, sea, and sky, about environmentally unhealthy conditions for humans due to human use of toxic substances, about damage to animal and plant habitats, and about protection of dwindling and endangered species.

The birth of a new movement of animal activists was sparked by the publication of Peter Singer's 1975 book *Animal Liberation*. This book is now considered the "bible" of the animal rights movement. The movement was fueled in the early 1980s by the laboratory raids that revealed animal abuse at some federally funded biomedical research institutions. It also gained strength from the work of philosophers such as Tom Regan, Stephen R. L. Clark, and Bernard E. Rollin, who criticized many current practices involving the treatment of animals.

Perhaps the most influential of the new organizations that emerged is People for the Ethical Treatment of Animals. In 1991 PETA claims a membership of 350,000, but it had only 100 members in 1980. Its 1991 assets approached the ten-million-dollar mark. In the same period, HSUS has increased its membership ten-fold—to about one million. Over the decade, many other new activist organizations developed and pressed pro-animal issues in state and federal legislatures and in the courts.

The range of animal issues taken up by these groups has grown. Virtually every use of animals by human beings has been under attack. It is not only animal experimentation but the condition of animals in the food industry, transport and slaughter methods, hunting, the commercial pet trade, zoos, and the use of animals in entertainment that are at issue.

The protests have brought some results. Among these can be counted the 1985 strengthening amendments to the AWA, the reduction in reliance on painful animal tests, and reduction in student exercises that cause harm or death to sentient animals. Also, a revolution is going on in the fur industry. Following years of public protests, the animal rights movement claimed a great victory when the Hudson Bay Company, a name synonymous with the fur trade for 300 years, closed its doors in 1990. Harrods of London, Nordstrom, and Lord and Taylor, along with many other department stores in several countries have closed their fur salons. Zoos have been a frequent target of criticism because of the sterile conditions of the concrete enclosures provided for the animals and the limited educational value of seeing caged animals. The 1992 closing of the historic London zoo, founded in 1826, is due in part to complaints from the animal rights movement, according to British press. Dolphin protection is another example. In 1989 Starkist, Chicken of the Sea, and Bumble Bee, which account for about 75 percent of the tuna fish sold in the United States, agreed not to buy from fishermen who set their purse seine nets deliberately around dolphins, causing the dolphins' deaths. Other nets that avoid these problems are available. This widely publicized change, resisted by the fishermen themselves, demonstrated the public's increased valuation of this non-human species that shows extraordinary abilities to communicate, recognize people and other dolphins, have relationships, learn, and per-

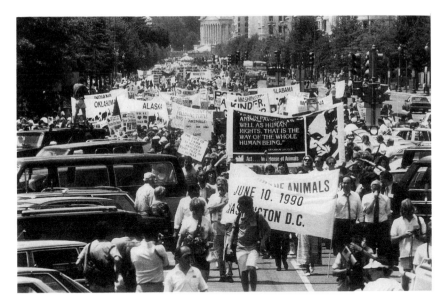

Figure 4.2 The animal rights parade in Washington, D.C. is an event attracting thousands of people from across the country who come to demonstrate their sympathy toward animals. Photo by Gerald Martineau—The Washington Post.

ceive pain. These changes can, I believe, be traced to changing public attitudes toward a more caring society.

People for the Ethical Treatment of Animals is the group that is most feared by those who are the target of their criticisms. PETA is threatening because of its close association with the Animal Liberation Front (ALF), the groups that conduct raids on laboratories. PETA's range of interests is expressed in a popular song in the Animal Rights Christmas Carols. Each Christmas day, PETA members gather outside the National Zoo in Washington, D.C. to sing pro-ALF anthems. One of them is: "On the 12th day of Christmas, the ALF set free 12 grateful turkeys, 11 lions roaring, 10 birds a-soaring, 9 pet shop puppies, 8 trapped coyotes, 7 crippled kittens, 6 blinded rabbits, 5 chimpanzees, 4 micropigs, 3 veal calves, 2 guinea pigs and a rat from a laboratory."

Street demonstrations by animal rights activists have now become a frequent occurrence. Some are protests and others are shows of strength. There have been parades in downtown Washington, D.C. where sympathizers from all over the country come to march. A typical one is shown in Figure 4.2.

Scientists join humane movement

A major change in the humane societies occurred when veterinarians and other scientists joined their ranks. In the early days, the 1950s and 1960s, this was unheard of. In the United States the first such appointment occurred in 1976 when Michael W. Fox, a veterinarian and ethologist, became the Scientific Director of HSUS. Fox has been an influential and articulate voice for humane causes, and this appointment was followed by others at HSUS such as Andrew N. Rowan, D. Phil. now at Tufts. Recently, HSUS has also established a Scientific Advisory Council comprising physicians, psychologists, and other scientists. Other humane organizations recognized that to have veterinarians and scientists as spokespeople vastly increased their credibility. ProPets had as its Director Michael A. Giannelli, Ph.D., a psychologist. In the UK, two examples are Michael Balls, D. Phil, Professor of Medical Cell Biology at the University of Nottingham, who is the Chair of the Trustees of the Fund for the Replacement of Animals in Medical Experiments, and Dr. Sheila Silcock, who is intimately involved with the RSPCA. Other scientists have formed their own organizations to address animal welfare/rights issues.

This involvement of scientists may reflect a social trend. Surveys have demonstrated an association between higher education and participation in the animal rights movement. For instance, a 1991 survey of a random sample of 1,400 readers of *The Animals' Agenda,* the leading animal rights magazine, with a circulation of 25,000 (Richards and Krannich, 1991), showed that 82 percent of those polled had received some college education as compared with 32 percent in the general population, 33 percent had postgraduate degrees as compared with 8 percent of the general population, and 39 percent had incomes above $50,000, against 5 percent in the general population.

The emergence of new organizations in the 1980s reflects this new involvement of professional persons in supporting animal welfare viewpoints. Among these groups are the Ethics and Animals association of philosophers started in the late 1970s; Attorneys for Animal Rights, originally started in 1979 and renamed the Animal Legal Defense Fund in 1984; Psychologists for the Ethical Treatment of Animals, started in 1983; the Physicians Committee for Responsible Medicine, 1986; the National Association of Nurses Against Vivisection, 1986; the Association of Veterinarians for Animal Rights, 1987; the International Network for Religion and Animals, 1987; and the National Society of Musicians for Animals, 1989.

Lawyers often play an important part in movements for social change. The Animal Legal Defense Fund, under the direction of Joyce Tischler and Steven M. Wise, has pressed reforms through court action. By 1992, the organization had 300 attorney and law student members throughout the United States who provide services *pro bono* to the animal protection movement.

In addition, a number of religious groups have started their own organizations. These include Christians Helping Animals and People; Buddhists Concerned for Animals in San Francisco, California; and the International Society for Religion and Animal Rights of Berkeley, California, among others.

1985 federal laws and their aftermath

The most far-reaching amendments to the Animal Welfare Act occurred in 1985 when the actual experimental procedures—previously exempt from control— became the subject of law. The passage of the 1985 amendments was pressed by the humane movement. Passage was significantly helped when the American Physiological Society and the Association of Professors of Medicine withdrew their opposition.

The current provisions covering laboratory animals are embodied in two laws. The first is the Improved Standards for Laboratory Animals Act passed in December 1985, which comprises amendments to the Animal Welfare Act. This was incorporated into the omnibus farm bill reauthorization, the Food Security Act of 1985 (P.L. 99-198). The second is the Health Research Extension Act of 1985, (P.L. 99-158), popularly known as the NIH Reauthorization Act. These laws and subsequent rulemaking govern the current conduct of animal research (see Animal Welfare Legislation, 1990).

The new legislation mandated that each research facility using animals establish an Institutional Animal Care and Use Committee (IACUC) with membership that includes one person not affiliated with the institution to "represent general community interests in the proper care and treatment of animals." This marks the first time that public members of IACUCs were required by law. Research protocols involving pain have to be reviewed by the IACUC, and investigators are required to consider alternatives to animal use and to consult with a veterinarian before beginning any experiment that could cause pain. Requirements also affect pre- and post-surgical care of animals, prohibition of the use of an animal for more than one major surgical procedure, and euthanasia practices.

Under these new laws, the NIH Guide is no longer a "guide" but is now the law. In the September 1986 edition, it was retitled the "PHS Policy on Humane Care and Use of Laboratory Animals by Awardee Institutions" and now covers all agencies of the PHS, not only the NIH. Importantly, this action adds the Food and Drug Administration and the Alcohol, Drug Abuse, and Mental Health Administration.

In 1985 three new concepts were introduced into the Animal Welfare Act: (a) that training shall be provided to laboratory animal personnel in the humane care and use of animals, (b) that the environment in which non-human primates are housed shall promote the animals' psychological well-being, and (c) that dogs shall be given exercise. The Secretary of Agriculture issued standards governing these provisions.

The first of these new provisions fared reasonably well. Institutions began to provide training for their personnel in animal handling, anesthesia, euthanasia, and what the concept of alternatives means. In-house programs were established, and lab personnel were encouraged to attend training sessions at scientific meetings. The climate changed appreciably. IACUCs began to be more alert to the qualifications of investigators to conduct traumatic procedures and to insist on training of the laboratory personnel who were not familiar with the techniques involved. The role of the veterinarian in providing this on-site training became increasingly important. A legal requirement that the experiments not be duplicative led to greater use of the computerized library resources at the increasingly influential Animal Welfare Information Center at the USDA and at the National Library of Medicine.

Psychological well-being and exercise

The other provisions fared less well. The Congressional requirements to promote psychological well-being of primates and to provide exercise for dogs—included in the Dole-Brown 1985 amendments to the AWA—proved highly controversial. Congress had left unclear exactly how they wanted the USDA to write the rules. Some researchers protested the inclusion of these requirements in the law, arguing that "neither the regulators nor the scientists who study primates can define a concept as vague as 'psychological well-being'" (King et al., 1988), that the scientific basis for these requirements was unclear (FASEB, 1989; Anonymous, 1989), and any changes would be too costly anyhow (Jaschik, 1990; Myers, 1990).

The first proposed rules, which were not even presented in draft form until March 1989, appeared under threat of legal action brought by the Animal Welfare Institute and the Animal Legal Defense Fund against the USDA for failure to act. These draft rules proposed that caged dogs should be released for exercise at least 30 minutes each day, and that a dog alone in a facility should receive "positive physical contact" from humans for at least an hour every day, (USDA, 1989).

The National Association for Biomedical Research representing researchers who were opposed to these proposals argued that the cost of compliance could run to $1,861 million (NABR, 1989). The USDA estimated the cost of compliance with these standards at $876 million for capital improvements over the next two or three years and an additional $207 million per year for operating costs (FASEB, 1989). At issue was whether the rules should be based on "performance standards" (supported largely by the biomedical community) or "engineering standards" (supported largely by the animal welfare activists). In the end, performance standards won out and were incorporated in a final set of standards which appeared in August, 1990.

What appeared finally was a much watered-down version of earlier provisions. Instead of setting specific standards, the regulations allow each laboratory to determine how it will improve treatment of research animals. A great deal of discretion is given to the supervising veterinarian and IACUCs. Each facility makes its own plan for exercising dogs and enhancing the environment for primates, in accordance with "currently accepted professional standards." The IACUC of each research facility has the responsibility of determining how well specific projects provide for the exercise of dogs and the psychological well-being of primates; the IACUC must approve all proposed research plans. Thus, the written plans for specific projects are especially important. The record of these plans, which show how the institution is addressing the issues, is maintained at the institution, and is open to USDA inspectors. The plans are not submitted to the USDA, and therefore are not available to the public under the Freedom of Information Act.

The final rules were generous to the biomedical community. As reported in *Nature,* Barbara Rich, a spokesperson for NABR, said that "For most research institutions, probably the majority, the new rules will mean no change" (Anderson, 1990). Anderson continues, ". . . if research facilities require little change, animal welfare can hardly be expected to substantially improve as a result. Performance-based rules, says William Cotreau of the Animal Welfare Institute, are like no rules at all. They're suggestions." The rules go into effect in 1994.

Former Senator John Melcher (1991), a veterinarian and the person responsible for adding the amendments regarding primate well-being, criticized the rule-making in a *Washington Post* op-ed piece. Currently, the caging commonly given to laboratory baboons does not allow the animals to walk, stand upright, or stretch their arms, all natural postures, he wrote.

A legal challenge was made. The Animal Legal Defense Fund and the Society for Protective Animal Legislation (the lobbying arm of the Animal Welfare Institute) brought suit against USDA alleging that USDA had failed to set standards on well-being and exercise, unlawfully delegating its job to the research constituency, the very constituency it is supposed to regulate. The court agreed. On February 25, 1993, Judge Charles R. Richey of the Federal District Court in Washington, D.C., struck down the Government's rules on well-being and exercise. USDA has failed to implement the 1985 law that Congress had passed, stated the court (Civil Action No. 91-1328). Furthermore, the court severely criticized USDA for having taken nine years to implement the law. USDA was ordered to promulgate new regulations on these matters "without unnecessary delay." Whether or not to appeal this ruling is now up to the decision of the newly appointed Secretary of Agriculture under the Clinton administration.

Despite the weak rulemaking, the inclusion of the key words *well-being* and *exercise* in the law is making a mark. Without the 1985 law, funding for projects to explore environmental enrichment of caged animals probably would not have been forthcoming. The NIH immediately started funding projects concerned with enrichment. At that time of passage of the legislation, the state of the art was such that the first studies involved adding a simple toy, like a ball, to the otherwise naked cage of a singly housed primate and observing the animal's reaction. But now, within a few years, far more elaborate enrichment schemes are being tested, and some are being incorporated into daily use. The literature has become extensive; people's imaginations have been stimulated.

Among the environmental enrichments now being explored are group housing;

58   IN THE NAME OF SCIENCE

structural changes such as the provision of more space, either by providing larger housing or by placing linking tunnels between two cages; the addition of up-rooted trees, poles, ropes and other swinging devices and climbing apparatus; the addition of manipulative devices such as chew toys, barrels and mirrors; and feeding enrichment through the choice of food (instead of boring chow) and the provision of foraging boards. All of these changes bring at least some variety into what was previously a sterile environment. Studies are now being done to record the incidence of abnormal behaviors in monkeys due to their poor environment (self-abuse, self-clasp, plucking hair, etc.) thus providing a measure that can be compared with improvements then made to comply with the law (Bayne et al., 1992). Surely as a result of these efforts there will be a reduction in the proportion of laboratory primates that are psychologically damaged.

Funding for implementation of laws

Funding for enforcement of the laboratory animal laws by the USDA has always been a problem. When the AWA was first passed in 1966, an appropriation of $300,000 was barely achieved. Slowly, annual appropriations rose to the 1989 level of $6.19 million despite attempts by the Office of Management and Budget to reduce them. In both 1985 and 1986, the Reagan administration recommended that no money whatever be allocated to administer the law and inspect the over 1,200 registered research facilities, as well as the 4,000 or so other premises of animal dealers and animal exhibitors that fall under their inspectorate. Lack of USDA personnel has also been a problem so that in 1989, for instance, there were 63 USDA inspectors to inspect 1,296 research laboratories.

In 1990, under the AWA there were 1,470 research facilities registered with the USDA. This compares with some 800 institutions that must comply with the PHS policy. Some overlap between the two groups exists. The academic and commercial institutions that either do not receive federal funding or that use species of animals that are exempted are still outside the provisions of any national policies. How many such institutions there are is unknown, but the number probably runs to several thousands.

Expanding coverage to rats, mice, and birds

The animal welfare community has long fought to have all species of animals used in experiments covered by the law. At issue has been the exclusion of rats, mice, birds, and agricultural animals from the Animal Welfare Act since it was first enacted in 1966. Initially, the USDA had enough on its hands just to get the law into operation. But as time went on, these exclusions became more glaring, especially as rats and mice comprise about 80 to 90 percent of all laboratory animals used.

After the passage of the 1985 AWA amendments, individuals and groups concerned about the welfare of animals exerted pressure to drop the exclusion of these species. The USDA resisted on the grounds of cost. Pressure continued, however, and the USDA finally ruled that, effective June 4, 1990, horses, sheep, goats, cows, and pigs when used for *biomedical or other non-agricultural research* are covered by the AWA. Still excluded are farm animals used in genetic engineering research to increase productivity for food and fiber purposes and also to produce various biologics and pharmaceuticals.

Including rats, mice, and birds within the AWA would have important repercussions in bringing additional facilities (especially testing and educational facilities) within the law and would tend to eliminate facilities whose owners would not want to have to comply with any law. For instance, community and other colleges, previously exempt, would now become subject to federal inspections because they maintained federally protected species.

After years of trying to persuade the USDA to amend the regulations and failing, the Animal Legal Defense Fund brought suit in 1990 to petition the USDA for a rulemaking to include rats, mice, and birds. The case was brought in the United States District Court for the District of Columbia.

In the first round of court hearings, the issue was whether or not the animal advocacy organizations had legal standing to sue. The USDA had moved to dismiss the complaint, claiming lack of standing on the part of the animal organization. But on April 1, 1991, the Court denied the USDA motion and acknowledged ALDF's standing to sue under the AWA. *Standing* is the requirement that a certain action has harmed the petitioner in a way that interferes with a legally recognizable right. It means that a citizen has a status or a right that enables the citizen to sue a government officer if, and only if, a substantive, legally-protected interest of the citizen has been invaded. ALDF along with the HSUS argued that their organizations were harmed because they cannot inform their members and the public about whether animal research facilities are providing humane conditions and treatment of these exempt species. This impairment of ability to inform the public, in the opinion of the Court, provides these organizations with standing to sue.

So the case proceeded to the next round. When the case was heard, the USDA argued that their objections to including these species were based mainly on costs and resources available. According to USDA estimates, 2,300 more facilities would have to be inspected and a 60 percent increase in field inspectors would be needed. They thought that this would double or triple the Animal and Plant Health Inspection Service's workload and would lead to declined enforcement of the AWA with respect to other animals.

The ALDF won its case. In a judgment issued January 8, 1992, Judge Charles R. Richey ruled that the USDA's exclusion of these species is "arbitrary and capricious" (U.S. District Court, 1992). The Court found the USDA's explanation of its refusal to include these species "troubling" because the USDA had concentrated so much attention on expenses and "only a few sentences [were] devoted to consideration of the impact of the proposed changes on the welfare of animals, which is, after all, the purpose of the agency's statutory mandate."

The Court ruled that the USDA is required to reconsider its denial of inclusion of rats, mice, and birds in the light of the court's ruling. So, after 26 years of the AWA, all species *may* be covered—but the USDA has appealed the Court's decision.

More on legal standing

Establishing legal standing is important. Similar battles over standing have been fought in other reform movements—for instance, in environmental protection cases. Christopher D. Stone, professor of law at the University of Southern California argued in a 1982 essay "Should Trees Have Standing?" that natural objects such as trees, mountains, rivers, and lakes should—like corporations— have legal rights. These arguments have been used by the Sierra Club and other groups. Stone traces the development of the idea of legal rights, reminding us that children, old people, women, aliens, and minorities have been without legal rights in many societies throughout human history. Although each new move- ment to confer rights on some new entity may have seemed, in Stone's words, "odd or frightening or laughable," legal rights have been extended to previously rightless people (and things) and have come to be recognized and valued in themselves.

Apart from the battles in court, bills have been introduced in Congress to give interested persons or groups legal standing to sue the USDA to compel enforce- ment of the AWA. These efforts have been strongly opposed by NABR and by the American Physiological Society, which condemn the idea of using citizens as "private attorneys general" (Jasny, 1988). According to Jasny's article in *Science,* these organizations fear that if such a bill were passed, "the flood of [resulting] lawsuits would halt the use of animals in medical research." Furthermore, oppo- nents contend that courts could be placed in the position of deciding such non- quantifiable issues as whether conditions were available to promote the psycho- logical well-being of primates or whether alternative, less painful experimental procedures could have been used by researchers.

In conclusion, it can be seen from these accounts that the range and complex- ity of issues before the legislature and the courts has expanded. There appears to be no lessening of the polarization of viewpoints.

5

Animal Subjects and Alternatives

How much current biomedical endeavor relies on animal experimentation? Among the 6,649 papers given at the 1989 Federation of American Societies for Experimental Biology (FASEB) meeting, nearly 60 percent dealt with experimental data obtained without the use of live animals (Zbinden, 1990a). FASEB does not cover all of the fields of biomedical research, but it is the major organization of basic medical science with a current membership of 33,000 research scientists. Zbinden's figures give some feel for what is going on at the moment. With this important consideration in mind—that animal experimentation is only a portion of the total biomedical endeavor—this chapter looks at that portion and reviews progress toward alternatives.

What is the scientific rationale for using animals as subjects of experiments? Why is it feasible to substitute different species one for another in biomedical experiments? The scientific reason is that, within the compass of living systems, there are generalizations that apply broadly. There is a unity in biology that is seen in the universality of cell theory, of common features in biological structure and function. A prime example is that the genetic code applies from the simplest virus all the way to humans. Universality is seen in the development of all vertebrate embryos consisting of a common program of blastula formation—a program that is characteristic of most invertebrates also. Indeed, it can be hard for the naked eye to distinguish between developing embryos of certain species; a bird embryo looks very much like a human embryo.

Reliance on animal experimentation presents a compelling ethical problem

61

because there are two directly opposing forces. Those species at the top of the phylogenetic scale are the most desirable experimental subjects because of functional similarity to humans. The closer the animal model is to human beings, the more likely it is to replicate the metabolic, physiological, pharmacologic, pathologic, neurologic, and psychological aspects of the human condition. On the other hand, these species are the least desirable because of their closer kinship to humans and their ability to suffer. Therein lies the ethical dilemma.

There are three broad categories of purpose of animal experiments—research, testing, and education. Unfortunately, USDA national data do not break down the information on experiments by purpose. Based on informed opinions from several experts, the best guesstimate is that about 40 percent of all animals used in experiments are used for basic research; 26 percent for drug development, evaluation, and toxicity assessment; 20 percent for product safety testing (other than drugs); about 7 percent for education; and about 7 percent for other purposes (see Figure 5.1).

In the Netherlands and the UK, data are collected according to experimental purpose. In the Netherlands, official 1987 figures show that 42 percent of all experiments are for the purpose of fundamental research, 47 percent for vaccine and drug production and testing, 6 percent for toxicity testing, 4 percent for education and training, and 1 percent for other purposes (Zutphen et al., 1989).

VARIOUS USES OF LABORATORY ANIMALS

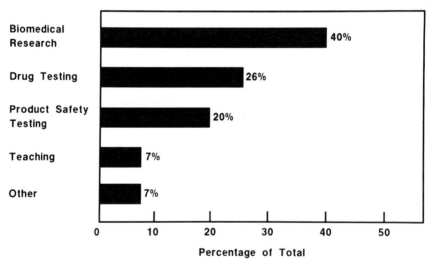

Figure 5.1   This graph is based on best estimates from informed sources. No actual data exists.

*Drug testing includes drug development, evaluation, and toxicity assessment. Source: Office of Technology Assessment, U.S. Congress, Background paper to project "Alternatives to Animal Use in Research, Testing, and Education," November 18, 1983.

Data are also broken down by major species used for research in the areas of (a) cancer, (b) cardiovascular diseases, (c) nervous and mental disorders, and (d) other human and animal diseases. In the UK, in addition to data according to general purpose, specific annual data are provided about the numbers of animals used in areas of great public concern—alcohol and tobacco research and cosmetic safety testing, for instance. Also specific data are provided by type of technique—application of substances to the eye, thermal injury, mechanical interference with brain or spinal cord, induction of psychological stress, physical trauma, LD50 (lethal dose 50 percent—administration of a toxic substance to determine the dose that causes 50 percent of the animals to die), and so on. This valuable information permits tracking the trends in the use of animals in these areas. Such information is not available in the United States.

For any biomedical experiment the selection of the living species to be used is significant. Wherever the ultimate goal is to apply the knowledge gained for human health benefits, (and this is true of much experimental use of animals, although not all), the ideal experimental subject in several respects (species relevancy and potential immediate therapeutic benefit) must be humans themselves; experiments conducted with human beings as subjects are essential.

Some human experiments are done *without* and some *with* prior animal experimentation. Among those conducted without recourse to prior animal testing are the development of many surgical and clinical procedures, development of diagnostic tests, epidemiological studies, and tests of protective measures to prevent onset of disease. A reform measure would be to add to this list those situations in which it is only ethical to use naturally occurring human clinical injury. This would apply in situations where it would be unethical to attempt to simulate such severe trauma intentionally in an animal.

Some human therapeutic procedures depend on the availability of animal tissues as replacement parts. Examples are pig heart valves, pituitary tissue, and other tissues obtained from food animals at slaughter. A highly controversial development has been the rare use of baboon hearts for human transplant. A baboon is so close to a human being in its sentience level and genetic composition that there is strong opposition to taking its life to extend a human life. This procedure stalled in its experimental stages and is unlikely to receive wide public sanction if continued.

In many lines of research, preliminary data are collected on non-human animals because of ethical constraints about using human beings. This often involves basic research on the pathophysiology and natural history of a disease, but it can also involve testing potentially useful interventions to combat the disease process. In current practice, it is only after assessment of animal tests of potentially useful new therapies have been done that cautious tests are conducted on a few human beings. If these show promise, only then will larger scale clinical trials be conducted to assess potential benefits over current therapeutic methods.

Many examples could be given of the value of testing on laboratory animals before human use. Although some members of the animal rights movement deny that human benefits have been derived from animal research, the evidence of benefits is irrefutable. Quite an extensive literature exists on this subject (Abee, 1989; AMA, 1989; Anonymous, 1985; Garattini and van Bekkum, 1990; Katterman, 1984; King et al., 1988; Miller, 1983; NAS Report, 1988; Sample, 1985; Spinelli, 1983). The usefulness of prior animal experimentation spans a wide range of human health issues including aging, AIDS, anesthesia, autoimmune diseases, genetic disorders, cancer, cardiovascular diseases, childhood diseases, diabetes, hepatitis, malaria, pulmonary diseases, organ transplantation, rabies, virology, and many more.

To mention only three: the use of sheep and other species has been critical in developing oral contraceptives; the use of dogs and other mammals has been critical in the development of treating blood disorders and the manufacture of modified hemoglobin as a blood substitute, critical for improving emergency care of those wounded in battle and other situations; the use of baboons in the development of therapeutic interventions for treating Parkinson's disease is another example.

The last example is described in more detail here because modeling this disease in monkeys is traumatic, replicating as it does the human condition. This research raises serious ethical issues and indeed, in Britain, these experimental procedures are ranked at the edge of what is permissible. When questions were raised, a recent UK policy was adopted to permit these studies to continue based on the absence of other currently known approaches.

Parkinson's disease, which usually occurs in people aged 50 or more, afflicts some half million people in the United States. It is a devastating, progressive neurological degeneration that results in death. There are mild and moderate forms that progress only slowly. Early symptoms include tremor and gradual loss of spontaneous movement. As the disease progresses, the more disabling it can become. Typical of the more severe symptoms are drooling, severe loss of balance, "frozen state" periods when the patient is completely unable to start movements, loss of mental abilities, and depression. There is no cure for Parkinson's disease, although the symptoms can be relieved with a drug called L-DOPA. This treatment grew out of a discovery 30 years ago that the disease results from the death of specific cells in a region of the brain that includes the substantia nigra, a term meaning black substance, so called because of the black pigmentation seen in this region. The effect of L-DOPA is to increase the neurotransmitter dopamine in the substantia nigra, thus facilitating relays of impulses between nerves and onward to the muscles. But L-DOPA has its limitations—for some patients it does not work, and in any case, it does not halt the progressive nerve cell death characteristic of Parkinson's disease; it just slows down the progress.

Until recently, Parkinson's disease was difficult to study because it apparently affects only humans. However, a rash of self-inflicted poisonings by drug addicts in the late 1970s gave scientists a clue for duplicating Parkinson's disease in animals. An epidemic of Parkinson's disease occurred among young narcotic addicts in the San Francisco Bay area who had purchased synthetic heroin made in a clandestine laboratory in San Diego. Later, a similar epidemic struck drug abusers in the Netherlands. By 1982, forty-three drug addicts had developed symptoms; eleven had died. The street drug was contaminated by a neurotoxic compound called MPTP (1-methyl-4-phenyl-1,2,3,6-tetrahydropyridine), a narcotic belonging to the Demerol family.

MPTP became the drug that, when tested in animals, revealed much of the basic pathophysiology of Parkinson's disease. In the early 1980s, MPTP was investigated in several species including rat, mouse, frog, leech, guinea pig, dog, and cat, but none of these is considered a useful model for a number of reasons. In some species no long-term motor deficit is seen, and in others the florid Parkinsonian syndrome does not develop. Monkeys, however, including cynomolgus, Rhesus, and squirrel monkeys, as well as marmosets and baboons, do develop the disease. They show the typical degeneration of dopamine-containing neurons. Probably the reason for this species variation is that monkeys' brains are second only to those of humans in the amount of black pigmentation contained in the substantia nigra. Initial responses of these animals to injections of MPTP include agitation, labored breathing, and calling out. Over the next few days the disease develops and then can become stable for years, depending on the species. The symptoms reverse rapidly with L-DOPA treatment. These animals become unable to feed themselves or to obtain water and may have to be tube-fed.

The monkey MPTP model has put scientists at a new threshold of research that has brought new hope to Parkinson's patients. Researchers at NIH, Yale University, and the University of Rochester have produced rapid recoveries in MPTP monkeys with monkey fetal tissue implanted into the substantia nigra. The implanted tissue survives, grows, and apparently produces dopamine in the monkey's brains. According to some reports, not only the implanted cells but also other brain cells begin to produce the needed dopamine. Based on these animal experiments, human tests with cell implants are now taking place in the United States, Sweden, and elsewhere. It is probably too early to draw conclusions about this line of treatment, but it seems worth exploring.

In this example, there is an intimate relationship between the animal experiments and the application of the results to relieving human suffering. But this is not always the case. Some agricultural research is not for the purpose of improving human health but of improving the financial rewards of the factory farmers; in some military experiments animals are used to physically carry the weapon or to test its lethality; some animal behavior and other research is conducted in which species variations make it implausible to apply the findings to human beings.

Total numbers and species of animals used in experiments: USDA data

Estimates are that the total number of vertebrate animals used each year in the United States is between 25 and 30 million. No national data exist on this, and estimates vary widely from 17 to 70 million.

Until 1990, USDA data on laboratory use covered only the following species: primates, dogs, cats, guinea pigs, hamsters, rabbits, and certain other species. Rats, mice, and birds have always been excluded, although this may change as a result of a 1992 court ruling (see details in chapter 4). Because data are limited, it is rather meaningless at this time to attempt to assess overall trends in animal use when 80 to 90 percent of all animals used are excluded. For what it is worth, the total numbers of AWA-protected animals used for the period 1973 to 1990 are shown in Figure 5.2 (actual numbers are given in Appendix A). The number of animals used ranges from a low of 1,378 thousand in 1975 to a high of 2,154 thousand in FY 1985, with 1,842 thousand used in 1991. There was an upswing

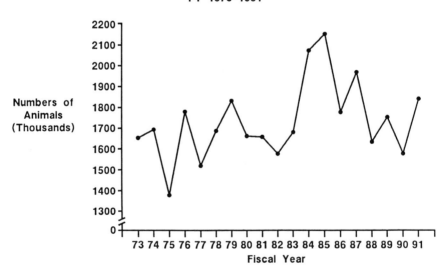

TRENDS IN TOTAL NUMBERS OF "AWA-PROTECTED ANIMALS" USED, FY 1973-1991

Figure 5.2 All years for which USDA data is available are included. "AWA-protected animals" means primates, dogs, cats, guinea pigs, rabbits, hamsters, and certain other species. Excluded for all years from "AWA-protected animals" are rats, mice, and birds. Agricultural animals—horses, sheep, goats, cows, and pigs—were first included in USDA data in 1990.

Source: APHIS, USDA.

in numbers of animals used during the peak years 1984 and 1985, and the USDA has no explanation for this (Richard L. Crawford, personal communication, May 24, 1991). Using only figures from 1985 on, some people have depicted these last few years as showing a decline in numbers of AWA-protected animals used. But this decline is not so impressive when the total span of years is viewed. All that can be said is that the increase in the mid-1980s has been somewhat halted.

USDA annually keeps track of the numbers of research facilities and sites where laboratory animals are used—an important piece of information in understanding trends in laboratory animal use. Both research facilities and sites have steadily increased over the years. The following figures from selected years illustrate the overall picture; facilities totaled 985 in 1975, 1,166 in 1983, and 1,474 in 1991. During this time, the number of research sites has almost doubled, going from 1,932 in 1975 to 3,495 in 1991. Within the last five years, over 700 new sites have been added—a dramatic increase. This increase in facilities and sites *might* be related to an increase in total numbers of animals used, but there is no hard data to substantiate or refute this reasonable possibility. Lacking, of course, are data on all species of animals used.

For comparison with other countries, in Britain, Canada, and the Netherlands, where all species of laboratory animals are counted, recent total use has been declining. In Britain, the 1990 total number of animals used for experimentation was 3.2 million (*Statistics on Scientific Procedures,* 1990). The breakdown by individual species shows that the percentage of total was mice 51 percent, rats 28 percent, and birds 8 percent (an aggregate of 87 percent), and others. Also, since figures are available for many past decades, overall trends can be tracked. Comparing the 1990 total (3.2 million) with the 1980 total (4.6 million), overall use has declined by 30 percent. This drop is primarily due to reduced use of mice and rabbits.

In Canada, the total number of animals used was 1.3 million in 1989, a 38 percent reduction since 1977 when the total was 2.1 million (CCAC, 1991/1992). Furthermore, Canadian data show that primate use has fallen from 4,744 in 1977 to 2,138 in 1989 (a 55-percent reduction). For other species also, such as dogs, cats, rabbits, guinea pigs, mice, and rats, there have been reductions of from 34 to 68 percent over the same twelve-year period.

In the Netherlands, just over 951,000 animal experiments were performed in 1990, 5.9 percent fewer than in 1989 and 10.5 percent fewer than in 1988 (*Frame News,* 1992).

In the United States, the USDA provides information broken down by six major groupings: primates, dogs, and cats (see Figure 5.3); and guinea pigs, hamsters, and rabbits (see Figure 5.4). Over the total period of years, the data do not show any decline in numbers of primates used. Figure 5.3 and Appendix A show that the numbers of primates have fluctuated from a low of 36,202 in 1975 to a high of 61,392 in 1987. Since 1987, there has been an annual decline, down to 42,620 in 1991, which is still not as low as the 1975 level.

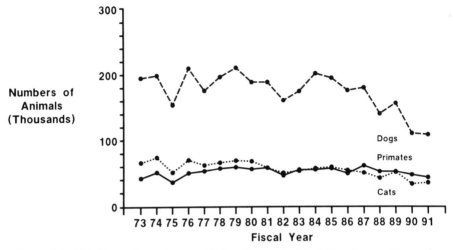

TRENDS IN NUMBERS OF PRIMATES, DOGS, AND CATS
USED IN EXPERIMENTS IN THE UNITED STATES, FY 1973-1991

Figure 5.3 This figure shows that overall, for all years depicted, there is no evidence of decline in primate use. Current levels in fact are higher than in some previous years. For dogs and cats, there has been a general trend toward decline over all years, the most significant being for dogs.

Source: APHIS, USDA.

Figure 5.3 also shows that the use of cats and dogs has fluctuated over time, but with these species there is some indication of a downward trend. The decline is greatest in dogs. Anecdotal evidence suggests that a shift to the use of other species (swine and rodents) is taking place.

Figure 5.4 shows that the data for guinea pigs, hamsters, and rabbits have fluctuated considerably over the years 1977 through 1991 and no consistent pattern is evident. There is a peak in guinea pig use in 1984–85. For all three species, figures for the last two years, 1990–91, are roughly equal to or are somewhat below the earliest years for which data are available. Since the peak in the mid-1980s, there is some suggestion of a decline. But in view of the great fluctuations in the past, this decline may not necessarily continue. Despite enthusiastic announcements that there has been a drastic reduction in the use of the Draize test (in which potentially irritating substances are tested in rabbits' eyes), only during 1990/1 did the use of rabbits fall below the all-time low of 1977.

A group called Investor Responsibility Research Center has made an analysis of the use of animals by pharmaceutical and household product manufacturers (Welsh, 1990). Under the Freedom of Information Act, they obtained from the USDA individual reports from various industrial facilities for the years 1986 to 1988, and they also constructed their own database. They reported that "Corpora-

**TRENDS IN NUMBERS OF GUINEA PIGS, HAMSTERS, AND RABBITS
USED IN EXPERIMENTS IN THE UNITED STATES, FY 1977-1991**

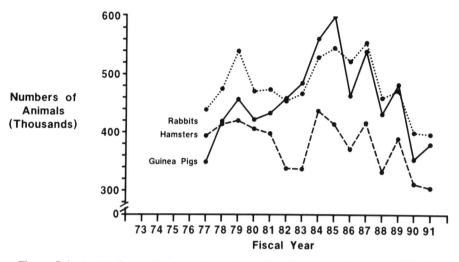

Figure 5.4   In this figure, the fluctuations shown for all three species are sufficiently great that caution must be exercised in assessing trends. Nevertheless, there is some suggestion that since the peak years of 1984 to 1985, there has been some decline in numbers. National data for the years 1973 to 1976 are not available.

Source: APHIS, USDA.

tions were most likely to use guinea pigs (40 percent), rabbits (29 percent) and hamsters (17 percent), while non-commercial facilities divided their use more evenly among rabbits (25 percent), guinea pigs (20 percent) and hamsters (11 percent). Cats and primates each made up 1 percent and dogs 6 percent of corporate animal use; for non-commercial use, dogs were 11 percent, primates 5 percent, and cats 4 percent" (pages 134–135).

Choice of species

The choice of species may be guided by good scientific reasons, as shown in a report of a recent NIH conference (Modeling in Biomedical Research, 1989). For instance, the rat heart is a good model for myocardial biochemistry because the biochemical processes are highly conserved, the hearts are small and easy to examine, and the animals are inexpensive. "On the other hand," the report continues, "rat hearts are of little value to an investigator who wants to know how myocardial blood flow is affected by stresses in the thick-walled ventricle or by changes in heart rate from 150 to 75 beats per minute because the rat left ventricle is very thin walled and its heart rate is about 450 beats per minute."

Good scientific reasons are not always at the heart of selection of species—

historical tradition also is a factor. Investigators learn techniques from their mentors, and once a pattern has been established, it tends to be perpetrated. To some extent, it is both economical and valuable scientifically to do so, but it significantly slows down the introduction of reforms.

Within the last few decades, pharmacologists have learned that among mammals there are considerable species variations in the degree and nature of response to drugs. So animal tests using several species rather than one are more likely to indicate the probable effects on humans. Before drugs are tested in humans, tests are commonly run on mice, rats, rabbits, dogs, cats, and maybe some non-human primates. There can be wide variations among species in the response itself and also in the relationship between dose and response, the frequency and type of adverse reactions, the mechanisms and sites of action, metabolic and excretion pathways, body storage patterns, etc. Under current law, testing of a new drug on several mammalian species must be done before clinical trials on humans can be legally started.

Despite these precautions of using several species, problems of untoward dangers of a new therapeutic procedure are never completely excluded. Put another way, it is never possible to be absolutely sure that the species chosen for study will replicate the human condition. These facts are well-appreciated by scientists; antivivisectionists are keen to dwell on them (see for instance Sharpe, 1988). The failure of animal testing to uncover adverse human reactions has been documented by Ryder (1989), who discusses the matter in some detail, noting the disastrous effects that overconfidence in animal tests has caused. In addition to these problems, individual variations in response between one human being and another can also lead to unforeseen disastrous results. But overall, most people believe that animal tests, although imperfect, are better than no tests.

There are other serious limitations of relying on a narrow spectrum of species. For instance, research on the aging process has traditionally relied on two rodents, mice and rats. Harvard biologist Steven Austad has said that this is "like trying to understand human psychology by interviewing two brothers" (Morell, 1990). Austad and others are now turning for their gerontological research to a curious menagerie that includes spiders, lizards, opossums, turtles, bats, Japanese quail—even platyfish. He and others predict a fundamental advance in gerontology as a result. In this case, the expansion to use lower species is not undertaken because of animal welfare concerns, but for scientific reasons.

Should there be more human research?

One of the proposals of the animal activists is that money should be deflected from animal experimentation into clinical studies of human patients, especially studies of substance abuse and mental disorders and studies of ways to apply already known preventive measures for cancer and heart disease. Regarding

RESEARCH MATERIALS USED IN NIH EXTRAMURAL RESEARCH PROJECTS
DOLLARS AWARDED, FY 1983-1989

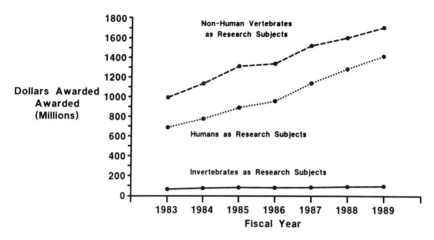

Figure 5.5 This figure shows that more money is spent on non-human than on human experimentation. Furthermore, there has been a increase in the dollars used for research in the two categories of research subject, non-human vertebrate species, and humans. The difference in expenditure between these two categories has remained relatively the same. In comparison, for research involving invertebrate species, there has been a relatively slight increase in the dollars expended.

NIH classifies "research subject" into the three broad categories shown here, non-human vertebrate animals, humans, and invertebrates. If a research project funded by NIH uses more than one of these categories, then the data are not counted. For instance, if a project involves use of humans and non-human vertebrates together in the same project, or non-human vertebrates and invertebrates together, then information on this project is omitted.

Source: National Center for Research Resources, NIH.

substance abuse, they argue that human addicts willing to enter rehabilitation programs immediately are often told to wait several months because of lack of clinical facilities, by which time they may have changed their minds. The suggestion made by the activists is that research on human victims of self-induced substance abuse would be preferable to animal research. Not only would there be immediate potential benefit to these individuals but also to the total population of human addicts because such research avoids problems of species variation.

NIH is the major funding agency for both animal and human research. Figure 5.5 shows that in the United States more money is currently spent on experiments in which animals are subjects than on experiments in which human beings are subjects. (This does not include money spent in human health care delivery, of course, which far exceeds the money spent on research.) In fiscal year 1989, according to NIH data, $1,701 million was spent on non-human vertebrate animal experiments (which includes non-human primates and all other mammals, birds, fish, amphibians, and reptiles) and $1,409 million was spent on research involving human subjects. Over the period 1983 to 1989, of the total expenditure, the proportion given to human experimentation has remained quite stable at 41 to 45 percent. (Figure 5.5 also shows funding for invertebrate studies, which will be discussed later.) Data showing how much is spent on primate studies, as distinct from studies using other species, is not available from NIH. This is regrettable because there is considerable public interest in tracking trends in primate use.

INFLUENCE OF PUBLIC ATTITUDES.   Public attitudes help protect certain species including those commonly encountered as pets (e.g., dogs, cats, horses), or particularly admired for their intelligence and beauty (e.g., primates or dolphins), or possessing beguiling attributes or juvenile characteristics (e.g., deer, seals, calves, pandas). On the whole, these species have a greater chance of humane treatment. Indeed, they may be singled out for special protection under the law. For instance, under British law from 1876 to 1986, scientists had to obtain special licenses to justify experiments on a dog, cat, or horse. In the United States, dogs and primates have been singled out for special legal provisions.

On the other hand, despite efforts by the animal rights movement to enlarge public concern for all species, some species continue to be less favored. Among these are mice, rats, pigs, and ferrets. Over the decades, trading in laboratory mice and rats has become big business, and there is no sign of its declining; recently, trade in laboratory "mini-pigs," "micro-pigs" and ferrets has increased. Anecdotal evidence suggests that investigators who used to conduct head-injury studies on baboons or spinal-cord-injury studies on cats are now using rats; other investigators have substituted pigs for dogs in their studies of cardiac arrest. As a sign of current trends, a speaker at a recent American Association for Laboratory Animal Science (AALAS) conference gave a paper called "Alternatives," and his message was that investigators should switch from dogs and cats to less-liked species such as pigs to avoid public attention. Although this is a distortion of the humanitarian meaning of "alternatives," this paper was greeted with approval by the attendees as being politically savvy.

Commercial breeders of laboratory animals exploit this approach by using the word *alternative* in their advertising copy. As examples, an ad that features laboratory swine and sheep is headed "The Better Alternatives"; "Your specific research needs—pigs—the inexpensive alternative"; and another touts ferrets as "an affordable alternative."

INFLUENCE OF VESTED INTERESTS.   A profitable business venture of supplying laboratory mammals has grown up over the last few decades—commercial developers have made it easy for investigators to obtain laboratory animals. Several species of mammals are bred in their millions. Choice can be made among many species by sex, age, and strain, and the animals can be shipped rapidly from the commercial suppliers to the laboratories. These animals are produced rather as in a factory in identical, easily replaced units, and marketed and transported with a certain uniformity. Scientists are beholden to these companies for providing a reliable source of health-standardized animals, and these suppliers have served a useful purpose in improving the quality and range of scientific research.

According to McArdle (1988), Charles River produces close to 16 million animals annually. It is not without significance that the most prestigious award given by the American Association for Laboratory Animal Science, whose primary constituency is veterinarians and technicians involved in animal experimentation, is the Charles River Award.

Another major laboratory animal supplier is Jackson Laboratories in Bar Harbor, Maine. Their advertisements state that they distribute over two million mice annually. They specialize in breeding and making available inbred genetically consistent strains of rodents, which have contributed in significant ways to the elucidation of biological processes.

Uses of invertebrate species

Animal welfare advocates have not shown much interest in the substitution of invertebrates for vertebrates. Yet especially in the use of animals in education (as opposed to research and testing), the substitution of invertebrate for vertebrate species could go a long way toward reducing ethical costs. This concept has appeared in a number of guidelines for the use of animals in education, but has not been put into practice in any noticeable way.

Invertebrate organisms have been used in certain areas of biomedical research. Invertebrates have many advantages: they are readily available in great numbers, relatively inexpensive, small in size so that less space is required for housing, and easy to care for. Moreover, their shorter generation intervals make them especially useful for research on aging and genetic inheritance. Much of the genetic work of the twentieth century has been done on *Drosophila* (fruit fly), which has a generation time of ten days.

There is a relative simplicity in invertebrate biochemical reactions and in the interactions of their systems. Researchers working on extremely complicated problems may start by trying to understand the basics in as simple an organism as possible and then go on to more elaborate systems. An example is "the worm project," which started in 1963 when Sydney Brenner set out to learn "everything there is to know" biologically about the nematode *Caenorhabditis elegans,* a tiny worm a mere millimeter long. "I would like to tame a small metazoan," is how he put it (Roberts, 1990). The Medical Research Council's Laboratory of Molecular Biology in Cambridge, England, where Brenner works, was the first of what are now about 100 labs around the world that have turned to the study of this nematode. This tiny worm has revealed a wealth of information about development of the brain. Currently, the biggest research project yet on *C. elegans* is a ten-year effort to decipher its complete genetic instructions. Brenner and other scientists are collaborating to work out the full nucleotide sequence, all 100 million bases. According to reports, this work is fast becoming the benchmark by which the human genome will be measured.

In 1989, NIH support for invertebrate biomedical studies amounted to $94 million (see Figure 5.5). There has been a steady increase in expenditure over the years commensurate with the steady increase in financial support for other areas of research. When represented as a proportion of expenditures for all research, expenditure for research using invertebrate animals has remained stable, ranging from 3 to 4 percent over the period 1983 to 1989. So, despite many inventive ways to exploit invertebrates for scientific purposes, nothing suggests that this research is likely to increase in proportion to the rest.

Alternatives: cells, tissues, and non-animal systems

Many alternatives to using whole animals are available. It is simplistic to regard alternative systems as being capable of fully replacing animals totally—at least with our current understanding. More commonly *in vitro* and *in vivo* approaches to biomedical problems need to go on side by side. (*In vitro* literally means within a glass or test tube but is interpreted to mean experiments that do not involve intact animals.) Body functions and reactions are so complex that using just one modeling system does not provide a complete answer to a scientific problem—a combination of methods is usually needed. For example, immunological responses can be dissected with *in vitro* techniques, but at a certain point they must be studied—and new therapies tested on them—in whole animals or humans simply because the whole of a biological response cannot be mimicked in a test tube. As another example, drugs are metabolized as they pass through the liver, and to examine the breakdown, storage, and excretion patterns involved in this biotransformation process, whole animal or human studies are needed. Typically, *in vitro* methods can be used to ask certain questions at the cellular or molecular level, whereas whole animals (including humans) are needed to answer questions at the organ and inter-organ level.

Thus, in defending their use of whole animals, scientists contend that many studies cannot be done without using whole live animals. Other examples are research on vision, brain function, the natural history of a disease, and drug effects on the heart or nervous system or on a developing fetus. Furthermore, certain organ systems and physiologic functions are so distinctive to mammals that no other human surrogate exists. An obvious example is the study of mammary glands—the subjects must be either humans or other mammals. These areas of study that are completely dependent either on human study or on whole live animal surrogates represent only a portion of the total animal use.

With this said, we can look at some of the *in vitro* approaches that are part of the scientific armamentarium. Among them are the use of human tissues derived from surgery or autopsy, tissue cultures, and non-animal systems such as mathematical modeling or computer simulation. These are the "replacements" that have been the primary focus of reformers. Some members of the public have come to believe that these techniques will be able to substitute for all animal experiments—a dream that the scientific community has strongly disputed as being unrealistic.

Human tissues, organs, and cells have all proved useful. They have a particular attraction because of the fact that they avoid the problems of species differences. Human blood, corneas, and fetal brain tissue have been utilized both for research and therapeutic purposes. Human umbilical cords provide tissues for study, including endothelial cells for tissue culture and membranes for the investigation of human labor processes. Also, the placenta is used to study laminin and other basement membrane proteins.

In recent years, the culture of cells and tissues, both human and animal, has reached a high level of sophistication and has been responsible for many new discoveries. Both normal and pathological cell culture lines have been useful in toxicological and cancer research. A significant change in the tide of animal use occurred in the late 1980s when the National Cancer Institute announced that it had developed a new *in vitro* screen, which has reduced its annual use of animals by 95 percent from six million to 30,000. The new system focuses on human cell tumor lines grown directly in test tubes and enables scientists to concentrate on more sensitive testing methods. The old system used mouse-based cancer screens and has now been phased out completely according to Robert Shoemaker, Ph.D., acting chief of the Information Technology Branch at NCI.

Because of the adoption of *in vitro* methods it is all too easy to assume that there must be some overall impact of reduction on the total use of animals. But this is not necessarily so, and in fact may be incorrect. An informed perspective on this matter is provided by Gerhard Zbinden (1990b) of the University of Zurich. He says that although *in vitro* methods are widely practiced, "the impact on the use of laboratory animals has been modest. The challenge of the future is to find out why so many animals are still needed to carry out scientific research."

Computer modeling is used extensively nowadays to simulate biological, chemical, and physical systems. Furthermore, by performing statistical comparisons across data sets and identifying relationships not already obvious, unforeseen relationships may be established. Also, of course, computers are used to disseminate information that has been generated from prior study of humans or animals, thus avoiding the needless repetition of a procedure by other scientists. Many data banks are now in use, including the Toxicology Data Bank, the Registry of Toxic Effects of Chemical Substances, and many others.

Computer and mathematical modeling has been part of the normal research endeavor for many years, but the motivating factor generally has not been saving animals' lives. This research selection probably has more to do with the investi-gator's special skills and the nature of the scientific problem, but in the areas of testing and education, computer and mathematical modeling does seem to be chosen because it saves animals' lives.

Resistance to alternatives

Evidence of resistance to the concept of alternatives is often seen. Sometimes the concept of alternatives is distorted by the presentation of only one aspect (re-placement), not all three aspects. This is done by both opponents and proponents of animal research. A few scientists present the case against replacement of animal experimentation and infer from these arguments that the concept of alter-natives as a whole is flawed. Such is not the case, since the refinement and reduction options remain applicable.

Critics of alternatives have held considerable sway at NIH. For instance, a frequent critic of alternatives is Frederick K. Goodwin, M.D., head of the National Institute of Mental Health, which is a part of the Alcohol, Drug Abuse and Mental Health Administration (ADAMHA). Goodwin is widely called upon by the scientific community as a speaker on animal experimentation issues; he received a public service award from FASEB for his activities in combating animal activists and promoting animal research. In 1990, at an annual meeting of the American Association for the Advancement of Science (AAAS), he argued that by adopting the three R's of reduction, refinement, and replacement, the biomedical research community creates the impression that scientists are "some-how apologetic about the use of animals," and that we are "going to try to eliminate" animal research as quickly as we possibly can (quoted in Anonymous, 1990). No such apology is necessary, he said, and it is undesirable from a political and public relations stand. Goodwin (1989) has also described the diver-sion of research funds into the search for alternatives as serious damage.

Echoing Goodwin, Robert Burke, M.D., Chief of the Laboratory of Neuro-control at NIH, at an NIH-organized conference said that "the Three R's translate poorly into policy and action . . . they suggest a collective apology by the scien-tific community for implicit wrongdoing. When we advocate the Three R's, we imply that we, as scientists, are currently doing something wrong, that we are a bit ashamed of being forced by necessity to do [animal research], and that we would stop if we could. We appear to defend research use of animals as a necessary evil" (Burke, 1989). Proposing refinements, according to Burke, sug-gests that current methods are "inadequate or unethical." He concludes by speak-ing of the "misleading baggage" of reduction and replacement and says, "In my view, it is intellectually dishonest and hypocritical to continue to advocate the original Three R's as a goal for science policy. It is also, without question, dangerous to give our enemies such useful tools with which to pervert the

scientific enterprise." These remarks appear in the proceedings published by
NIH. It is one thing for such inflammatory remarks to appear in publications of
advocacy groups, and quite another for them to appear in publications of the
Office of Animal Care and Use of NIH.

However, as a counter to these influences, other scientists are fully supportive
of alternatives. Indeed, an NIH conference in August 1992 is entitled "The
Humane Care and Use of Laboratory Animals" and is subtitled "Reduction,
Refinement and Replacement in the Field and Laboratory." This is one of a series
of conferences NIH holds each year in conjunction with host universities whose
faculty are largely responsible for the program. This one is at Idaho State University and their scientists apparently want to foster the three R's.

Funding for alternatives

Despite this coolness toward alternatives within some parts of the scientific
community, the adoption of alternatives has nevertheless thrived, primarily because funding for alternatives has been made available. In the discussion that
follows, three types of funding are described: (1) targeted funding for alternatives; (2) non-targeted, indirect funding that does not have the specific objective
of promoting alternatives but that is helpful toward achieving these ends; and (3)
in-house funding.

Targeted funding by reform groups

A sure way to get a job done is to announce that specific funding is targeted for
it. Although the amount of money available for developing alternatives is comparatively small compared to the overall research budget, an increasing number
of research scientists are receiving such funds.

The initiative to provide this funding came from several antivivisection societies. Later, animal welfare groups, foundations, corporations, and governments
joined in. A chronological history of these events is provided in Appendix B
along with information on sources of funds, see page 275 et seq.

Traditionally, antivivisection organizations had maintained a hostile distance
from scientists, so it was a significant move when, in the early 1960s, they
started to fund biomedical investigators. Some dedicated and highly respected
scientists, determined to pursue the goals of reducing and replacing the use of
animals, have done the actual work, and their involvement of course has been
indispensable. Among these scientists are Joseph Leighton, M.D., professor and
Chair of the Department of Pathology at the Medical College of Pennsylvania,
who developed the CAM Assay (chorioallantoic membrane of a chick) as a
Draize alternative; and Björn Ekwall, M.D., professor of toxicology at the
Swedish University of Uppsala and Erik Walum, Ph.D., professor of neuro-

chemistry at the University of Stockholm, who run the Multicenter Evaluation of *In Vitro* Cytotoxicity, which evaluates non-animal product tests. Those named are among the scientists who have received funding from the American Fund for Alternatives to Animal Research, but many others could be mentioned.

There were benefits in both directions from this new interchange. Not only did this funding encourage the sort of research techniques that reformers wanted, it also helped to change attitudes both within the biomedical community and in the public. The concept of "alternatives" over time has become a respectable goal held not only by outside pressure groups but also by some scientists.

To some extent barriers were broken down. Scientists started to associate with antivivisectionists and humane society people—something that could have courted censure from their colleagues previously. They presented their research results at meetings sponsored by humane groups, and antivivisection groups started to report in some detail in their literature the scientific work they had sponsored. As a result, some members of the public became more educated about the conduct of science. A focus of such funding has been the development and validation of alternatives to the Draize and LD50 tests and other toxicology testing. More recently, another growing area is funding for computer models and other alternatives to replace the harming and killing of animals for educational purposes.

Reform groups pressed for corporate funding from Revlon, Inc. and The Cosmetic, Toiletry, and Fragrance Association—as described in Chapter 10—and this resulted in the establishment of two academic centers: in 1980, the In Vitro Toxicology Laboratory at The Rockefeller University devoted to research on alternative toxicity tests, first headed by Dennis Stark, D.V.M., Ph.D., and since June 1991 by Michael D. Hayre, D.V.M.; and in 1981, the Center for Alternatives to Animal Testing at The Johns Hopkins University, headed by Alan M. Goldberg, Ph.D. The mission of both centers is to conduct research to develop alternatives to animal use in testing. In 1989, another academic center was established, the Center for Animals and Public Policy at Tufts University School of Veterinary Medicine, headed by Andrew N. Rowan, D. Phil., and part of its mission is to explore alternatives in toxicity testing. Initial funding for the Tufts Center was from the Environmental Protection Agency; now corporate funding has been added. These three academic centers pursue all three R's in their programs.

On the other hand, antivivisection organizations tend not to pursue all three alternatives. They concentrate on replacement alternatives, which may bring in their wake a reduction in numbers of animals used; they will not fund refinements. The American Fund for Alternatives to Animal Research is typical. As a hypothetical example, AFAAR would not fund development of a more humane method of restraining monkeys to eliminate traditional immobilization chairs. Efforts were made when AFAAR was first established to encourage the organization to include all three R's, but they failed. What AFAAR does fund is non-animal methods (such as computer simulation), or studies that involve use of human tissues (such as placenta), tissue culture techniques, and other *in vitro* systems.

Similarly, The Dr. Hadwen Trust for Humane Research in England has a 1991 policy that states in part, "it is a basic principle of the Trust's policy that research which requires the use of living animals in any way, even though the ultimate aim may be to replace their use, cannot be supported. It is appreciated that in order to demonstrate the validity of a new technique some may feel the need to continue temporarily with a procedure using animals, but support from the Trust may not be used for this purpose. The Trust will not fund the purchase or maintenance or animals for any purpose." Hence, development of a new animal model using a snail to test anesthetics to substitute for a widely-used rat model in pain research would not be supported because inevitably this would require comparison of the two systems and thus use of rats.

Recently, The Hadwen Trust has gone even further. Reflecting the concern of their members who point out that to derive a cell culture can sometimes mean harming an animal (captivity or death), they have announced they will no longer offer grants for research that uses animal cells or tissues of any sort. This, they state, reflects recent progress in the culture of human cells.

Toward the end of the 1980s, a few animal welfare groups, foundations, corporations, and governments entered the picture, and they fund all three R's. These include the privately funded Doerenkamp-Zbinden Foundation and Parks Foundation, and the Dutch Platform for Alternatives (a consortium of several government ministries, pharmaceutical companies, and animal protection organizations), and many others. See Appendix B for details.

NIH-targeted program

The Health Research Extension Act of 1985 required NIH to establish plans for research into methods of biomedical experimentation which "do not require the use of animals, which are likely to reduce the number of animals used, or which would produce less pain and distress than methods currently in use." Accordingly, in January 1987, NIH made its first announcement of the program, which involved all NIH institutes (NIH Guide for Grants and Contracts, 1987). No funds were set aside, as happens with some program announcements.

I had to use the Freedom of Information Act to obtain details about what has been funded under this NIH grant program. Over the three years 1987 to 1989 a modest seventeen awards have been made. The breakdown is as follows: 1987—seven awards totaling $1,077,000; 1988—five awards totaling $490,000; and 1989—five awards totaling $890,000. Very little that is new has been stimulated. Many of these seventeen awards have been for development or use of nonmammalian models, including projects on frogs, mollusks, octopuses, squid, insects, and earthworms. As shown in Figure 5.5 and discussed earlier, such research has been supported for many years by NIH, and the dollar amounts have remained stable relative to other types of research. Many of these seventeen are a subset of those included in Figure 5.5.

Other awards made under this alternatives program support mathematical modeling and computer studies. Again, there is little evidence that NIH would not have supported this type of work in any event. Only one project seems to cut new ground for NIH. In 1988, this program provided core support of the Johns Hopkins Center for Alternatives to Animal Testing. It seems unlikely that this award would have been made without the 1985 Congressional directive.

Although one of the stated goals of the program is to help develop methods in biomedical research that will "produce less pain and distress in vertebrate animals than models currently used," as of 1992 no awards have been made that directly fulfill that goal—refinement projects are not in evidence. Overall, the impression is that, meritorious as the seventeen funded projects are, this program has done little new to support alternatives.

Non-targeted, indirect funding

In its 1986 report, the Office of Technology Assessment (OTA) made an analysis of funding sources for alternatives under a broad interpretation of what this covered (U.S. Congress OTA Report, pages 259–272). This interpretation encapsulates the biomedical community's perspective. OTA included projects likely to improve either the humaneness of the animals' living conditions or the skills of the laboratory personnel in conducting animal experiments (such as training in anesthesia and euthanasia methods and humane techniques); projects that reduce or eliminate animal pain or stress; studies of animal anesthesiology, pain perception, and other aspects of pain research; and all aspects of improvements to enhance the environment, social enrichment, and expression of the animals' normal behavioral repertoire. Thus, funding for research on environmental enrichment for primates and on exercise of dogs would be counted as "alternatives funding."

The OTA report rightly points out that most funding for alternatives has occurred incidentally through federal funding of basic research in the physical and biological sciences rather then through targeted funding. Among the examples it cited are the development of new methods in computer simulation and non-invasive imaging, and developments in biotechnology and cell culture. The purpose of these grants is not to reduce the need for animals, but they may have this effect indirectly.

For many years, NIH has provided funding for the renovation of animal facilities (also included under OTA's interpretation of alternatives funding). Renovation has made possible the accreditation of facilities that otherwise would not have qualified. Better facilities add to the animals' welfare and lead to healthier, less stressed animals that can add to the reliability of research results by reducing the confounding variables that come with inferior husbandry. However, from the point of view of those like Tom Regan who has said he does not want to see better cages but empty cages, improvements in animal facilities do not qualify as alternatives.

According to the NIH Laboratory Animal Facility Improvement Program, the following dollar amounts have been awarded:

1985	$ 8,571,000	1989	11,131,000
1986	3,820,000	1990	10,931,000
1987	9,849,000	1991	11,100,000 (estimated figure).
1988	11,778,000		

(Source: NIH. Personal communication from Don C. Gibson, February 25, 1991).

Compared to the amount of money spent for vertebrate animal research, NIH grants to improve animal facilities represent less than one percent. Typical are the figures for 1989 when NIH spent $11 million on animal facilities compared with $1,701 million on vertebrate animal research. This does not give the whole picture because to some extent research institutions contribute their own, non-federal dollars to animal facility improvements.

In-house funding

Another way to promote activity in a specific area is to provide in-house funding, an established practice within government, industrial, and private research labo-ratories. Most notable in this respect has been the response of industry. As part of their public relations efforts, several companies involved in the production and testing of cosmetics, pharmaceuticals, and household products announce these expenditures annually. For instance, Proctor and Gamble announced that they have spent over 14 million dollars to develop alternatives since 1986. Also, Johnson and Johnson state that during 1989, in their total programs (in-house and other), they have spent over $4.3 million "on the development of and/or utiliza-tion of *in vitro* alternative test methods" (John E. Willson, personal communica-tion January 14, 1991). Colgate Palmolive's 1989 Report of Laboratory Research with Animals states that the company has invested more than $3 million in alternatives research since 1983. Other examples could be cited.

A broad interpretation of what funding of alternatives means might include training of laboratory personnel in humane techniques. The 1985 Congressional mandate requires that "each research facility shall provide for the training of scientists, animal technicians, and other personnel involved with animal care and treatment . . . shall provide instruction on 1) the humane practice of animal maintenance and experimentation; 2) research or testing methods that minimize or eliminate the use of animals or limit animal pain or distress."

Although such training was not entirely absent before the 1985 law, now that it is mandated new expenditures have occurred. Each institution devises its own method of complying with the law. A typical course lasts a few hours, although in some institutions it may be longer. Such training teaches laboratory personnel about anesthetic use and euthanasia methods and introduces them to the concept of alternatives. At The University of Texas M. D. Anderson Cancer Center, for example, the training courses include the following topics: husbandry, euthanasia, government policies, operation of the IACUC, the veterinary services available, alternatives, and the animal rights movement. It is difficult to determine just how much money has gone into these endeavors, but all research facilities that fall under the AWA are probably devoting some funds to training purposes.

In summary, the use of animals currently comprises a major part of the biomedical research endeavor; it has a rational basis but raises ethical concerns. Efforts to introduce alternatives to animal experimentation have been pioneered by citizen groups, and now the concept of alternatives has gained acceptance in industry and in federal policies. These events have surely had an impact in promoting humane attitudes. Finally, there is evidence that the numbers of animals used in experiments has already peaked in the United Kingdom, Canada, and the Netherlands. But for the United States, data are so incomplete that it is impossible to make such a statement.

6

Protocol Review

The 1985 amendments to the Animal Welfare Act mandated for the first time that experimental protocols involving animals be reviewed for humane concerns. How is protocol review conducted? What do Institutional Animal Care and Use Committees look for, and how can the degree of harm to an animal be assessed or minimized? This chapter addresses these issues.

The mechanism of IACUC review was fashioned after the review of experimentation using human beings as subjects, but followed some decades later. For both Institutional Review Boards and IACUCs the committees are selected by the local institution, membership must comply with mandated representation, the charge is to ensure compliance with certain policies, and reports of committee activities must be made at regular intervals to the overseeing federal agency.

Charge of the committee

Nationally, IACUCs were not functioning effectively before the 1985 legislation. Richard L. Rissler, head of the Animal and Plant Health Inspection Service, USDA, estimated that 39 percent of the USDA-registered facilities (475 of a total of 1291) either had no IACUCs or had non-functional committees before the law was passed. Among the 61 percent that did have an IACUC, the committees were mainly concerned with checking cage sizes for compliance with USDA standards and estimating costs for maintaining animals so that these could be charged against grants. Review of experimental procedures was rarely part of their charge, and even if it was, the committees acted largely as rubber stamps.

An indication that committees were ineffective in overseeing the conditions of animal experimentation came from an NIH study, the results of which were published in 1984 (NIH Guide for Grants, 1984). Undertaken under the pressure of proposed federal legislation, this study found that animal care committees are "generally not as active as their charters (organizational descriptions) had depicted them." Furthermore, NIH site visitors were "disappointed to find that the animal care committees frequently seemed less than fully assertive." This is governmentese to say that these committees were inactive and had little clout.

The 1985 law sought to change this. It requires IACUCs to review "practices involving pain to animals, and the condition of animals." In addition, the September 1986 Public Health Service policy is specific about protocol review. It states that IACUCs shall review relevant sections of PHS grant applications to ensure that (a) procedures with animals will avoid or minimize discomfort, distress and pain to the animals, consistent with sound research design; (b) appropriate sedation, analgesia, or anesthesia is used; (c) animals that would otherwise experience severe or chronic pain or distress that cannot be relieved will be painlessly killed at the end of the procedure, or, if appropriate, during the procedure; (d) laboratory personnel are appropriately qualified and trained in the procedure they are using; (e) methods of euthanasia are consistent with those prescribed by the American Veterinary Medical Association; (f) "procedures involving animals should be designed and performed with due consideration of their relevance to human or animal health, the advancement of knowledge, or the good of society"; (g) the animals selected are of appropriate species and quality and are the minimum number required to obtain valid results; (h) methods "such as mathematical modelling, computer simulation, and *in vitro* biological systems should be considered." In accomplishing these tasks, the IACUC either approves, disapproves, or modifies the proposed animal experiment.

Attitudes of investigators

Investigators had not been accustomed to having their protocols reviewed for animal welfare; it was a new challenge. Traditionally, the biomedical community had held that review should only be of animal *care* (i.e., husbandry) and not of animal *use* (i.e., experimental procedures). Until 1985, policies, and therefore procedures for accrediting and funding, tended to reflect this attitude. Animal husbandry conditions were open to inspection, but review stopped at the laboratory door.

At first, many in the biomedical community strongly resisted the notion that research design and actual experimental procedures should be subject to formal review for animal welfare concerns. For instance, in 1984, the Federation of American Societies for Experimental Biology (FASEB)—with some 27,000 members at that time—objected when NIH proposed to use the term "Animal Research Committee" to describe the institutional oversight committee in the new PHS policy. FASEB said that the use of the word research "invites the interpretation that the committee should become involved in experimental design considerations" (Krauss, 1984). NIH subsequently changed the name to Institutional Animal Care and Use Committee in the new 1986 PHS policy. The word "use" remains in the committee title despite the FASEB objection and clearly refers here to experimentation.

A reluctance to accept protocol review has been evident in a number of quarters. Protocol review is viewed by some to be an invasion of academic freedom and unnecessary bureaucracy (Traystman, 1987; Williams, 1987). Also, investigators have questioned the ability of any broadly constructed committee to pass judgment on the animal procedures used and the significance of their work. As IACUCs have become better established and have increasingly involved more and more faculty members, these concerns have diminished but have not disappeared.

How is animal review conducted?

Current regulatory policy requires that the number of animals used should be the minimum necessary to produce valid results and that pain and distress to laboratory animals should be reduced to the minimum necessary. Federal policy directs the IACUC to review proposals to see that investigators incorporate these principles into their research.

In practice, a committee should see that the following information is supplied by the investigator and made available to all members of the committee:

1. A clear description of the investigator's field of inquiry in comprehensible, nonscientific jargon is essential for effective review. All members of the IACUC must understand what is being reviewed.
2. Information must be broad enough in describing the research so that the committee can attempt to weigh its expected contribution to knowledge against the potential harm to be inflicted on the animal.
3. Information on the animal procedure must be precise in detail so that the actual procedures can be assessed. The investigator should report the justification for the experiment, why an alternative that does not involve harming a sentient animal has not been chosen, the numbers and species of animals used, dosages of anesthetics and analgesics, exact experimental procedures to be used, the expected reactions of the animals, details of the possible adverse effects and the severity and length of time that such effects will be expected to last, what procedures will be taken to avoid or alleviate adverse effects, and euthanasia methods.

In 1992, a much-needed manual of advice was issued on committee practices. Entitled "Institutional Animal Care and Use Committee Guidebook," it was developed on an initiative from Applied Research Ethics National Association

(ARENA) and is distributed by both ARENA and NIH. The level of IACUC involvement in attempting to reduce or avoid animal use is "not clear cut" in federal policy, the guidebook states. "The decision to require a modification of proposals to take these considerations into account requires an assessment of the necessity of a given procedure. This can be a decision for which the IACUC is inadequately equipped insofar as the committee cannot expect to cover all aspects of scientific and technical expertise for all proposals which they will be asked to review. However, certain general questions should be answered in the proposal; the onus should be on the investigators to justify and explain their experiments. . . . If there is no alternative to the use of the specified animals, an evaluation of the research must be attempted. The higher the level of the anticipated distress the stronger must be the justification of the value of the research.

"Often the IACUC will lack the scientific expertise to perform the relevant evaluation. Also consideration of social value will be difficult when society itself has not made such determinations. This limits the IACUC's ability to make absolute judgments, but the committee can still have a valuable impact by simply raising the consciousness of investigators to the need for careful preparation of the justification they supply."

Assessing harm to the animal

An essential element for clear communication between the investigator and the committee is that each knows how much animal pain or harm is involved. An effective way of quantifying pain is requiring that the investigator use a pain classification system. Table 6.1 presents a pain classification system used by several institutions. This simple system ranks the ethical costs from zero or minimal in category A to great in category E. The word *pain* is used loosely to cover both pain and suffering and other harms. In Canada, this classification system is called "Categories of Invasiveness," which is a better term. Since levels of pain are a continuum, the scale suggests a distinction between categories that is sharper than it is in reality. The particular circumstances in which a procedure is conducted (for instance with or without use of drug or non-drug methods for relief of pain, the expertise of the investigator, etc.) can strongly affect the degree of animal pain or harm. This does not invalidate the concept of a pain scale but does suggest the utility of modifying it by adding specific examples that represent the conditions of the particular experiment.

The rationale for using a pain classification system is that without knowing how much animal pain is involved, any assessment of the justification of an experiment cannot even begin to be made. The 1992 NIH/ARENA Guidebook quoted earlier states that "the higher the level of the anticipated distress the stronger must be the justification of the value of the research." If this assessment is to be made, then the level of "distress" needs to be identified. (In this, as in

TABLE 6.1   Categories of invasiveness in animal experiments

Category A
Experiments Involving Either No Living Materials, Live Isolates, or Most Invertebrate Species.

Examples: the use of tissue culture and tissues obtained at necropsy or from the slaughterhouse; the use of eggs, protozoa, or other single-celled organisms; use of invertebrate species with a simple nervous system.

Category B
Experiments that Cause Little or No Discomfort or Stress.

Examples: experiments involving invertebrates with complex nervous systems; vertebrate studies involving the short-term and skillful restraint of animals for purposes of observations or physical examination; injection of non-toxic material by the following routes: intravenous, subcutaneous, intramuscular, intraperitoneal, or oral, but not intrathoracic or intracardiac (Category C); acute non-survival studies in which the animals are completely anesthetized and do not regain consciousness; approved methods of euthanasia following rapid unconsciousness, such as anesthetic overdose, or decapitation preceded by sedation or light anesthesia; short periods of food and/or water deprivation equivalent to periods of abstinence in nature.

Category C
Experiments that Cause Minor Stress or Pain or Short-Duration Pain.

Examples: vertebrate studies involving cannulation or catheterization of blood vessels or body cavities under anesthesia; minor surgical procedures under anesthesia, such as biopsies, laparoscopy; short periods of restraint beyond that for simple observation or examination, but consistent with minimal distress; short periods of food and/or water deprivation that exceed periods of abstinence in nature; behavioral experiments on conscious animals that involve short-term, stressful restraint; noxious stimiuli from which escape is possible.

Note: During or after Category C procedures, animals must not show anorexia, dehydration, hyperactivity, increased recumbency or dormancy, increased vocalization, increased aggressive-defensive behavior, or demonstrate social withdrawal and self-isolation, or self-mutilation.

Category D
Experiments that Involve Significant but Unavoidable Stress or Pain to Vertebrate Animal Species.

Examples: vertebrate studies involving major surgical procedures conducted under general anesthesia with subsequent recovery; induction of anatomic or physiological abnormalities that will result in pain or distress; applicaton of noxious stimuli from which escape is impossible; prolonged (several hours or more) periods of physical restraint; induction of behavioral stresses such as maternal deprivation, aggression, predator-prey interactions; procedures that cause severe, persistent, or irreversible disruption of sensorimotor organization; the use of Freund's Complete Adjuvant; production of radiation sickness.

Note: Procedures used in Category D should not cause prolonged or severe clinical distress as may be exhibited by a wide range or clinical signs, such as marked abnormalities in behavioral patterns or attitudes, the absence of grooming, dehydration, abnormal vocalization, prolonged anorexia, circulatory collapse, extreme lethargy or disinclination to move, and clinical signs of severe or advanced local or systemic infection, etc.

Category E
Procedures that Involve Inflicting Severe Pain Near, At, or Above the Pain Tolerance Threshold of Unanesthetized, Conscious Animals.

Examples include the use of muscle relaxants or paralytic drugs such as succinyl choline or other curariform drugs used alone for surgical restraint without the use of anesthetics; severe burn or

continued

TABLE 6.1   (continued)

Category E
continued

---

trauma infliction on unanesthetized animals; toxicity testing and experimentally induced infectious disease or other induced conditions that have death as the endpoint; attempts to induce psychotic-like behavior; killing method not approved by the American Veterinary Medical Association or the Canadian Council on Animal Care, such as strychnine; inescapably severe stress or terminal stress.

Note: Category E experiments are considered highly questionable or unacceptable irrespective of the significance of anticipated results. Many of these procedures are specifically prohibited in national policies, and their use may result in withdrawal of federal funds and/or institutional USDA registration.

These categories of invasiveness are depicted in a step-wise scale of increasing ethical cost. The examples of procedures for each category provide a guide of how such a scheme is being used currently by research institutions. The examples are based on a combination of sources; (a) Orlans, F.B., 1987, Research Protocol Review for Animal Welfare, *Investigative Radiology* 22:253–258, and (b) Canadian Council on Animal Care, Categories of Invasiveness in Animal Experiments, Revised 1989.

---

other official documents dealing with animal welfare policies, the word "distress" is used in preference to the stronger words of "pain" or "harm.")

Use of a pain classification system is not mandatory in the United States as it is in some other countries (for instance in Canada, the UK, and the Netherlands). As described in chapter 9, efforts have been made by the Department of Agriculture to introduce a pain classification system into U.S. public policy, but these have so far failed. However, among the American institutions that voluntarily use a pain classification system are the M. D. Anderson Hospital, University of Texas System Cancer Center; Auburn University; the College of Physicians and Surgeons of Columbia University; the New York State Department of Health, New York; University of Wisconsin; Roswell Park Memorial Institute of Buffalo; San Jose State University; Uniformed Services University of the Health Sciences; the University of Cincinnati Medical Center; the University of Colorado Health Sciences Center; the University of Michigan; the University of Nebraska Medical Center; and the University of Virginia.

Several of these institutions have modified Table 6.1, citing their own selection of examples, as encountered in their own research programs. This adaptation is beneficial because it gives the classification system relevance and immediate applicability to the local situation and provides important guidance to the investigator. A number of IACUC members have reported enthusiastically to me about the educational value of adapting Table 6.1 to their own needs. In practice, many IACUCs have found that this classification is surprisingly easy to apply and greatly facilitates protocol review because it provides immediate information to an IACUC about the intensity of review the project will need.

There are problems with using a harm scale that should not be ignored. In the U.K., where experience has already been gained in using a harm classification system nationally, some problems have been identified. David B. Morton, professor of Biomedical Science and Ethics at Birmingham University, points out that the same procedure carried out by two different scientists could turn a severity level from mild into one of severe according to the investigator's level of competence. Therefore a system must include training and competence assessment if the scheme is to be satisfactory. Furthermore, there needs to be some nationally accepted standardized protocols because techniques can hide extremes of animal suffering (for instance with use of Freund's Adjuvant, raising antibodies, or removal of blood where the severity would depend on volume removed, the frequency, the route, and even the animal species). Finally, says Morton, the classification for any procedure must be validated with independent retrospective analysis if any scheme is going to be accepted by all concerned (David B. Morton, personal communication, March, 1992). These problems must be addressed if a nationally accepted pain scale is to be adopted.

A harm classification system is not set in stone—rather it is a constantly evolving system. Over time, the various systems in use (described in chapter 9) have been refined by modifying the examples provided to illustrate the various categories. Scientists in many countries have contributed to this process, in particular the Canadians who, more than anyone else, have had the longest experience. Furthermore, information gained from new research into methods of recognizing and assessing animal pain and harms from behavioral indicators have been incorporated into pain classification systems.

Investigators to classify pain level of their work

IACUCs that use Table 6.1 (or a modification thereof) usually require investigators to classify their own projects as part of formal submission of the protocol for committee review. Both the duration and intensity of pain should be assessed, as required in the sample protocol form shown in Table 6.2. Assessment of pain level at different stages of the experimental procedure may be necessary because it can change over time. For the purposes of filling out a protocol form, the highest level of pain is to be recorded. The sequence of events is that an investigator prospectively assesses animal harms, writes down that assessment, receives concurrence or modification of that assessment from an IACUC, and after the completion of the experiments retrospectively sees if that assessment was correct (as in a renewal, for instance).

In practice, investigators often underestimate the amount of animal pain involved in proposed procedures, so it is important that the committee review the investigator's classification for concurrence both before the work is started and again retrospectively to check for accuracy of prediction. This is commonly done. If the predicted pain was wrong, then the ethical judgment might also be affected and the protocol should be re-reviewed. This active involvement of

TABLE 6.2 Extract from model protocol form—description of procedures involving animals

	Yes	No
Indicate CCAC [animal pain] level of invasiveness (A through E)		
Checklist—all items must be checked		
The project will use conscious or recovered animals	☐	☐
Animals will suffer pain or stress because of the project	☐	☐
If "yes" indicate:		
Intensity: ☐ Low ☐ Moderate ☐ High ☐ Severe		
Duration ☐ Seconds ☐ Minutes ☐ Hours ☐ Days		
Clinical or behavioural changes, or signs of toxicity may occur	☐	☐
The project will involve the animals in:		
(a) Prolonged physical restraint	☐	☐
(b) Food and/or water deprivation	☐	☐
(c) Severe variations in environment	☐	☐
(d) Severe sensory deprivation	☐	☐
(e) Surgical procedures without anaesthesia and/or postoperative analgesia	☐	☐
(f) The use of immobilizing agents/muscle relaxants without anaesthesia	☐	☐
(g) Electrical shock stimulation	☐	☐
(h) Infliction of burns, fractures or, other severe traumas	☐	☐
(i) Prey killing or fighting experiments	☐	☐
(j) Predator prey studies	☐	☐
(k) Unanesthetized death as a direct result	☐	☐
Will the project be used for student instruction?	☐	☐
Will the project be used for conference/seminar demonstration?	☐	☐

This extract is from the protocol form (revised January 22, 1992) used by Queen's University, Kingston, Canada. It flags specific procedures that the committee will review particularly carefully for justification and possible refinement. In addition to checking these items, the investigator must provide a detailed description of the project. CCAC = Canadian Council on Animal Care.

investigators and the committee in assessment of the degree of animal harm focuses their attention on one of the most important issues of the review process.

Design of protocol form

For a vast majority of protocols, what is provided on the protocol form may be all that the committee ever sees. A committee can obtain additional information from the investigator, but the form is the key link in the flow of information.

By looking at the form used, it is often possible to assess the degree of commitment of the committee to its job. Some forms are so cursory that it is apparent that the committee is functioning as a rubber stamp. The information supplied is insufficient for making informed judgments. On the other hand, other forms are well-drafted for their purpose; investigators are asked specific questions and detailed information is required about any questionable procedures. Some committees go even further and provide guidance to investigators on questionable procedures.

Most institutions that use the pain classification system categorize the procedure according to the maximum level of pain the animal is ever likely to endure.

But the University of Ottawa refines this by requiring the investigator to state the pain category that is anticipated at three time intervals; during the experimental procedure, post-procedure, and during convalescence.

A number of conscientious committees also request information about particularly traumatic procedures, (see Table 6.2). As another example, Cornell University asks investigators specifically if the procedure involves any of the following: moderate to severe malnutrition, neurophysiological preparations, induction of psychotic behavior, injection of any agent that induces inflammation or necrosis (i.e., bradykinin, Freund's Complete Adjuvant, and certain infectious agents). Other examples could be given. These listings are useful in highlighting procedures likely to be viewed with special concern.

Increasingly IACUCs are asking questions about the competence of an investigator to carry out a particular scientific technique or procedure. Among others, the University of Michigan and the University of Nebraska include such a question. Assessing competence has implications not only for scientific merit but also for animal welfare. Back in 1984 a survey asked "Should IACUCs assess the qualifications of investigators to do certain procedures?" One in five of the scientist respondents thought it was of no importance and not the committee's job to inquire (Orlans, 1987). If asked the same question today, probably fewer would hold such a view.

Expedited review

Committees that use a pain classification system often incorporate some form of expedited review. For example, experiments falling within categories A or B are either exempt entirely or reviewed only by a subset of the full committee membership. As the categories advance through C, D, and E, the intensity of review must be increased.

Expedited review for those projects involving the least animal pain is attractive for reducing the work load of a committee, but it can be abused. Indeed, animal welfare advocates have been leery of endorsing pain classification systems because of potential misuse of expedited review. For example, the Progressive Animal Welfare Society (PAWS) publicly objected to the category 2 classification, defined as "some discomfort or distress," given by a named IACUC to a project involving heart transplants in dogs (PAWS, 1988). Because of the classification, this project was exempt from discussion by the full IACUC unless such a request was specifically made by a member of the committee. This particular committee used a classification system on a 1 to 4 scale of increasing severity of the procedure; only those projects falling in categories 3 "potentially significant distress or pain" and 4 "potentially severe pain" were automatically subject to full committee discussion. According to PAWS, in a one-year period several hundred category 1 and 2 projects had received "offhand but official" approval through the committee's inaction. PAWS, whose court action had forced these committee meetings to be held in public, complained that this IACUC assigns 98 percent of its projects to categories 1 and 2.

Applying the alternatives of replacement and reduction

In Table 6.1, a replacement is anything that fits in Category A—use of lower organisms, cell cultures, tissues from slaughter or autopsy, or non-animal systems such as computers or mathematical modeling. A recommendation from an IACUC to replace an animal experiment with a non-animal model would be highly exceptional and perhaps has never happened even in the most effective committee. Furthermore, rarely, if ever, would an IACUC recommend a change in subject species to one lower on the phylogenetic scale. Committees tend, almost automatically, to accept the investigator's justification for choice of species.

IACUCs do occasionally recommend a reduction in numbers of animals. Indeed, according to the NIH/ARENA Guidebook, among the justification questions addressed by IACUCs, the need for a given number of animals is probably "the most common."

The use of naturally occurring pathologic states is a replacement that ought to receive greater attention than it currently does. Instead of induced pathologic conditions, it may be preferable to study naturally occurring clinical cases, which may be either human studies or client animal studies in veterinary research. Some conditions that, if induced, would cause a conscious animal to be either near, at, or above the pain tolerance threshold are not ethically permissible. For these studies, the use of naturally occurring clinical material with active therapeutic intervention may be the only solution. Examples could include any severely traumatic condition, such as head injury, severe burns, and so on. Rarely in research are such replacements with clinical cases used, but they are beginning to be used in veterinary education, as discussed in Chapter 12 on the use of animals in education.

Refinements

Many refinements of technique that would reduce animal harm are ready for application in biomedical research. Currently, the most common refinements recommended by IACUCs are those involving improvements in use of anesthetics and analgesics. Also, an increasing number of committees are formulating in-house policies and distributing packages of information for investigators about recommended (or required) refinements for certain common procedures. These in-house policies go beyond the requirements of federal policy and have been very successful in practice. What is needed in the future is national guidance on refinements of commonly encountered procedures. Some examples of refinements currently being recommended follow.

Early termination of study

In studies of cancer, infectious or other debilitating disease, or in toxicologic studies, using an early endpoint based on clinical criteria and supported by autopsy findings can provide more information with less suffering than using death as an endpoint. Such provisions are included in national policies of Australia and Canada, and also in guidelines of the U.K. Coordinating Committee for Cancer Research. In 1990, an official U.K. report on experiments said that "it is *standard practice* [in the U.K.] to reduce the severity of the project by setting as early an endpoint as possible to avoid unnecessary suffering" (emphasis added). The 1992 NIH/ARENA Guidebook states that the "*routine* use of death as an endpoint should be discouraged. Endpoints other than death must always be considered and should be used wherever the research objective makes it possible" (B-2-9, page 24).

Limitation of tumor size

In the last few years, there has been increasing acceptance of a policy of limiting tumor size in cancer studies. Some years ago, before such policies had been developed, animals such as mice sometimes were left until tumors grew to a size greater than the animal's own body. Animals dragged these burdens around, and sometimes were unable to move to water or food and died as a result of dehydration. M. D. Anderson Hospital, a major center for cancer research, has an in-house policy that limits tumor growth to 10 percent of body weight. A large tumor causes significant stress and pain to the animal and is unnecessary for the purpose of the experiment. This policy reflects the recommendations from an international workshop of cancer researchers (Kallman et al., 1985).

Physical restraint procedures

Restraint of animals, especially non-human primates, has been a contentious issue of long standing. When NASA first flew rhesus monkeys in space, in order the keep an animal from floating around in a weightless state, this conscious animal was bolted down to its seat with permanent screws through its pelvis. Some animals died under these traumatic conditions. Later, NASA switched to the more humane method of tethering devices combined with specially designed soft jackets.

Immobilization chairs for primates in which the animal's limbs and head are clamped into place are still used, but nowadays more care is taken with the length of time the animals are left there. Also, substitutes are now recommended, such as behavioral training of the animal to obtain its willing cooperation, telemetry, or use of soft slings, soft jackets, or tethering devices with backpacks. The special precautions that must be taken to ensure the well-being of primates when any physical restraint is used are addressed in the policy of the University of California San Francisco (UCSF policy, 1984).

Freund's complete adjuvant

Freund's adjuvant is an emulsion, used to immunize animals for research purposes, that sets off an inflammatory reaction resulting in intense pain under certain circumstances. In the past, repeated injections of this adjuvant typically were made in the footpads of rabbits, and this could result in ulceration and inability to walk. National policy has been developed on this matter by the Canadian Council on Animal Care, and in-house policies are used by UCSF and the University of Texas Medical School in Houston. In general, these policies prohibit certain routes and sites of injection and recommend others as acceptable (see details in chapter 8 under "Unacceptable Procedures").

Acute versus chronic experiments

As a substitute for chronic experiments involving conscious animals that may last days, weeks, or months, acute, short-duration experiments of a few hours or less can be conducted on animals rendered incapable of perceiving pain. For example, an animal can be fully anesthetized, the experiment conducted, and the animal killed without its ever regaining consciousness. Alternatively, a decerebrate animal (an animal also incapable of perceiving pain and time-limited for survival) can sometimes be used.

Prolonged water deprivation

As a final example of a refinement that would decrease the ethical cost of an experiment, the use of prolonged water deprivation as an inducement for an animal to do a task will be examined. This will be described in greater detail than the preceding examples inasmuch as raising questions about this procedure is on the cutting edge of what some mature IACUCs are debating. The story is told as it unfolds before an IACUC, and indeed as it really happened; the only addition is that some relevant policies have been added. This account illustrates how a conscientious IACUC goes about its business. In this case, I was brought in as a consultant.

The procedure involves adult rhesus monkeys, *Macaca mulatta,* which were required to perform certain visual discrimination tasks as part of a project intended to investigate the development and alleviation of strabismus (cross-eyes) in children. The visual discrimination tasks involve the animals' watching a screen and selecting various "answers"; the animals need inducement, otherwise they will not cooperate for any substantial length of time. As an inducement, the monkeys were deprived of water for 22 out of every 24 hours for each of the five test days in any one week. After the 22-hour water deprivation period, each animal was placed in a restraint chair and tested for a period of an hour to an hour and a quarter. During the test period, one drop of water was given as a reward each time the monkey performed a required task. During the remaining 45 to 60 minutes of the 24-hour period, the animals were allowed as much water as they needed. On the sixth and seventh days of the week, the animals were also allowed free access to water. The cycle was then repeated.

When this procedure came up for review, the IACUC questioned whether such a long period as 22 hours of water deprivation was either necessary for the protocol or tolerable for the animal. The committee required the work to be stopped temporarily while additional information was sought.

The investigator was angry at the suspension of his experiments. He claimed that a 22-hour period of water deprivation was common practice among investigators and that any change in protocol would interfere with his baseline data collected for more than six years. He said that the animals seemed to be in tolerable condition, that they maintained satisfactory body weight, and that none had ever died from water deprivation. He claimed that other investigators who currently use such periods of deprivation had encountered no problems.

The committee's response was threefold: (a) that the procedure was standard practice did not necessarily indicate that it was desirable or justified; (b) the claimed interference with baseline data was an untested assumption since alternatives had not, at that point, been tested; and (c) the animals' failure to die was an unacceptable criteria because life can be sustained under intolerable conditions.

The committee reviewed this protocol at several meetings, gathering additional information at each step. Eventually, notwithstanding the investigator's objections, the committee finally disapproved the water deprivation aspect of the study. The IACUC concluded that prolonged water deprivation was not justified for several reasons: (1) although the animals appeared to be in satisfactory physical condition, they were subject to unjustifiable mental suffering; (2) the animals' thirst had no relevance to the subject of scientific investigation—this was not thirst research, thirst was being used merely as an inducement to perform a task (there was a consensus among committee members that some water deprivation would have to be permitted in thirst research); (3) reasonable alternatives that would induce the animals to perform the tasks exist.

The committee explored what reasonable alternatives exist. They learned that, given free access to water and food, animals will work well for rewards of high preference foods or drinks that are not part of their normal laboratory fare.

Rhesus monkeys will work well for rewards such as mandarin oranges, yogurt, Gatorade (a commercially available fruit drink), or malted milk. (For the animals' general health, these nutritionally balanced rewards are better than others such as sucrose pellets or marshmallows). The investigator was advised to redesign his protocol along these lines.

An analysis of the information that helped the committee arrive at this decision is given below. The sources were expert opinions, literature search, and statements of national policy.

Expert opinion

The committee solicited expert opinion from a number of primatologists, psychologists, physiologists, other scientists, and relevant professional scientific associations. A wide range of opinion emerged, from immediate objection to tolerance regarding this protocol. A response typical of those who objected was that there is "no rationale for this water deprivation at all." Several scientists wondered whether human beings could deal with 22 hours a day without water for five days a week. Primatologists as a group tended to show particular sensitivity to animal welfare issues involved. They, and others, concluded that the monkeys would suffer severe distress from the long period of thirst followed by drop by drop water administration and said they would disapprove this procedure. Several experts questioned whether the daily dehydration would affect the monkeys' vision and therefore the researcher's results. Many offered constructive advice regarding alternative procedures, suggesting the use of rewards instead of extreme thirst.

On the other hand, support for the procedure was voiced. For instance, a spokesperson for a professional association of psychologists, after having sampled opinions from association members, reported, "There was no sense [among these scientists] that there was anything wrong with this regimen, not at all." One expert who personally used a similar procedure said, "animals adapt to drinking only once per day, and there is no cause for concern over this protocol."

Among those experts who were tolerant of the 22-hour deprivation, several suggested that the animals be evaluated at the start of the experiment to be certain that they are in good health, and then monitored continuously. Each individual animal should be checked for continued good health judged by stability in weight, stable performance in the experimental protocol, signs of dehydration, signs of stress (using such indicators as disturbance in level of normal activity, changes in normal sleep/wake cycles, etc.). These experts recommended that the monkeys should be removed from the study if their health begins to deteriorate.

In summary, the preponderance of opinion to approve or disapprove this procedure was hard to assess. It depended on how many experts of which disciplines the committee wanted to contact.

In discussion with the experts, the committee debated whether the investigator should be asked to substitute food deprivation instead of the water deprivation because animals can withstand food deprivation with less stress. However, the committee abandoned this idea because of the general principle that rewards should be used in preference to punishments wherever possible.

The experts' information about using high preference foods and drinks as rewards played an important role in the committee's final decision. A significant fact was that this information emerged only from communication with experts. Neither the scientific literature nor policy statements provided such information. This underlined the importance of exploring many avenues of advice.

Literature search

The scientific literature search was of little assistance. The committee asked the investigator to provide publications to substantiate his claim that this pattern of water deprivation is not deleterious to the animals. Although similar procedures are used by others, the investigator could provide no published research articles where the humaneness or justification of the procedure was discussed.

Nor could any accounts be found in the literature of the effects on animals of prolonged and repeated daily periods of water deprivation. Single prolonged periods of water deprivation conducted for thirst research confirmed the concerns, voiced by some experts, that cellular dehydration should be recognized as a potential confounding factor in interpreting the researcher's results.

Committees like to know what other committees have done when faced with a similar situation. In what is probably the first endeavor to compile data on IACUC decisions, Rebecca Dresser, J.D., (1989 and 1990) reported on a study of IACUCs that agreed to review identical hypothetical protocols she had given them. In one of Dresser's protocols, six squirrel monkeys were to be deprived of water five days a week except for one randomly timed thirty-minute period daily. The thirty-one committees that participated in this study "typically wanted evidence that monkeys would be adequately hydrated and often asked whether the investigator could substitute a positive reinforcement or food deprivation, which is viewed as less detrimental to the animals." One committee immediately disapproved that section of the protocol and others wanted additional information. For instance, one committee required that the investigator justify the need for water deprivation; another wanted documentation that water deprivation is safe and required the investigator to describe the monitoring plan to ensure against dehydration; another wanted information on how nutritional needs of the animals would be satisfied during water deprivation because they would be unable to eat when their mouths were dry from severe thirst. As one would expect, these committees did not show uniform judgments, although there is certainly a sense that prolonged water deprivation raised significant concerns among them.

Policies

The original IACUC also sought guidance from mandated policies. Current United States public policy does not address the issue of water deprivation as part of a research protocol. The 1990 Australian Code of Practice for the Care and Use of Animals for Scientific Purposes is, to my knowledge, the first policy to specifically address this issue. It states that severe withholding or restriction of water (or food) "should produce no continuing detrimental effect on the animal (page 30). . . . Behaviour can usually be modified using procedures that involve no more than a physiological stress, e.g., thirst within the range of the normal experience of the species (page 27)." Thirst therefore should not exceed that which is normally experienced. The Canadian Council for Animal Care's national policy unreservedly states, "Water deprivation should be used only when thirst is the specific subject of the study" (CCAC, 1980).

Voluntary codes from some professional organizations would call into question 22 hours of water deprivation. For instance, the guidelines of the American Psychological Association state that "procedures involving extensive food or water deprivation should be used only when minimal deprivation procedures are inappropriate to the design and purpose of the research" (American Psychological Association, 1985). In another context the guidelines state that "psychologists should adjust the parameters of [aversive] stimulation to levels that appear minimal."

The investigator was confronted with this statement, but he said that if he used a lesser period of water deprivation such as six hours, then the monkey refused to perform the required tasks after a relatively short period of time. The investigator said he needed a one-hour or more test period in order to collect what he considered to be a satisfactory volume of results each day. Obviously, the investigator's decision was based on convenience to himself—namely, the faster accumulation of data—and not on benefit to the animals. Several policies have provisions which state that when there is conflict between investigator convenience and welfare of the animal, then the welfare of the animal should take precedence, (see, for instance, those of the Canadian Council for Animal Care, 1980).

The committee found that, in its totality, the information from experts, from the literature, and from policy statements tended to substantiate their original concerns. They finally came to a firm conclusion that this procedure could not be approved. This did not block the total experiment; it meant only that this particular method of inducing the animals to do tasks was disapproved, and a less stressful alternative was required.

The experimental setting of this particular example (performing visual discrimination tests) is irrelevant to the ethical issues raised and the to applicability of the policies cited about water deprivation. Thus, irrespective of the experimental setting, the ethical requirement to substitute a less traumatic refinement wherever possible applies.

7

Community Members on Animal Review Committees

It was an unprecedented move in 1985 when Congress decreed that Institutional Animal Care and Use Committees include a community member. For the first time, it was required that members of the public would have a say in day-to-day decisions of approving or disapproving specific animal experiments. Before 1985, only 26 percent of existing IACUCs had voluntarily included a community member, according to Charles R. McCarthy, Director of the Office for Protection from Research Risks (OPRR), NIH. In the future, it was going to be 100 percent.

The humane movement—that is, organizations whose major focus is on protection of animals—was responsible for first proposing to a receptive Congress that community membership be required on all committees.

The term *community member* means what it says although in common parlance it is often used rather loosely. Terms such as community, public, lay, unaffiliated, non-institutional, and non-scientific member, are sometimes used as if they were interchangeable, although some of these terms mean quite different things. The rationale for including such members lies in the consensus that, where federal funding is concerned, decisions concerning social values should be made in a forum that includes societal involvement. Congress wanted to make clear that scientists are not free to do whatever they wish to animals—decision-making should not rest solely in their hands.

Scientists could not cavalierly dismiss this proposal for community members and retain credibility with Congress. Nevertheless, the specter of having a disruptive antivivisection or animal welfare member in their midst with decision-making power appeared as a real threat. When this proposal first appeared in a congressional bill, the biomedical community did not directly challenge the appropriateness of citizen input; rather, some of its members argued that a non-aligned member might disclose information detrimental to the institution. The academic community was fearful that community members might leak information to the press with a view to embarrass their institutions, or worse yet, to animal rights activists who might then raid the laboratories or otherwise sabotage the work. Pharmaceutical companies were troubled about possible breach of trade secrets and providing "intellectual property" to rival companies. Of course, this was a risk they faced with their regular employees and, in any case, a federal law already existed that forbids the release of trade secrets. But "a great deal of hard work had to be done to prevent the issue [of breaking confidentiality] from becoming a major danger to enactment as some of its proponents doubtless wanted it to be," said Christine Stevens, one of the major proponents of change. Since the passage of the law, there has been no episode, to my knowledge, of any community member's breaking trust.

At the time, intense battles were fought over the exact wording of how the community member should be described in the law. The American Physiological Society (APS), which held an unusual position among scientific associations of supporting the general thrust of the 1985 amendments, was cautious. The Society's official history of that period states, "Of most concern to the Society was identification of the Institutional Animal Care Committee's 'nonaffiliated member,' who, according to [proposed] legislation, was to represent 'concern for the welfare of animal subjects.' Not only did this portray a public image that researchers and educators do not have concern for their laboratory animals, but it also implied that the nonaffiliated person must be an animal welfare protectionist. The Society had been an early proponent of institutional animal care committees with a nonaffiliated member, but not on those terms" (Brobeck et al., 1987).

A minority view, espoused by radical antivivisectionists, opposed the inclusion of community members entirely. The United Action for Animals, a national group noted for its hard-hitting attacks on animal research, opposed the 1985 legislation saying, "This scheme [to appoint lay members to IACUCs] is window-dressing, aimed at lulling the public . . . if [the lay members] oppose an experiment, they're simply outvoted. . . . It is our view that no self-respecting lay person would agree to serve on such a committee" (United Action, 1984).

After much wrangling, the wording finally agreed to and which became law was that each institutional committee shall have a minimum of three members of whom at least one person (a) shall represent "general community interests in the proper care and treatment of animals", (b) shall not be affiliated in any way with the facility, and (c) shall not be a member of the immediate family of a person affiliated with the institution. One person could fulfill all these requirements.

According to the provisions of the AWA, other required persons on the committee are a veterinarian and a scientist. The PHS policy is basically similar; it requires a committee of not less than five persons, including (a) a doctor of veterinary medicine, (b) a practicing scientist experienced in research on animals, and (c) "one member whose primary concerns are in a nonscientific area (for example, ethicist, lawyer, member of the clergy)", and (d) "one individual who is not affiliated with the institution in any way other than as a member of the IACUC, and is not a member of the immediate family of a person who is affiliated with the institution." Again, one member may fulfill more than one requirement. Thus, in neither the AWA nor the PHS policy is it specifically stated that the community member shall represent organizations concerned with animal protection.

In contrast, the national policies of some other countries—Germany, Denmark, Switzerland, and Australia—provide explicitly for participation of animal welfare groups in decision-making. Under the 1986 German law, the national oversight committee has twelve members of whom one-third are experts from national animal welfare organizations (Wiemer, 1989). This one-third is chosen by the federal ministry from lists put forward by animal protection groups. Under the 1987 Danish law, the ten-person national oversight committee includes four persons proposed by animal welfare organizations, and in Switzerland animal welfare interests must be represented in the cantonal boards that approve applications for experiments. The Australian Code encourages appointment of persons "selected on the basis of membership of an animal welfare organization" to serve on institutional oversight committees (Australian Code, 1990).

In the United States, appointment to IACUC membership is made by an institution's chief executive officer. This means that the community has no say in who is to represent them.

In 1987, public protest broke out in Boston because the Dana-Farber Cancer Institute, one of Boston's premier medical research centers, chose as its community representative Annaliz Hannan. As executive director of the Massachusetts Society for Medical Research, Hannan was politically active in opposing greater public control over the use and care of laboratory animals, and she was reappointed to a second term. The Massachusetts Society for Medical Research, founded in 1982 to lobby for and publicize the medical community's position on animal care issues, lists Dana-Farber as one of its financial contributors. After the protests, Dana-Farber officials checked with NIH about this appointment and found that they were within their rights according to PHS policy. However, they did appoint an additional outside member.

The Cambridge ordinance

The Dana-Farber incident added fuel to the fire of an active group of animal welfare advocates, the Cambridge Committee for Responsible Research, headed by a computer scientist at MIT, Gul Agha. At that time, the laboratories using animals in the city of Cambridge included MIT, Harvard, one other university-related facility, and ten private companies. The reform group pressed for the appointment to IACUCs of people whose perspective clearly favored animal welfare—representatives of humane societies and the like.

Rival advocacy pressures became so great that the mayor appointed a three-person Blue Ribbon Committee. The members were an animal advocate lawyer, Steven M. Wise; a physician and chair of MIT's IACUC to represent the research community, John M. Moses; and a neutral veterinarian, Stuart E. Wiles. Their charge was to investigate the oversight and state of animal research and testing facilities in Cambridge. After two years of study, they reported to the city council in 1989 (Blue Ribbon Committee, 1989). They found that of the thirteen IACUCs in Cambridge, two did not have a public member at all, and among the others, not one included a public member with any connection with an animal protection organization.

In the report, Wise pressed for passage of a city ordinance that would allow animal welfare groups to prepare a list of candidates for service on IACUCs and that would require selection from this list. His rationale was that since animals lack the ability to give consent to what is done to them and lack a voice of their own, some specified animal advocate should be part of the oversight committee. By comparison, Institutional Review Boards that regularly review research on a vulnerable category of subject (those who cannot intelligently consent, mentally disabled persons, prisoners, children, and fetuses) must have at least one member primarily concerned with the welfare of these subjects. This system has worked well, according to Wise. Animals, unable to consent, are as vulnerable as these human subjects and need an advocate primarily concerned with their welfare.

However, representatives of the Cambridge research institutes were strongly opposed to giving animal groups such authority. In the Blue Ribbon Report, Moses, who presented the views of the research community, argued that the selection of an IACUC member from a movement that promotes the dissolution of animal research would be self-defeating. Such an appointment would result in counter-productive disruption of committee effort. The development of meaningful exchange, candor, and cooperation between research scientists and the IACUC that are important for successful IACUC oversight would be eroded by the presence of an animal rights activist, the researchers said.

Although many contentious issues were involved in the debate over this ordinance, including banning of the LD50 and Draize tests, the nonaffiliated member issue was the most controversial. But finally in 1989, the Cambridge city council unanimously passed an ordinance that specifically prohibits a person who is "aligned with an antivivisection organization" from serving (City of Cambridge, 1989). However, the ordinance requires that the nonaffiliated person should be "knowledgeable about animal welfare philosophy and about the purpose of scientific research." So the door is open for persons aligned with animal welfare organizations to serve.

As of July, 1991, no person identifiably associated with an animal welfare organization has been appointed to any of the now 23 IACUCs in Cambridge (Commissioner Stuart E. Wiles, personal communication, July 23, 1991). Wiles, whose job requires him to approve community member appointments, says he would welcome lists of animal welfare advocates from which institutions could choose their nonaffiliated members.

No national data are publicly available about how many committees use their community member slot for an animal welfare or animal rights advocate. It is my impression from a reasonably exhaustive search for information that the situation in Cambridge is not unusual; indeed it may well be the norm. The community slot is commonly filled with clergy, lawyers, ethicists, local business people, biology teachers, and even scientists from other institutions rather than animal welfare advocates. The PHS policy specifically mentions clergy, lawyers, and ethicists as possible candidates, thus promoting such choices.

It is noteworthy that at least two institutions have announced policies that provide for animal advocacy voice on IACUCs. These are (1) the Wisconsin Regional Primate Research Center whose policy states, "Advocates of animal rights, along with scientific peers, will be appointed by the Director to participate with full voice and vote (Wisconsin, 1982); and (2) the University of Southern California whose policy requires a committee "composed of an inter-disciplinary group of faculty most of whom are not in animal research, the Vivaria Director, a public member representing the animal advocate community, a public member representing the community-at-large, and at least one graduate student" (USC, 1991).

Even without a formal policy to that effect, some institutions have gone beyond the letter of the law in appointing humane society representatives. Persons likely to be critical of animal research are usually given rigorous interviews by institutional officials before appointment. One antivivisectionist philosopher who was interviewed three times and finally did gain appointment described this process as "three versions of the Spanish Inquisition." A typical question that can be expected is "Are you an antivivisectionist?" and much may hinge on the response.

The results of such appointments have been mixed. Sometimes they have worked well, and a few humane society representatives have written or spoken positively about their experiences (see Peck, 1987, Hutchinson, 1985, 1988). In some cases, matters have gone badly and the member has been fired or has resigned in protest, as reported in the press and animal rights literature (for instance see Roy, 1990).

Surveys on role of community member

Widely varying accounts of how community members had fared led me to make two informal telephone surveys, first of persons who have served as community members of IACUCs who represent the animal advocacy constituency, and second of chairpersons of IACUCs.

My sampling of experiences had several purposes: (a) to probe how the role of the community member is perceived from each of these two perspectives; (b) to provide a profile of animal advocates chosen to serve on IACUCs and to record their experiences and assess their impact; and (c) to gather information on IACUC procedures and gain insight into what to expect from IACUC review. The results of each survey will be reported in turn.

Interviews with animal advocate members of IACUCs

To be included in the sample, the person had to be either an active member or staff member of a humane association or animal rights group. As a group, these persons probably include the most vocal animal advocates, those most critical of the status quo, and those most politically active concerning animal legislation and policy. This focus on their experiences in no way implies that some other members of the committees (both nonaffiliated and institutional members) do not hold strong animal welfare or animal rights opinions—some do. The survey was conducted in 1991.

The first step was to obtain the names of persons who filled the criteria. This proved to be a difficult task. Some of the most obvious sources could not be approached. NIH's OPRR has on file the names, position titles, and credentials of all IACUC members. This information is not publicly available because NIH must protect the privacy both of the institutions and of the individuals. Also, research institutions were not asked to reveal the names of their community members because they also consider this to be sensitive information.

Names were obtained in several ways: through personal contacts, from information provided by animal welfare and animal rights organizations throughout the country, through computer networking, and through announcements at humane society meetings. It was surprising how few leading humane and animal rights organizations knew of such persons. The small number of names that were found after a diligent search suggests that nationwide, members of humane and animal welfare groups are seldom appointed. A total of sixteen persons who fulfilled the criteria were interviewed.

The results are presented in two ways. First, seven personal stories, selected on the basis of recentness of IACUC service, and variety and range of issues emerging, are recounted that represent the views of the persons interviewed. Second, some summary comments are given. Because of its anecdotal nature, this survey makes no claim to be a representative national sample. In those situations where there was conflict between the community member and the institution, the institution's perspective is not presented because interviews about these events with institutional officials were not part of this study.

Number One—director of animal shelter

Number One holds an associate degree in applied science, and is the only nonaffiliated member of the nine-person committee, all of whom serve one-year terms. He felt some resentment from some of the scientific members of the committee, but for the most part relationships were good.

The committee meets monthly to review between three to eight protocols in approximately two hours. Before the meeting, each committee member receives all materials (approximately three to eight pages per protocol) and previous minutes. He regularly spent several hours prior to the meeting reviewing the materials and making enquiries of others to help him comprehend the science. In the year of his service, about 10 to 20 percent of all protocols were modified to reduce the number of animals or the degree of likely pain. Mainly he abstained from voting but did occasionally vote no on projects he felt were duplicative of work already done. He spoke up on projects that he considered would not meet with public approval and tried to vote from a public perspective. Apart from himself, there were three or four other members of the committee who would on occasion vote no and he was impressed with the overall concern for animal welfare on the committee. Projects with negative votes would be deferred for revision by the investigator until the committee's objections were met.

He established an excellent relationship with the institution's veterinarian. The veterinarian could not be too aggressive in pointing out animal welfare problems because there was a limit to how much he could "rock the boat," but he would tell Number One of the problems he had identified, and it would be up to Number One to raise these for discussion at the meeting.

The committee spent no time discussing the social value of any work and none on self-evaluation of committee activities. The most difficult issue for Number One was that the committee had no formal institutional policy document spelling out the parameters of its functions and powers.

Although Number One would have liked to continue his service, his appointment was not renewed, and he believes this non-renewal was related to the occurrence of laboratory break-ins nearby.

Number Two—local humane society staff person

Number Two was one of three community members appointed to a one-year term on a trial basis, none of whom initially had voting rights. The other nine committee members were given three-year appointments and the right to vote. (The institution has now removed these discriminatory practices.) She felt intimidated at first and encountered hostility from one committee member who made it obvious that community members were not welcome; all other members were friendly. After the trial period, she was appointed to a three-year term with a vote, and went on to serve a total of more than five years.

Each member was provided with full written protocols for review, and decisions were by majority vote. Each committee member turned in written comments on each proposal, so although no single composite minority report was filed, any negative comments became part of the written record. Lacking scientific background, she found considerable difficulty in understanding the protocols, and although some improvements have been made, this remains a problem.

Out of the twenty protocols reviewed each year, two or three received some negative votes but none were stopped. Her greatest problems have been with approving experiments on primates that received brain implants and on rats that were suspended by their tails to simulate microgravity.

She felt she did not change anyone's opinions; nevertheless, she was favorably impressed with the committee. She is currently the public relations staff person of this institution and attends the IACUC meetings as an *ex officio* member.

Number Three—local humane society staff person

Number Three, who identifies with the animal rights movement, was appointed to an open-ended period of service on an IACUC. She was one of two community members, the other being a retired professor of that institution. In addition there were thirteen other members, all of whom were involved in some way with animal experimentation. Number Three found that the protocols were never written in a form that was comprehensible to a non-scientist such as herself, but she was given permission by the chair to seek help from scientists whom she knew. Over time, some effort was made to ameliorate the language problem, but the issue remained.

When she joined the committee, there was no committee discussion of any protocol, but gradually she began to ask questions and to promote some animal-welfare-related exchange. In the two years in which she served, the committee reviewed over three hundred protocols. She tried to make her vote from what she described as a "general populace" position (what she believed society would approve) and she voted no on about a third of the protocols, always filing a minority report. During this period, only two other no votes were cast by other committee members. The protocols she objected to most were those that (a) did not provide proper information, (b) involved the LD50 Test, and (c) involved considerable animal suffering, such as repeated electric shocks as part of undergraduate teaching. The vote was by majority, so no protocols were rejected.

On the protocol form to be filled out by the investigator, there was a question about whether or not an alternative that did not require the use of animals was available. Routinely, the investigators answered "Not applicable." She believed this to be an inadequate response. She recommended that the protocol form should only include questions that the committee is serious about getting a response to; otherwise they should be omitted.

She felt great hostility from the chair and from one other person, but not from the others. She felt she was a lone voice, up against all the researchers on the committee. She spent a great deal of time reviewing the protocols before the meeting and writing her minority reports. On occasion, the rest of the committee edited her report before it entered the files. Her attempts to bring about discussions of the social merits of some animal experiments were disallowed. On the positive side, she felt she made a significant contribution to the facility inspections by insisting that they be thorough. But overall, she judged her committee service to be "the most painful experience of my life."

After considerable harassment, she resigned in protest. In her letter of resignation she said that unlike any other committee member, she had had to battle for her right to vote as she wanted on protocols—the chair had directed her to abstain rather than vote no. She further stated that she had been publicly defamed by an IACUC member at forums where she was not present to defend herself.

Following these unhappy events, several animal welfare and animal rights groups immediately submitted names of several nominees for community member to this institution. Most nominees held a Ph.D. in biology or other scientific credentials. All were rejected. Some weeks later, the institution established criteria that had to be fulfilled for nomination of IACUC community members. One criterion was that persons "must support research with animals so long as it is conducted according to applicable animal welfare laws and regulation."

Number Four—local humane society board member

Number Four is a veterinarian in private practice who volunteered to serve on an IACUC of a research facility that had been criticized by animal rights groups. He knows that he is "hated" by some local animal rights advocates because he has "joined the opposite side." He reports to his humane society board in a general way about his activities on the IACUC and the board supports the positions he takes. Out of the committee of fifteen persons, he and a clergyman are the two community members. He has served two years now of a four-year term.

The committee meets six times a year and reviews over five hundred projects a year. The institutional veterinarian classifies all projects into four categories. For class 1 (training) and class 2 (minimal pain), the IACUC members receive one page of sparse information (name of protocol and investigator)--some 100 or so for each meeting. For class 3 (higher levels of pain), full written protocols are given to all members, a subcommittee pre-reviews them and reports to the full committee in writing. Class 4 protocols are those that are determined by a subcommittee to involve an unacceptable level of pain and are therefore disallowed. Whether there have ever been any class 4 protocols is not known by the community member because no information on their existence or contents is reported to the committee.

No class 1 or 2 projects have ever been rejected. Maybe 10 to 15 percent of the class 3 protocols have received some negative votes, but they were all approved after modification. This community member has voted several times against protocols, as have others, and negative reports are recorded in the minutes; no minority reports are filed.

On one project, the vote was seven against and eight in favor, and it went through as approved. Those who had voted negatively were reassured by the chair that, since only a fraction of proposed protocols succeed in getting funded, the chances were that this would not, and therefore would not be done. No subsequent report was made to the committee on whether or not the project did get funded.

Number Four says his biggest problem, even though he is a veterinarian, is that he cannot understand the science in some protocols. He speaks up mainly about primate and cat behavior projects that involve maintaining the animals in darkness and that the investigators claim have relevance to learning disabilities in children. He judges experiments on their potential social worth, and some projects he thinks are "totally worthless" because he cannot see the relevance of them to the human condition. In these cases, he always votes no.

Committee service has not been exciting, he says, but he is favorably impressed with the effort that the institution makes to comply with humane standards. One benefit of being an IACUC member is that he is permitted to attend the university's courses free of charge; he has been pleased to receive free continuing education.

Number Five—national humane society part-time staff

Number Five, who had worked as an animal technician in the past, was appointed for an indefinite term of office and is the only nonaffiliated member on a committee of twenty-one persons. She served for four years until outside circumstances required her to leave. The IACUC had the same chairperson throughout this period, and there was little turnover of other members.

The committee met once a month for about two or three hours and reviewed approximately thirty protocols per meeting. The community member is required only to attend, and receives no information of substance in advance. There are four classes of experiment: those involving (a) no pain or negligible pain, (b) low-level pain, (c) moderate pain, and (d) a high level of pain. Those falling within the first three classes, which constitute about 99 percent of all proposals, are reviewed solely by the institution's two veterinary staff, who are members of the committee and who are the only ones to see the material submitted by the investigator. Other committee members receive sparse information (protocol title, name of investigator, and numbers and species of animals used) compiled by the committee administrator, a secretary. If the veterinarians have a modification to recommend (most commonly adjustments in anesthetic use), this will be verbally reported to the full committee. These revisions are always accepted, usually with little or no discussion.

The class d experiments—about six to eight protocols per year—involve a high level of pain or significant stress and receive fuller review. For these, the veterinarians select two members of the committee (both scientists whose research areas are close to that of the investigator) to act as primary and secondary reviewers. These two persons and the veterinarians are the only ones to see the complete protocol forms. Number Five has never been asked to be a reviewer and has never seen a full submission of an investigator. She had no objections to this. She was very satisfied with her term of office and regrets that she was unable to continue.

Number Six—local humane society staff person

Number Six was appointed to a one-year term, renewed for a second year. There are a total of twenty committee members of whom two are nonaffiliated members, the other being a professional business woman. There is a real effort to rotate the membership of the committee with no one exceeding two years of service.

The committee meets once a month to review an average of about 200 protocols a year. The meetings usually last a full day, including lunch and dinner, but may continue for twelve hours. Number Six finds the atmosphere collegial; she has been a welcomed member and enjoys getting to know the others. Before the meeting, all committee members receive everything that the investigator has submitted, usually between eight and ten pages per protocol. This includes a "lay abstract," which is well done. At the first two meetings Number Six did not understand what was going on and felt intimidated due to her non-academic background. But now, although comprehension of the science remains a great challenge, she receives good help from other committee members. During the last twelve months, six protocols have received some negative votes. No minority report is ever filed. The vote is by majority, so these projects proceeded. During the almost two years that she has served, two protocols have been stopped because of disapproval by the committee. Both were teaching projects, one of which had received nationwide negative publicity.

Number Six believes she has made a useful contribution to the committee. Although there have been "no major steps" toward more humane experiments, she believes she contributes a sense of balance and public accountability. Her greatest hardship has been facing the antagonism of the local animal welfare or animal rights community who reject her as a "collaborator."

Number Seven—active member of an animal rights group

This lawyer, who holds a bachelor's degree in science and is not an antivivisectionist, was appointed at the suggestion of an animal rights group which had been
asked to nominate a representative. He has so far served over four years of an
indefinite term. Number Seven is the only nonaffiliated member on a committee
of nineteen. Not until he had served four years was there any turnover, and then
half the membership was changed.

The committee meets once a month and reviews approximately 200 protocols
per year. When Number Seven first joined the committee, IACUC members
would receive the face page only of the four-page form for each protocol to be
reviewed. This would arrive the day before the meeting. He repeatedly protested,
claiming that he could not make a meaningful review. Out of the total committee,
now there are now three people (himself, a chosen reviewer, and the veterinarian) who receive complete information, which may be anything from four to
twenty-five pages for any one protocol. His copies arrive two weeks before the
meeting, and he is conscientious in spending several hours in his review before
the meeting.

In committee discussion, the most common problems refer to the dose of
anesthetic or the number of animals. He has voted no a few times during the last
twelve months, for instance on drug addiction studies. Everyone else always
votes yes to everything. But all protocols go ahead over his negative vote, which
he finds dispiriting. His most significant victory resulted from a personal meeting
with an investigator whom he persuaded to reduce the number of cats to be used.

He recognizes that he has not effected much change, but he believes he helps
to keep the committee "honest" because his presence forces the rest of the
committee to look at things more carefully.

Conclusions from community members' stories

Based on this anecdotal information, some summary observations are offered.
People who serve as community members tend to be well-educated, holding
doctoral, master's, or baccalaureate degrees and having skills that have placed
them at the middle or top managerial levels of humane societies. In the selection
of community members, there is no apparent predominance of either sex. Several
persons experienced hostility and sometimes intense attacks from other members
of the committee. Community members who are most satisfied with their term of
office on the committees are those who have an appreciation of science and, in
the words of one person, "can access the culture." To be effective, they need to
be able to withstand role ambiguity and to deal with group pressures. Community
members need excellent communication skills, an ability to present a reasoned

view with dignity and without hostility to persons who do not agree with them. They must be satisfied with having only moderate or minor impact on the committee and seeing only occasional disapprovals of protocols. Their overall impact of contributing balance and some measure of public accountability to the proceedings must suffice. For this, they must be prepared to devote a considerable amount of their time.

Among the 16 institutions represented in this sample, committee procedures vary widely; some are open to serious question. Sometimes the provision of protocol information to committee members is deficient, making meaningful review impossible. Problems of incomplete information and lack of timeliness were both encountered with some frequency. In several instances, community members had to struggle to assert their rights on these matters. On the positive side, institutions are repeatedly revising their standard protocol forms in order to improve the quality of information provided by the investigators. Expedited review is sometimes taken to an extreme (as at the institution where 99 percent of the protocols are reviewed by the veterinary staff who alone had access to the protocols). From this survey, it appears that the discriminatory practices found in the early days against community members, such as no vote, have been largely abandoned. (But Mench and Stricklin (1991) even at this date still advocate these measures when the institution has "reservations" about the noninstitutional member.)

Many committees in this sample appear to have no established term of office for members; turnover is sluggish. The chair and other members frequently serve for four or more years of open-ended appointments. Such practices can be detrimental because the educational experience of serving on an IACUC is thus limited to relatively few persons. Also, the opportunity for the committees to be exposed to fresh ideas is reduced. It tends to weaken the defense of the IACUC to outside criticism. Few committees included student representation, although some community members commented favorably on this practice.

A sense of frustration in effecting any change is high on the list of complaints of the community members interviewed; many felt the IACUCs were "rubber stamps." It is striking that community members were usually alone in voting against any protocols. In every case, their negative votes are overridden. Only rarely were no votes cast by any other member, and disappointment was expressed that reservations about certain experiments were not voiced by other committee members. Minority reports are exceptional.

From these reports, the consensus is that it is very rare for any animal experiment to be disallowed completely. Some experiments are deferred for a period of time for problems to be resolved, but start up again later. Of all those eleven persons who were asked how many experiments were completely stopped during their total period of committee service (average 3.5 years, range 1 to 5), about half said none, about a quarter said one, and another quarter said two or three. In at least two institutions, information about this disapproval was given to the funding agency or overseeing authority.

Disapproval rate may not be a reasonable measure of a committee's effectiveness. A philosopher who is co-chair of a particularly well-functioning and mature IACUC told me that on their committee, disapprovals rarely happen; instead, a more common resolution would be limited pilot studies using a minimal number of animals and done under strict veterinary supervision. This committee has many well-worked-out written policies on problematic commonly used procedures (such as orbital bleeding, hybridoma procedures, etc.). These policies are now well-known among investigators and the researchers have therefore largely stopped submitting many types of projects that would raise a red flag.

Members of IACUCs who are also animal advocates are in an ambiguous position. Those who cross the line to work within the system risk rejection by other animal advocates and also rejection by other members of the committee. Whatever they do, they are criticized by someone. If they are too complacent, they are viewed as collaborators; if they are too stringent, they are viewed as obstructionists. The isolation of being at odds with other committee members takes its toll; also, some community members suffer considerable emotional pain because of the stress of having such direct contact with animal experiments that they know will proceed despite their objections.

The alternative of "refinement" of experiments is the most common revision; many protocols are modified in some way. Lessening animal pain, primarily through modifying the use of anesthetic or analgesic, is the most prevalent modification. The implementation of these modifications falls heavily on the institutional veterinarian, who can face a challenging job if there is an uncooperative investigator. Reductions in numbers of animals may occur, but rarely. Replacements probably never occur in the context of research, but may occur occasionally in the use of animals in education.

A commonly stated opinion among the survey respondents was that the value of being a community member lies not so much in the specific reforms effected but in being a constant reminder to the institution of the outside world. Some spoke of the "crucial role" that community members play since they are the most likely people to bring up social and ethical issues for discussion. Whether or not ethical discussion should take place at all in IACUCs has been something of a contentious issue among IACUCs nationally. In general, scientists can be comfortable with discussion of anesthetic selection and dosage but not with discussion of the limits of justification of infliction of animal pain in the name of science. Indeed, raising ethical issues can be threatening to those who fear that generalizations would be made, and that an entire class of experiments, or even animal experimentation as a whole, would be challenged for social worth. The mainstream view has been that this Pandora's box should be left firmly closed.

The law is not explicit about addressing ethical concerns. It suggests that the social merit of an experiment is a permissible consideration, but nowhere is it stated directly that it is the IACUC's responsibility to make this assessment. In any case, ethical concerns often go beyond the law. Just how ethical discussion can be fostered in IACUCs deserves serious attention. Since non-scientist members and students appear to be more likely than others to raise such issues, a start would be to numerically increase such representation. Also, a non-scientist as chair or co-chair would likely to beneficial. Some IACUCs have already taken these steps. Another helpful avenue would to be introduce instruction on the ethical issues of animal experimentation into the regular course work for investigators who will use animals as subjects. Efforts in this regard have barely begun.

The range in committee practices revealed in this survey shows how well some committees are performing in comparison to others. The best committees, which engage in meaningful review and self-assessment, can serve as a model to show how much can be achieved within this system.

Survey of chairpersons

To provide a different perspective, I interviewed ten chairpersons of IACUCs by telephone in early 1992, obtaining their names from inquiries among scientists. Selection was not based on any exclusionary factors other than no overlap with the first survey. All who were approached agreed to answer a standard set of open-ended questions about their perspective on the role of the community member. Two chairpersons also voluntarily commented that they welcomed this type of survey because it was important to get the word out about the role of community members.

All the chairpersons were scientists: physiologists, biochemists, psychologist, and so on. They were not asked if they personally conducted animal experiments. The length of service varied; seven were serving unexpired terms that ranged from two to nine years, with a heavy cluster around five years; two had served terms of three or four years that had recently ended; one had served less than one year but had had several previous years of IACUC service.

All chairpersons thought that community members serve an important function, that their committee has fulfilled or more than fulfilled the intent of Congress in this regard, and that no changes regarding community membership of IACUCs are necessary. Details of the pooled responses are reported below.

The Intent of Congress

There was complete consensus that congressional intent in mandating community representation was to broaden the perspective of the committee beyond that of the institution. A good many mentioned that the community member's presence was to provide assurance to the community that all animal experiments were appropriate and necessary and deserved community endorsement.

Beyond that, viewpoints differed. Several chairpersons mentioned that the intent was to let the community know what is going on in their community. Just how this outward flow of information was being achieved was unclear since there is no mechanism for it. Two respondents specifically said that the community member should inform outside people if anything is wrong. Some thought that Congress had intended the community representative to "speak up for the animals," others that Congress had not intended any particular advocacy or expertise in animal welfare. One respondent thought that having a community member was "primarily a PR move."

Selection of a community member

The most common method of selecting a community member was by word-of-mouth, primarily from suggestions from current IACUC members, but occasionally from other members of their institution. Sometimes retired faculty were approached based on an interpretation of the law that non-affiliated meant not *currently* employed at that institution. In two cases outreach efforts were made by requesting names from local SPCAs and animal shelters and by posting notices on bulletin boards of such organizations as the Chamber of Commerce, Council of Churches, and women's clubs.

An underlying assumption was that antivivisectionists were unacceptable. One chairperson said outright that they never considered having "an animal welfare person"—making no distinction between welfarists and antivivisectionists. Such persons had sought membership, he said, but had been rebuffed. It would be "disruptive and contrary to the function of the committee." Most of the time, less direct words were used. For instance, I was told that the community member should "not be a devil's advocate," should have "no excess emotional baggage," should have a "flexible attitude" and be "non-confrontational." Two chairpersons mentioned that they had sought a person with knowledge about animal welfare, one saying that he "didn't want a pushover" and therefore directly sought a member of the local SPCA.

A wide range of other desirable attributes were mentioned such as being well-educated, fair-minded, and having professional standing and credibility in the community. Availability was a key factor, and since employed persons had problems of daytime availability, retired persons were frequently sought. Two chairpersons said they wanted only theologians or ethicists, preferably those who had previous experience of service on an Institutional Review Board.

Half of the respondents volunteered the information that non-attendance of their community member had been a real problem and most expressed dismay at this. However, one said he interpreted non-attendance as a "sign of confidence" by the community member "that the committee was functioning well."

Although the question was not asked, several chairpersons volunteered information about their current or past community members' profession. The list included two retired clergy and one currently employed administrator of a theological college, a retired physician, a retired businessman, a president of a business association, three representatives of humane associations, a veterinarian, a high school science teacher, and an ethicist.

Significance of the presence of a community member

Six of the ten respondents believed that the presence of a community member of their IACUC had had beneficial effects. Primarily, their presence brings awareness of the "outside world" and stimulates discussion about how the public would view a particular animal experiment, especially those experiments that involve considerable animal pain. As one person put it, "Science can become mured because animal experimentation becomes commonplace, so you need an outsider to keep the scientists alert to the community." The benefit, they said, was that an outsider's presence makes investigators explain what they are doing and why, and makes scientists more introspective about their work. Some noted that community members tend to speak up on ethical issues such as balancing the suffering of the animals against the good to society.

An absence of effect was noted by four respondents. One explained this by saying that they had a good committee to begin with, so the community member did not improve it. One explained it a different way; he said he "feared the committee is a rubber stamp for what the scientists want to do."

Any changes needed?

The question posed was "Are there any changes needed (a) on your committee or (b) nationally regarding community members serving on IACUCs?" "None" was the typical answer although many said they had not thought about the issue. One person was adamant that one community member was enough—"We need no more." Another wanted his committee to have an alternate, so that when the primary community member could not attend, the alternate would come instead. He said he was "uncomfortable when the community member was not present."

A few thoughtful comments were added by some about the need for educational materials (brochures, handbooks, and the like) to help community members understand their charge. Although not needed by all community members, some would benefit. (In fact, some materials are available. See Animal Welfare Institute, 1987; Canadian Federation of Humane Societies, 1985; USDA, 1989.) Also, a couple of chairpersons said it would be beneficial if community members attended conferences where IACUC topics are discussed (such as those of NIH, the Scientists Center for Annual Welfare, and Public Responsibility in Medicine and Research). One person thought that although no more regulations are needed, it would be helpful if NIH and USDA clarified the purpose and functions of an IACUC and explained the philosophy behind having a community member.

General conclusions

In comparing the results of these two informal surveys, some stark differences are apparent. Chairpersons of IACUCs are generally well satisfied with the role of their community member. Community members who represent the animal advocacy community may or may not be satisfied. Those persons from moderate animal welfare organizations may be quite content with their role; others— largely those from the animal rights movement—are highly critical.

These probably irreconcilable disparities in viewpoint emerge from widely differing expectations of what an IACUC should do, what functions it should serve. Disapprovals and modifications of protocols that the animal rights movement want are unlikely to be effected by this route. Even though increasing the proportional representation of community members would probably be beneficial, the overall result would not be dramatically changed.

Over the long haul, IACUCs have only limited power. Some improvements in the humaneness of animal experiments will certainly take place, such as insistence on greater use of anesthetics and approved euthanasia methods and getting rid of certain student exercises. IACUCs can and do prevent animal experiments from being conducted that would be embarrassing to the scientific community. Realistically, more cannot be expected.

Limited impact has also been the experience of Institutional Review Boards. Useful as these committees have been from an educational viewpoint, they have not been the major mechanism for change in protecting the rights of human subjects. A leading bioethicist, LeRoy B. Walters, who has studied and participated in the development of IRBs since the early 1970s, said that as he was reading the above accounts of what was happening in IACUCs, he recalled how IRBs functioned in their early days. There had been similar problems of unacceptable committee practices (no vote for the community member, lack of access to the material for review, etc.) and limited reforms. This view was supported by several other bioethicists who are experts in human experimentation issues who also read a draft of this chapter. They said that the IRB review process will weed out those activities that would bring harm to the medical profession, but not much more.

In human experimentation, other avenues of greater importance for reform have been (a) the recommendations of the 1978 National Commission for the Protection of Human Subjects; (b) the NIH Study Section reviews, which have become increasingly more alert to ethical issues; (c) the publicity surrounding national bodies that hold open meetings like the one that oversees the NIH gene therapy project; and (d) legislation. I believe the comparison will stand in the animal experimentation field.

Serious consideration should be given to the establishment of a national commission on animal experimentation issues with representation that reasonably reflects current social attitudes. Such a commission could thrash out some of the ethical concerns that are voiced by some members of the public, including the limits of primate research, use of purpose-bred animals, and the encouragement of alternatives. It could make policy recommendations on the specific functions of IACUCs and elucidate the role of community members—issues that are still poorly defined.

8

Animal Pain Scales in Public Policy: An International Perspective

In his book *Alternatives to Animal Experiments*, David H. Smyth, emeritus professor of physiology at the University of Sheffield, described a new concept—a scale for replacing animal experiments (Smyth, 1978). This scale ranged from Stage 1, in which there is no involvement of animals, through increasingly stressful animal use up to Stages 7 and 8, which include "all the controversial procedures" that cause substantial animal pain. He suggested that efforts to find alternatives be concentrated on procedures in categories 7 and 8 "instead of putting equal effort into finding alternatives to all animal experiments, whether they are painful or not."

People rapidly built on his ideas. The Swedish Medical Council worked out a six-step pain category system that was adopted as Swedish national policy in 1979 and was used by the newly established Swedish regional ethical committees in their protocol review. In the same year, the Netherlands also adopted as national policy a simpler, three-step pain scale (minor, moderate, and severe). The Dutch policy provides various illustrative examples: blood sampling, vaginal smear sampling, force feeding of innocuous substances, and terminal experiments under anesthesia are rated "minor" pain; frequent blood sampling, insertion of indwelling catheters, immobilization or restraint such as the use of primate chairs, skin transplants, caesarean section, and immunization with incomplete adjuvants are rated "moderate"; collection of ascitic fluid, total bleeding without anesthesia, production of genetic defects such as muscular dystrophy, carcinogenicity research with tumor induction, immunization in footpad with complete adjuvants, and induction of convulsions are rated "severe."

118

As can be seen from these example, the phrase "pain scale" is something of a misnomer. The word *pain* is being used rather loosely. Much more is involved—animal pain, harms, and adverse states in general are being described. In order to categorize a particular procedure, typical questions to be asked are, What is the degree of surgical invasiveness? and, How sick is the animal and how abnormal is the animal as a result of the procedure? For the purist, a better term would probably be "animal harm scales."

The categorization systems used in Sweden and in the Netherlands have served as models for other countries. In 1986, Britain adopted a four-tier "severity banding" and investigators are granted project licenses to conduct experiments at one of the three lower bandings of mild, moderate, and severe—a novel method of controling what is permitted. Any procedures that would fall into the fourth band (beyond severe) are prohibited (David B. Morton, personal communication, March 25, 1992).

In the United States, the Swedish pain scale gained attention when Karl Johan Öbrink, M.D., professor of physiology at Uppsala University, presented a paper at the first conference organized by the Scientists Center for Animal Welfare (SCAW) in 1981 (Öbrink, 1982). This center adapted the pain scale and, after wide circulation for comment by American scientists, the results were published (Orlans, 1987). SCAW's five-category pain scale has certain educational advantages over other systems because it includes a bottom level A below "low" and a top level E above "severe." Lacking an equivalent to a category A, other category systems cannot be used to convey the concept of replacement techniques. Also, lacking a top-level equivalent to category E, other systems do not completely convey the concept of procedures that are unacceptable irrespective of their scientific merit.

The Canadians adopted a scale based on that of SCAW in 1987 and revised it in 1989 (CCAC, 1989a). New Zealand included both the Swedish and SCAW's pain scales in their 1988 guidelines for animal ethics committees. The National Health and Medical Research Council of Australia (1991) has designed its own classification system of experiments.

In the United States, efforts to adopt a pain scale nationally have so far failed. Two early efforts proved premature. The first was made in 1983, when Joseph S. Spinelli, D.V.M., of the University of California, San Francisco, recommended that the Swedish pain scale be included in the revisions of the PHS Guide. He made this recommendation in testimony to the committee charged with the guide's revision. The idea was rejected.

The second effort was made in 1987 when a pain scale very similar to SCAW's was officially proposed by USDA as part of the rule-making under the Animal Welfare Act (Federal Register, 1987). But too many objections were raised during the 1987 public comment period and not enough people spoke up in its favor, so the idea was dropped from the final version.

Among the public comments, a major objection was that a pain scale exceeded congressional intent. Typical of other objections are the following. "[The schema] is the wrong approach. The categories . . . only confuse the issues and interfere with the ability of the [IACUC] to carry out its mandate. . . . The schema proposed makes no distinction between [tolerance and threshold] levels of pain and the alleviating effects of anesthetics and analgesics in each of the examples used" (John D. Loeser, President, American Pain Society, 1987). "We believe this provision is totally inappropriate and unworkable and should not be part of regulatory review" (Jean E. Brenchley, President, American Society for Microbiology, 1987).

Negative comments about pain scales had an effect in Sweden as well. In the mid-1980s, the Swedish pharmaceutical industry managed to persuade the responsible federal agency to abandon pain scale use. According to an informed source, a major reason may have been that the pharmaceutical companies' animal experiments frequently fell in the highly invasive categories and therefore were subject to considerable scrutiny by the ethics committees; this was not what the companies wanted (personal communication from Lars Wass, M.D., Swedish National Board of Universities and Colleges, July 6, 1990). After ten years of use, the pain scale was dropped when a new Swedish law was passed, effective January 1, 1989.

Other systems of classifying animal experiments have been proposed. One was specifically designed for the use of animals in education (Orlans, 1980); others, for general application, can be found in Shapiro, 1987, and the New York Academy of Sciences, 1988. None of these has been widely adopted.

New schemes for assessing harms to animals are being developed. The latest is a more inclusive approach embodied in the "Scheme for the Assessment of Potential and Likely Cost to Animals in Research Involving Animal Subjects" (Smith and Boyd, 1991). Proposed by the Institute of Medical Ethics in the U.K., this scheme offers a numerical basis for rating the following factors: the quality of the research facility, the quality of laboratory personnel who care for the animals, the severity of effects of husbandry and scientific procedures, provisions for amelioration of adverse effects, the numbers of animals, and overall costs imposed on the animals. Smith and Boyd provide an accompanying scheme to assess the "benefits," including evaluation of the project's potential benefits (the value of its hoped-for outcome); assessment of the quality, validity, and necessity of the methods proposed; and an overall assessment of the project to judge whether the potential benefits will be realized given the proposed scientific approach.

Another scheme to aid in decision-making as to whether the experiment should be allowed to proceed has been proposed by David Porter (1992) of the University of Guelph, Ontario, Canada. Like the Smith and Boyd proposal, this system also aims to evaluate the benefits of animal experiments and the harms to animals that are likely to result. Parameters used in this judgment include the aim of the experiment, the realistic potential of the experiment to achieve its objective, the degree and duration of pain likely to be involved, the number of animals, and the quality of animal care, among others.

In the national policies of Britain and some other countries, the concept of weighing animal harms against the scientific worth of an experiment is written into public policy. For instance in issuing any license, the British Secretary of State is specifically required to "weigh the likely adverse effects on the animals concerned against the benefit likely to accrue." Also, the Australian code of practice requires that the Animal Experimentation Ethics Committees make an ethical decision to approve or not approve "by considering the scientific value of the project weighed against the welfare aspects" (Anderson, 1990). This utilitarian concept of weighing "goods" against "harms" is described in some detail in an article by Patrick Bateson, F.R.S., professor of ethology at the University of Cambridge (1986).

The national policies of the United States do not include such statements, but the concept is beginning to gain acceptance. For instance, the 1985 voluntary guidelines on animal use prepared by the American Psychological Association state: "The scientific purpose should be of sufficient potential significance as to outweigh any harm or distress to the animals used" (APA, 1985).

Unacceptable procedures

Another important concept, that of totally unacceptable procedures, can be conveyed with a pain scale. It is reasonable to consider that some procedures on laboratory animals are beyond ethical justification and therefore unacceptable irrespective of any scientific knowledge that might be derived. Category E in Table 6.1 denotes such procedures.

Category E includes legally prohibited procedures—which vary from country to country—and other procedures judged to be unethical. Of the legally prohibited procedures, in the U.K. two examples are the using living animals to gain manual skills other than in microsurgery and harming animals in experiments conducted in elementary and secondary schools. The 1987 amendments to West Germany's Law for Protection of Animals prohibit the experimental use of animals in the development and testing of weapons, and in the safety testing of tobacco products, washing powders, and decorative cosmetics.

In the United States certain experimental procedures are outlawed. The PHS policy states, "Surgical or other painful procedures should not be performed on unanesthetized animals paralyzed by chemical agents" (PHS Guide, 1985). Under the PHS policy the provisions of the American Veterinary Medical Association's policies on euthanasia must be followed, and certain methods of killing are "absolutely condemned." These include the use of agents such as strychnine, nicotine sulfate, and curariform drugs (AVMA, 1987). Up until at least 1987, it was a practice in some U.S. veterinary schools to demonstrate the lethal effects of strychnine poisoning in conscious dogs. These practices have since stopped.

Canadian national policy is similar to that of the United States with respect to euthanasia methods, but goes much further regarding experimental procedures. CCAC policy first enunciated in 1980 and restated in 1989 declares, "the following experimental procedures inflict excessive pain and are thus unacceptable: (a) utilization of muscle relaxants or paralytics (curare and curare-like) alone, without anesthetics, during surgical procedures; (b) traumatizing procedures involving crushing, burning, striking or beating in unanesthetized animals" (CCAC, 1989b).

Over the course of time, additional procedures have been added to this list. Use of Freund's Complete Adjuvant (FCA), a procedure used to stimulate antibody production to bacteria, bacterial toxins, and numerous chemicals in order to obtain blood serum with high antibody levels, is a case in point. A common practice has been to inject FCA into the footpads of rabbits with the result that the feet become inflamed; since several feet were injected, the animals were unable to walk, and in extreme cases, thereby unable to obtain water or food. The procedure was used often enough to warrant devising a national policy to prevent its recurrence.

Such a policy—the first of its kind—was issued by the CCAC in 1990. The policy states that Freund's Complete Adjuvant "must never be given either intravenously or in repeated doses. FCA should not be used in horses. . . . FCA should not be injected in the feet of rabbits." Severe restrictions are also placed on the use of FCA in other rodents such as rats and mice. It is possible that universal use of a pain scale by Canadian IACUCs had hastened the development of this reform since the initiative came about because some Canadian IACUCs had repeatedly identified injection of FCA into the footpads of rabbits as falling in category E, thus alerting the scientists to action.

Certain procedures, although not prohibited by national policy, are judged to be in an unacceptable category because of in-house policies. These may either be formal, written policies (on primate restraint procedures or tumor burden size described in chapter 6 under Limitation of Tumor Size) as have been established at some research facilities, or less formal ones as established by IACUC decisions. Examples of the latter are found in Rebecca Dresser's 1989 study of decision-making by some thirty voluntarily participating American IACUCs. Dresser prepared a number of hypothetical protocols and each participating IACUC reviewed them and reported their decisions. One protocol involved the injection of Freund's Complete Adjuvant into the footpads of mice; Dresser reports that this "would simply not be permitted" by a number of the committees. As another example, she reports that a significant number of committees took an "extreme position that no scientific project would justify the lengthy restraint period" of keeping squirrel monkeys in restraint chairs for twenty-four hours a day for up to ten weeks without relief (Dresser, 1990). So, in practice, category E is in everyday use.

An agenda for future reforms for the U.K. of what procedures should be banned has been voiced by Michael Balls, professor of cell biology at Nottingham University and Chair of the Trustees of Fund for the Replacement of Animals in Medical Experiments. He states; "I think that there are some uses of animals which should not be permitted in ANY circumstances, irrespective of potential benefits, including the following:

• experiments aimed at the discovery of "safe" smoking materials;
• the induction of anxiety and depression through "social deprivation" (e.g., in monkeys) or "learned helplessness" (e.g., in dogs);
• the use of aversive stimuli (e.g., electric shocks) in "behavioural training" in psychological and behavioural research;
• the use of wild-caught members of threatened and endangered species;
• ANY experiments on chimpanzees, our closest relatives, which possess many qualities once thought to be uniquely human" (Balls, 1988).

Some scientists have been unwilling to acknowledge that unacceptable procedures are part of current biomedical science. Perhaps they have felt that any concession on their part would throw suspicion on the acceptability of a much wider range of animal experiments. The very concept of there being a category E bites at the core of the general controversy.

Pain scales as a basis for national data collection

Another practical use of a pain scale is in national data collection on animal experiments—an essential part of public accountability.

The Dutch government's method of reporting is among the best because a meaningful pain scale is used, and therefore trends in reduction and refinements in animal use can be properly assessed. Reporting includes the number, purpose, species, estimate of degree of discomfort, and source of cats and dogs used in experimentation (use of pound animals is not permitted). The 1977 Dutch law requires that the degree of pain be ranked according to minor discomfort, moderate discomfort, and severe discomfort according to one of four durations—less than one day, one to seven days, seven to thirty days, and more than thirty days. Because there can be problems in deciding how to classify certain procedures, the government agency for administration of the law organizes regular conferences, three or four times a year, to discuss these issues with representatives from research institutions in order to further unity of opinion.

The Dutch method of reporting national data makes available information that the public wants. As seen in Table 8.1, over the period 1985 to 1987 there was

TABLE 8.1   The Netherlands: percentage of animals used in experiments
involving pain, 1985–1987

	1985		1986		1987	
Minor discomfort	52.8		53.5		57.5	
Moderate discomfort	19.9		22.7		20.7	
Severe discomfort, less than 1 day	10.6		6.5		8.1	
Severe discomfort, 1–7 days	12.5	27.4	13.7	23.8	10.4	21.8
Severe discomfort, 7–30 days	1.9		3.2		2.9	
Severe discomfort, more than 30 days	2.4		0.4		0.4	

The Dutch data collection system uses meaningful severity bands of pain and also provides details on the duration of severe pain. For severe discomfort, figures are given broken down into four groups ranging from less than one day to more than 30 days, and as a total for all durations. Numbers are rounded to the nearest decimal place. The actual number of animals used on which this percentage data is based is: 175,088 for 1985; 852,038 for 1986; and 760,052 for 1987.

Source: "Statistics. Animal experimentation in the Netherlands" for the years 1985, 1986, and 1987. The Veterinary Public Health Inspectorate, Rijswijk, The Netherlands.

some achievement made with respect to refinement. The percentage of animals subjected to severe discomfort was reduced from 27.4 percent in 1985 to 21.8 percent in 1987. Furthermore, severe discomfort lasting more than thirty days was dropped from 2.4 percent in 1985 to 0.4 percent in subsequent years. During this period, the total numbers of animals used in experimentation also progressively declined.

The British reporting system is like that of the Netherlands in providing useful information on animal pain. Recent figures show that there has been a decline in the number of procedures involving animals from 5.2 million in 1978 to 3.2 million in 1990. The proportions between projects involving substantial, moderate, and mild pain have remained approximately the same over the period 1987 to 1990. For 1990, proportions were as follows: of all the project licenses in force, 2 percent involved substantial pain, 49 percent involved moderate pain, and some 41 percent involved mild pain, (the rest, 8 percent, were unclassified, that is, the procedures were carried out under anesthesia from which the animal was not allowed to recover) (Animal Procedures Committee Report, 1990). The severe pain category consisted of substantial surgical procedures with anesthesia and subsequent recovery of consciousness, LD50 tests, and cases where infectious or other diseases were induced in animals, either as unprotected controls in a study of a potential therapy or in studies of disease diagnosis.

Furthermore, the British statistics give a detailed breakdown by purpose of experiment and type of procedure. They clearly demonstrate that the *control* of animal pain during experimentation has significantly increased. Several procedures involving considerable trauma have decreased numerically over recent years. These include exposure to ionizing radiation, induction of psychological stress integral to the procedure, and physical trauma to simulate human injury (Statistics of Scientific Procedures, 1989, 1990).

Deficiencies of the USDA pain scale and statistics

The statistics gathered by the USDA provide the most inclusive look at animal use now available in the United States, but eighty percent or more of the animals used (rats, mice, and birds) have been excluded from the AWA and therefore are excluded from official statistics. This makes it impossible to assess trends in total numbers of animal used.

Trends in progress toward refinements are difficult, if not impossible, to assess from USDA data because the way data is presented on animal pain is not serving current needs. Historically, it was a significant step in 1973 when the USDA started to collect national statistics on animal use. At that time, there was a need to emphasize and encourage the use of anesthetics and analgesics. Accordingly, it was established that reports from animal research facilities were to be filed under three levels of pain and discomfort—level 1 being pain and discomfort associated with routine procedures such as blood sampling and injections that require no anesthetic or analgesic (roughly the same "low" level as in other countries); level 2 including procedures that would cause pain greater than routine procedures, but pain that is ameliorated by the use of appropriate anesthetic, analgesic, or tranquilizing agents; level 3 including procedures that involve pain greater than routine procedures, but pain that cannot, for scientific reasons, be ameliorated by the use of appropriate anesthetics, analgesics, or tranquilizing agents. This reporting system is still in use.

The statistics broken down according to these three pain levels for the years 1986 to 1990 are presented in Table 8.2. This shows that the percentage of animals used at each of these pain levels has remained fairly constant over the last five years. (An exception is the aberration in the figures for levels 1 and 2 in 1988 for which there is no known explanation.) Anecdotal evidence suggests that there has been an increase in use of pain-relieving drugs, but this does not show up in the statistics. The figures for level 3 suggest that there has been no reduction in numbers of animals that suffer pain and do not receive anesthetics.

These data do not provide an adequate picture because the focus of the classification system is on use or non-use of anesthetics, not on the overall level of pain for the animal. From current data it is impossible to distinguish between "moderate" and "severe" levels of pain since levels 2 and 3 include a mixture of these levels. With level 2, the fact that an anesthetic is used does not mean that the procedure is therefore painless. Furthermore, with level 3, the fact that an anesthetic has been omitted provides little information on the level of pain that the animal is exposed to; it could be low, moderate, or high. Thus, it is not possible to track national trends toward reducing pain that animals experience.

TABLE 8.2   United States: numbers and percentage of animals used in experiments according to pain level, fiscal years 1986–1990

	1986	1987	1988	1989	1990
Level 1					
no pain, no drugs	1,056,934*	1,146,503*	583,617*	1,019,350	920,330
(percent of total)	59%	58%	36%	58%	58%
Level 2					
pain, with drugs	608,308	692,247	961,271	619,219	586,145
(percent of total)	34%	35%	59%	35%	36%
Level 3					
pain, no drugs	113,161	130,373	90,400	116,587	89,624
(percent of total)	6%	7%	6%	7%	6%
Total	1,778,403	1,969,123	1,635,288	1,754,456§	1,578,099§

See text for discussion of the numbers presented here, where it is argued that very little can be deduced from this data. The percentage figures (which have been rounded to the nearest whole number) have been derived from two charts in the USDA annual reports to Congress, namely Chart 1 of 1988, and Chart 3 of 1990. The total numbers have been compiled from other USDA sources, not Charts 1 and 3 mentioned above. The numbers marked * have been derived by subtraction from the relevant totals for that year. Because numbers shown in this figure have been collected from various USDA tables, some slight discrepancies have occurred: in the columns marked §, the numbers in the subtotals when added together do not exactly tally with the total figure given.

Source: APHIS, USDA.

The three pain levels devised in 1973 made sense at that time but have outlived their usefulness. Nowadays, a different focus is needed. There is reason to believe that the IACUCs are now largely fulfilling the task of alerting investigators to the need to use anesthetics. Now, the focus needs to be on achievement of refinements. The amount of pain or harm inflicted on animals is now the focus of public attention.

Fuller information would result from the use of a pain scale that represents the amount of pain irrespective of the use of pain-ameliorating drugs. USDA officials are sensitive to this need for change: in 1987 they proposed adoption of a pain scale similar to that of Table 6.1 but were rebuffed. In October, 1992, The Humane Society of the United States submitted a *"Petition for Changes in Reporting Procedures Under the Animal Welfare Act"* to the USDA. The petition argues for several reasonable reforms in statistical reporting including adoption of a pain scale similar to that in Table 6.1. This issue is yet to be resolved.

Adoption of a pain scale for public policy brings with it certain limitations. Assessing animal pain involves considerable subjectivity, and the pain assessment provides only one dimension of a multidimensional issue—assessing the total amount of harm to animals. It does not account for the number of animals experiencing pain, the number of lives taken, and the possible harms resulting from unsatisfactory animal husbandry or from causes other than the procedure itself, but the use of this recommended pain scale is a step toward assessing animal harm.

Additional recommendations in national data collection

An additional recommendation is that the *purpose* of each procedure should be part of the information gathered. What proportion of animal experiments is conducted for medical research and what is done for non-medical purposes? Other categories are military research (to develop and test weapons and to do research into methods of treatment of injuries resulting from military weapons), agricultural research (to increase yield for commercial purposes for the food trade and, in some cases, to improve the human condition), veterinary research (aimed specifically at the benefit of the subject animal), testing, and education. This information may be burdensome for the reporting institutions to provide, but with increasing computerization of IACUC records, the task is made easier. It is worth the effort to enlighten the public.

Also, greater detail is needed on primate experiments because this information is of keen public interest. The total number of each species used (chimpanzees, baboons, macaques, etc.) as well as the purpose of experiment and the pain level by species should be reported.

The example of chimpanzees serves to illustrate the importance of having data on primates broken down by individual species. Chimpanzees are an endangered species and there is a real threat of extinction. Currently, the annual report from the USDA provides no information on chimpanzees, and the information is therefore virtually impossible to track.

Furthermore, I would argue for separate reporting of the numbers of animals and the numbers of procedures. This is significant because animals are not always killed at the end of a single procedure; primates in particular may be used for several different, unrelated procedures and even "recycled" by being passed to another laboratory because of their monetary value and the rarity of some species. A truly informative reporting system would count both the numbers of animals and numbers of procedures, if not on all species at least on primates.

Finally, increased educational efforts with respondents are needed to achieve greater uniformity in data compilation between institutions. Regular meetings between responsible government officials and respondents to clarify instructions could improve reliability.

In summary, it is recommended that national statistics be compiled so that all species used are reported; that breakdown figures be provided by species numbers and numbers of procedures, experimental purpose, and highest pain level endured irrespective of efforts to ameliorate the pain; and that improvements be made in the uniformity of reporting.

9

Pain, Suffering, and Death: Warm- and Cold-Blooded Vertebrates, Mollusks, and Insects

This chapter deals with the controversial issue of which species of animals do or do not have capacities to perceive pain and to suffer adverse mental states such as fear or suffering. To gain insight into this issue, not only is the research on pain perception across species lines assessed, but also analysis is made of many official policies, both nationally and internationally, as to whether or not they require use of anesthetics and humane killing procedures. The topics discussed in this chapter are definitions of adverse states, pain perception in warm-blooded vertebrates, systems of measuring animal pain, adverse mental states in all vertebrates, and pain perception in cold-blooded vertebrates and invertebrates.

In recent decades, scientific understanding about the nervous systems of humans and other animals has vastly expanded. The work of neuroscientists, physiologists, psychologists, animal behaviorists, and ethologists has demonstrated in animals capacities that previously were thought to be uniquely human. These capacities include language and complex communication systems, culture, consciousness, use of tools, the practice of deceit, reasoning ability, pain perception, and suffering. Because of recent research, it is now recognized that the perception of pain and the capacity to suffer extend further down the phylogenetic scale than was previously thought.

The phylogenetic scale provides a developmental history of a group of animals—a phylum being the main division of the animal kingdom. The developmental history is a continuum, so the phylogenetic scale cannot be represented by a straight line of events in time. Rather, the sequence of evolution emerged as a tree with many branches, as Darwin depicted.

The vertebrates are distinguished from invertebrates by having a backbone and a centralized nervous system with a brain and spinal cord. They comprise the mammals, birds, reptiles, amphibia, and fish. Mammals include the primates (apes, including *Homo sapiens*, and monkeys) and cetaceans (whales and dolphins), among others such as rodents.

The invertebrates do not have backbones, and their nervous systems are not centralized but rather consist of interlinking nerve clusters (ganglia) throughout the animal's body. Among the invertebrates are the mollusks, insects, worms, sponges, and protozoa. (Under the "modern" classification system, protozoa are classified as a separate kingdom.)

Definitions of adverse states

There is considerable controversy over the definition of adverse states. The American Veterinary Medical Association warned that "[d]etermining precisely whether an animal is in a state of discomfort, pain, or distress or is suffering is difficult. . . . Many terms involve mental states that are impossible to distinguish with precision, even in human beings. However, this lack of precision does not mean that certain domains of experience and perception that are generally recognized between individuals and across species lines cannot be determined" (AVMA, 1987). Most of the following definitions are based on those provided by the AVMA panel on animal pain.

Pain

The AVMA defines animal pain as an unpleasant sensory and emotional experience perceived as arising from a specific region of the body and associated with actual or potential tissue damage. Pain is distinguishable from moods such as sadness or body feelings such as hunger, which may be felt as arising from the body but not necessarily a particular body region.

The AVMA report continues, "Pain is a perception that depends on activation of a discrete set of receptors (nociceptors) by noxious stimuli, eg, thermal, chemical, or mechanical. Further processing in neural pathways, eg, spinal cord, brain stem, thalamus, and cerebral cortex, enables noxious stimuli to be perceived as pain." Thus, there is nociception and then feeling. The multidimensional aspect of pain is important. Human pain has at least three components: (1) *nociception,* the body's detection and signaling of noxious events; (2) *pain,* the conscious perception or recognition of the nociceptive stimulus; and (3) *suffering,* the affective, behavioral, or emotional response to the pain—referred to as the motivational-affective response. The same three components underpin the working definition of pain in animals (Rose and Adams, 1989).

Pain perception varies according to site, duration, and intensity of the stimulus and can be modified by previous experience, emotional states, and perhaps individual differences.

A pain-detection threshold can be established as the lowest intensity of a stimulus that is perceived as painful or that induces a response. A pain-tolerance threshold is the highest intensity of a stimulus that will be tolerated voluntarily. An animal may perceive a hypodermic puncture as painful, but may tolerate the injection if it is coupled with a food reward. Seemingly, the pain-detection threshold is uniform across species lines, whereas the pain-tolerance threshold may be more species-specific and subject to modification.

(AVMA, 1987)

Suffering

Suffering is an unpleasant emotional response usually associated with pain and distress; it is an inability to adapt or cope that causes mental anguish. It is not a sensory precept such as pain or temperature. It is akin to severe distress, which is defined below.

Among the best sources of information is *Animal Suffering*, a book by Mary Stamp Dawkins (1980a), the Mary Snow Fellow in Biological Sciences of Oxford University. Animal suffering can result from disease, starvation, exhaustion, and adverse mental states arising from the deprivation of exercise, companionship, or stimulation, or from frustration of other psychological needs, she says. Dawkins cites as short-term causes of suffering some capture and transportation methods used on animals, and as long-term causes the loss of social companions, as when animals are held captive in isolation. Relief of suffering may involve removing or changing some aspect of the internal or external environment, or giving the animal an opportunity to avoid, escape, or control some aspect of its environment. Suffering "carries overtones of mental experience like fear, pain or a generalized longing for freedom, which are difficult enough to gauge in our own species, let alone in others" (Dawkins, 1980b).

A number of scientists avoid the use of the word *suffering* because they feel it is "too emotional" and associated too intimately with critics of animal experimentation. In the United States, the use of the word *suffering* is avoided both in mandated policies on humane use of laboratory animals and in voluntary guidelines prepared by professional associations. It is as if animal suffering did not exist. Whenever the PHS policy speaks of adverse mental states, the word *distress* is used—denoting a less intense state—not *suffering*.

Similarly, the word does not appear in the revised bylaws of the Scientists Center for Animal Welfare, a group established in 1978 to promote animal welfare within the scientific community. After ten years of existence, this organization changed its course and its bylaws, expunging the word *suffering* from its charter. Whereas the originally-stated goal of the organization was to improve animal welfare by "reducing unnecessary suffering of all kinds, including pain and fear but also emotional, social, and behavioral deprivation and other forms of physical and psychological distress," the 1988 revision of the bylaws deleted every mention of the word *suffering*. Board members said that using the word suffering was too inflammatory and likely to dissuade scientists from joining.

However others, including Jane Goodall, the world-famous primatologist, consider the word *suffering* to be an acceptable word to describe certain mental states of laboratory-held chimpanzees. Dawkins finds the word *suffering* to be reasonable to describe the condition of agricultural animals in current intensive farming practices. In the British Act of 1986, the word *suffering* is frequently used in the context of scientific procedures.

Distress

Distress is a state in which the animal is unable to adapt to an altered environment or to altered internal stimuli. In the acute form, distress can be relieved by tranquilizers; but sustained distress does not respond to drug therapy and can be relieved only by environmental change and behavioral conditioning. The AVMA panel notes that prolonged or excessive distress may result in harmful responses, such as abnormal feeding and social interaction behavior.

Anxiety and fear

Anxiety can be defined as an emotional state involving increased arousal and alertness prompted by an unknown danger, which may be in the immediate environment. Anxiety is a generalized, unfocused response to the unknown. Fear is a focused response to a known object or previous experience. To illustrate these differences, the AVMA notes that a dog may tremble in a veterinarian's examination room during the first visit because of anxiety as to what may happen. On the second visit, the dog may whine or try to escape from fear of a remembered event.

Discomfort

Discomfort is experienced when a small change in the animal's adaptive level of homeostasis is required. This change is not sufficient to cause pain or distress.

Pain: its occurrence across species lines

Pain researchers Stephen G. Dennis and Ronald Melzack (1983) state, "Distinctive behavioral responses to intense stimulation are displayed by virtually all animal species down to the protozoan, suggesting that rudimentary painlike behavior emerges at a very low level of organismic complexity." Pain, an important adaptive survival mechanism, appeared early in evolution. Detrimental stimuli such as heat, electrical current, chemicals, or mechanical compression or restraint evoke responses in a wide variety of motile organisms (including bacteria). But it is argued that the fact that an organism withdraws on contact with a noxious stimulus does not necessarily mean that it has perceived pain—it could just be a stimulus triggering a response, not pain. Just where the dividing line comes between species that do and do not perceive pain is controversial. It is known that the physiological mechanisms of pain perception are similar throughout the vertebrate animals. In invertebrate animals, creatures that lack a spinal cord and thalamus, the integration of perception occurs in other ways not fully understood.

Various biochemical reactions are associated with pain sensation and perception. If cells around the peripheral nerve endings are damaged or stressed, a substance is released that causes the nerve to discharge. This substance, thought to be bradykinin, is present not only in peripheral nerves but also in the dorsal horn of the spinal cord. Also, other substances such as histamine and various prostaglandins appear to play a role. As the pain sensation passes up to the thalamus, another peptide, substance P, appears to be involved. Substance P occurs in all mammals, birds, and frogs so far investigated, and also in fish (RSPCA, 1980, p. 9).

In 1975, Hughes described other substances involved in pain mechanisms, the endogenous opiates, peptides which are now collectively known as endorphins. The endorphins that actually bind to receptors in the brain are called enkephalins and they produce analgesia—that is, they serve to reduce pain.

There is substantial evidence that opioid peptides are involved in the modulation of nociception and of behavioral responses to aversive and stressful stimuli in mammals. Recent research has established that opioid peptides occur in all classes of vertebrates. It was a revelation when, in 1979, four Swedish workers demonstrated that these substances are found in earthworms (Alumets et al., 1979). This finding created a stir in scientific circles because it expanded the current views about pain perception in invertebrates. It has now been discovered that opioid peptides occur in a number of invertebrate phyla, including Mollusca (snails, slugs, and the cephalopods such as octopi and squid) and Annelida (segmented worms). These findings have contributed considerably to the understanding of pain mechanisms, although a complete understanding of the distinguishing features between a pain response and a purely nociceptive response has yet to be achieved.

Pain in warm-blooded vertebrates

Starting at the top of the phylogenetic scale, the manifestations of human pain are easily recognized. Because the expression of feelings has a large element of universality, the manifestations of pain in individual humans, whatever their race, culture, or habitation are similar worldwide. Manifestations of human pain include flexor reflexes to withdraw from the noxious stimulus, crying out, production of tears, moaning, writhing, facial grimacing, struggling, convulsions, and fear at the prospect of repetition. Longer-term responses include learned avoidance or learned aggression, and changes in sleep patterns, feeding, drinking, and social contacts. Pain can usually be relieved with anesthetic and analgesic drugs.

Similar expressions in response to pain are found in other animals, especially those species closest to us, other mammals, and these expressions have many common characteristics. For instance, mammals usually cry out when hurt: humans cry and scream, dogs whine or whimper, cats meow, rats squeak at an unusual pitch, and primates may scream or grunt when moving.

The type of vocalization can carry information about the character of the emotional expression. For instance, researchers have analyzed spectrographically the cry associated with pain and have found it to have unique characteristics that are common to that species. The pain cry in human babies, for instance, can be clearly differentiated from that associated with hunger, discomfort, and stress (Levine and Gordon, 1982). These scientists note that a similarly unique pain cry is exhibited by non-human primates that receive painful stimuli.

Birds have "alarm notes" that they use to startle a predator, and which may be associated with fear. According to some authorities, it appears that some species of birds do not make any sound when subjected to a painful stimulus although rigid data on this is lacking.

Manifestations of suffering (as distinct from pain) are also shared between humans and other close species. For instance, the suffering of a drug-addicted individual who is deprived of needed heroin is expressed in a similar fashion in human beings, non-human primates, and dogs. The extreme mental agony of drug withdrawal is clearly evident from behavior, bodily positions, and vocal and facial expressions.

What hurts a human being hurts another mammal, and the hurt appears to be of a similar kind and degree. In technical terms, the pain-detection threshold is relatively similar throughout the mammalian species, including humans (AVMA, 1987). This has important implications with respect to the development and testing of new pain-relieving drugs, which are commonly pretested on laboratory mammals before being tried on humans. In the past, many scientists thought that animals experience a lower quality or degree of pain than humans and that therefore in situations where anesthetics and analgesics would be used in humans, they would not necessarily be needed in animals. But now, this notion is being discarded.

Within recent years, the similarity in pain perception between human and other vertebrate animals has been written into a number of national policies. For instance, the 1985 PHS policy states, "Unless the contrary is established, investigators should consider that procedures that cause pain or distress in human beings may cause pain or distress in other [vertebrate] animals." Similarly, the Australian 1990 Code of Practice states that investigators "must assume that animals experience pain in a manner similar to humans. Decisions regarding the animals' welfare must be based on this assumption unless there is evidence to the contrary." Hence indications for analgesia and anesthesia should parallel those accepted for human and veterinary practice, according to Warwick Anderson (1990) of Monash University, Australia. He continues, "[A]ll involved in the use of animals, including [IACUC] members with no biological training, should feel able to make a decision (about whether or not an animal is in pain) on each project. 'Would this be painful to me?' is already a widely used rule-of-thumb; the [1990 Australian policy] revision strengthens this common sense position."

Systems for measuring animal pain

How to assess pain is a critical issue for laboratory personnel. Starting in 1985, a number of systems have been developed to quantify how much pain is experienced based on behavioral manifestations (Morton and Griffiths, 1985; Morton, 1990; Barclay et al., 1988; and Wallace, et al., 1990; Manser, 1992). Morton and Griffiths, whose work has been widely acclaimed in the veterinary and biomedical community, described species-specific signs of pain in rats, rabbits, guinea pigs, dogs, cats, and monkeys. They also developed a scoring system based on behavioral signs involving posture, vocalizing, temperament, and locomotion, and also clinical signs of the cardiovascular, respiratory, nervous, and musculoskeletal systems. Morton later suggested using a chart for scoring the appearance of the animal (thirteen parameters), its response to handling (six parameters), and its body weight (three levels of severity) (Morton, 1990). The score is used as a basis for providing either alleviation of the pain, or in some cases euthanasia. The 1985 paper by Morton and Griffiths and the 1990 paper by Morton should be required reading for all investigators who experiment on animals. It is essential that laboratory personnel be trained in the recognition of adverse states.

Using a scheme similar to that of Morton and Griffiths, some Dutch workers have reported their assessment of discomfort from gallstones in mice (Beynen et al., 1987). Using nine parameters such as behavior, stance, hair coat, response to palpation of the upper abdomen, and so on, they assigned scores to individual mice, of which some did and others did not have gallstones. They reported that the mice with gallstones experienced pain continuously.

Another system of scoring is the "Disturbance Index" developed in 1988 by Barclay et al. for the Universities Federation for Animal Welfare (UFAW). The index is determined by monitoring changes in the normal exploratory behavior of an animal that has been placed in a new environment. This method generates a statistic that indicates the extent to which the animal's behavior has been changed, and this statistic allows different experimental procedures to be compared. UFAW recommends that investigators determine the Disturbance Index for procedures of unknown severity and then select the most humane method.

Wallace and co-workers (1990) have taken another approach by allocating a numerical score to each of several components that contribute to the severity of the procedure. The sum of the scores is called the "Severity Index." The scoring system considers (1) whether the animal is conscious throughout the procedure, (2) if an anesthetic is used, the duration and complexity of anesthesia and the potential risk, (3) procedures involved in the preparation of the animals, (4) type and duration of restraint, (5) differing tissue sensitivities, (6) the risk to a particular organ, (7) the risk to the animal's survival, and (8) the potential to cause pain, distress, and deprivation both during and as a consequence of the procedure.

Broom (1986) has described the indicators of long-term adverse states, which he calls "poor welfare." These indicators are based on the extent of the individual animal's effort to cope with an environment and whether it fails or succeeds.

A 1990 report of a working party of the Laboratory Animal Science Association provides a system for assessing severity as minimum, intermediate, and high—corresponding to the severity bands used in British law on laboratory animals. A procedure is ranked by scoring various components such as whether or not the animal is conscious throughout the procedure, the use of restraint—its duration and whether it is continuous or discontinuous, tissue sensitivity, organ risk, mortality, assessment of level of pain, distress, deprivation of normal physiological function or activity, and other factors. The final score is tallied after assessment of these components, and ranked accordingly—the higher the score, the greater the severity. As examples of how the scoring system works, the report assigns the following indexes of severity for these procedures: intraperitoneal injection—4; collection of blood from the orbital plexus in conscious animals—11, and in anesthetized animals—4; parabiosis (the joining together of experimental animals by surgical operation)—24; cardiac puncture with anesthesia—6; and adrenalectomy—8.

The availability of these new indexes for assessing pain and harm in animals should help laboratory workers to acquire greater sensitivity to animal pain. Improved recognition and relief of pain would not only bring about better animal welfare but also may enhance the reliability of the scientific results because the presence of pain or stress may confound the validity of the results. As Flecknell (1985/6) points out, pain has adverse effects; for example, animal movement is restricted and food and water intake are depressed. Pain has been shown to cause widespread vasoconstriction and to perpetuate the metabolic changes induced by surgery. Sources of stress to an animal (such as heat, cold, noise, crowding, light, darkness, temperature, air quality, surprise, fear, infection, disease, trauma, restraint, methods of handling, and a host of other variables) can seriously affect the experimental results (Bustad, 1987; Morton, 1990).

Key policy concerns of pain and death

Public policy reflects concern about pain in laboratory animals (a) by requiring use of anesthetics and analgesics, and (b) by stipulating acceptable methods of killing. In 1976, the AWA strengthened the provisions for requiring use of anesthetics and analgesics in the United States. This stimulated interest in proper dosages and selection of appropriate anesthetics and analgesics for use during surgical procedures and post-operative care. Some influential scientists, such as veterinarian Franklin M. Loew of Tufts University and pain researcher Lloyd Davis of the University of Illinois, advised laboratory personnel that when in doubt about whether an animal is in pain, err on the side of administering pain-relieving drugs. For the first time, animal pain became the subject of scientific conferences; textbooks devoted to the physiology and relief of animal pain were published; research was stimulated to develop new anesthetics specifically for certain laboratory species.

The 1980s also marked a new interest in euthanasia methods for animals, and the AVMA set up a task force to revise their earlier version of recommended practices. The report that emerged in 1987 covered species commonly encountered in veterinary clinical practice (domestic pets and agricultural animals) and also in biomedical laboratories.

By now, it is well recognized in national policies that warm-blooded vertebrates feel pain and that humane death is a requirement. In agricultural animals and birds, however, policies on these matters are less well established, and on some points are controversial.

Policies on agricultural animals

The PHS policy and USDA regulations cover agricultural animals only when used in biomedical research and not in "food and fiber" research (i.e., research commonly conducted in agricultural science departments of academic institutions). However, there is a certain grey area between the two types of research because animals used in biomedical research may be housed in farm conditions, and clear-cut distinctions in application may be lacking, as in some nutrition research.

In 1988, quite permissive guidelines were devised by a consortium of organizations representing the academic agricultural science groups and the animal food industry (Guide for the Care and Use of Agricultural Animals, 1988). In general, these agricultural guidelines are simply descriptive of current commercial agricultural practices, the standards of which fall well below standards of care for laboratory animals. In commercial practice the goal is to reduce labor and increase efficiency of production. The means for production place restrictions on the activity and behavior of the animals. In this guide, policies on pain relief are relatively poorly developed. The guide does not condemn overcrowding, or excessive confinement of animals; nor does it offer guidance for introduction of more humane practices.

This guide is now used by IACUCs to establish criteria for their review of protocols involving "food and fiber" agricultural research and is accepted national policy for accrediting purposes for schools of agriculture by the American Association for Accreditation of Laboratory Animal Care. The 1992 NIH/ARENA Guidebook for IACUCs states that the welfare concerns of agricultural animals used in biomedical and food and fiber research "should not differ," but the relevant policies do differ. For institutions that have one centralized IACUC reviewing animal experiments in all academic departments, as happens, it certainly confuses the issue to have one set of standards for pigs or cows kept in one area and another set for the same species kept in another area.

Policies on birds

Scientific research using birds as subjects falls into three main areas, (a) biomedical and behavioral studies using captive birds (where purpose-bred pigeons, quail, and chickens are commonly used), (b) wildlife studies (free-living birds of all species), and (c) agricultural science research (domesticated hens, turkeys, etc.). Historically, policies were first established for group (a) birds, then for group (b), and most recently for group (c).

Under the 1985 PHS policy, only captive laboratory birds are addressed, and not much attention is given to them other than requiring certain cage sizes. Under USDA regulations, the AWA has excluded birds (but see chapter 4 on the 1992 court ruling requiring inclusion of birds).

The need for nationally accepted standards for wild birds and certain other wild species became evident after passage of the 1985 strengthening revisions in the AWA. Then, for the first time, field research protocols became subject to IACUC review. But these committees found they were working in a vacuum. No nationally accepted humane standards had ever been prepared for field research in the United States. Furthermore, birds were not well covered in the 1987 AVMA euthanasia recommendations, so ornithologists were in need of some national standards. At the same time, there was a need for standards for research on other free-living species.

Accordingly, the National Science Foundation, the federal agency that funds wildlife research, charged the relevant professional associations to establish guidelines, and four sets were prepared. They covered birds, wild mammals, fish, and amphibians and reptiles (Field Research Guidelines, 1987, 1988, numbers 1–4). These guidelines marked a new phase in upgrading federal regulations.

The bird guidelines are exemplary in their specificity and humaneness. This first-time effort provided advice about experimental manipulative procedures, humane handling, marking, and killing of wild birds. The key issues of anesthesia and euthanasia are dealt with in detail. The guidelines require anesthesia for major manipulative procedures such as surgery. Specific anesthetic agents are recommended and references given to textbooks on avian anesthesia.

In general, there is a paucity of information about pain perception in birds, but the fact that pain and chronic distress can exist in birds is acknowledged in these guidelines. The word *pain* occurs a number of times, and *chronic distress* is mentioned. This is noteworthy because guidelines prepared by other professional organizations for other animal groups avoid these terms, as will be discussed later.

The bird guidelines point out that avian surgery is very different from mammalian surgery. In part, the differences are due to avian structure, especially the air sacs and flow-through respiratory system. Most birds show little evidence of pain or discomfort from punctures and incisions over much of the body but exceptions are the head and beak, scaled portions of the legs, and the vent area. Also, pinching or pulling of the skin is painful (Field Research Guidelines, Auk, page 31a).

The wild bird guidelines provide very specific instructions about bird euthanasia (in comparison, the agricultural guidelines are silent). The wild bird guidelines note that the AVMA panel on euthanasia gave sparse advice for killing birds and state that healthy birds should not be killed at the end of an experiment, but should be provided with opportunities for continued, comfortable existence; however, those birds that are in "chronic distress or pain" should be killed. Detailed information about recommended methods is provided, and nonrecommended methods are identified. Inasmuch as this information was not available before, it is proving useful not only to ornithologists, but also to biomedical laboratory personnel.

In summary, the bird guidelines make it clear that pain and significant distress surely exist in birds and require investigators to observe strict standards with respect to both relief of pain and methods of death.

Pain in fetuses and neonates

Humane concern extends to avian embryos, and several IACUCs are currently facing this issue. Avian embryos are not covered by national policies on laboratory animals in the United States. The Office for Protection from Research Risks at NIH has interpreted "live vertebrate animal" in the PHS policy to apply to avians (e.g., chick embryos) only after hatching (The Public Health Service Responds to Commonly Asked Questions, 1991).

But IACUCs at a number of institutions are having to make decisions about invasive projects on bird eggs done by professional scientists, and there is little guidance on the matter. There is an unproven possibility that these embryos may feel pain, at least in the period near to hatching time when their nervous systems are well-developed, albeit not complete. Some IACUCs are currently working out in-house policies on this matter, but none to my knowledge has so far been formulated.

Historically, concern about avian embryos first developed because a popular biology project for teen-age American students is to cut windows in birds' eggs in order to watch development. In addition, these novices in scientific skills sometimes inject toxic substances into the eggs, thus interfering with normal development. The avowed purpose is to show that toxic substances can be dangerous during fetal development. If the birds are allowed to hatch, as they often are, then the chicks are likely to be deformed and to suffer a lingering death. Such projects are relatively easy to do and provide sure-fire results, so they have been popular in junior and senior high school science fairs.

The Canadian Council on Animal Care was the first to address this issue (CCAC, 1972). This policy states that, in pre-college level *classroom projects* involving birds' eggs that have been subjected to any manipulative procedures, the embryo must be humanely destroyed at least two days prior to normal hatching time. Later, the Canadians adopted even more stringent rules for *science fairs* (as opposed to classroom projects) in that such projects were completely prohibited (CCAC, 1975). These rules remain effective today.

In the United States in 1980, the voluntary guidelines of both the National Science Teachers Association and the National Association of Biology Teachers (NABT) required that embryos of manipulated eggs be destroyed several days prior to normal hatching time. (Revised NABT policy current in 1992 bans such manipulative procedures). Later, in 1989, the Institute for Laboratory Animal Resources of the National Academy of Sciences adopted similar provisions (ILAR, 1989). The International Science and Engineering Fair rules have no such provisions, even by 1992—they merely require that such projects be supervised, but as has been repeatedly shown, supervision is not enough in itself to ensure humane standards.

In contrast to the United States, both Australia and Britain include fetal forms in their animal protective laws for professional scientists. The Australian Code requires that procedures involving vertebrate embryos (both bird and mammalian) be reviewed by IACUCs (Australian Code, 1990). The Code states, "When fetal experimentation or surgery compromises the ability of the neonate to survive and be without pain or distress, it must be killed humanely before or immediately following birth unless such pain or distress can be relieved" (page 31). Furthermore, the policy states that birds eggs "must be destroyed before hatching, unless hatching is a requirement of the experiment. The [Animal Experimentation Ethics Committee] must approve the arrangements made for the hatchlings." In Britain, the protected animals are defined as any living vertebrate except man (Home Office, 1986). Fetal, larval, and embryonic forms are protected only from the stage in their development when (a) in the case of a mammal, bird, or reptile, half the gestation or incubation period for the relevant species has elapsed; and (b) in any other case, they become capable of independent feeding.

In 1986, a European Directive on this mater was issued by the European Council. Article 2(a) states that "animal," unless otherwise qualified, means "any live non-human vertebrate, including free-living and/or reproducing larval forms, but excluding foetal or embryonic forms" (European Council, 1986). Such directives apply to the twelve member states of the European Community and when ratified are laws; breach of these laws can be brought before the European courts. As of October, 1992, this particular directive is still awaiting ratification in several countries.

In the United States and elsewhere, fetal surgery has been practiced on sheep and other mammals in order to pave the way for human surgical procedures to correct embryonic defects. Although mammalian fetuses are themselves not protected under American laws, the mothers are. Thus, any projects involving animal fetal surgery would have to be reviewed by IACUCs, at which point the fate of the fetuses would probably be considered. Overall, there has been increasing attention to the relief of pain and the welfare of fetuses and neonatral animals in laboratory practices.

This follows along the same lines of the increasing attention to the relief of pain in human newborns. Historically, pain has been downgraded not only for animals, but also for human children and newborns. It was over the issue of circumcision that the controversy over pain perception in human newborns emerged in the mid-1980s. Traditionally, circumcision has been done without benefit of anesthesia despite the fact that the babies cry and show other behavioral signs of pain, such as facial expressions, breathholding, and body movement. At an NIH conference, a nurse challenged this omission. Her remarks caused something of an uproar, challenging as it did accepted practices, but she had supporters. The medical literature took up the issue (Anand and Hickey, 1987; Fletcher, 1987; Berry and Gregory, 1987). A revealing survey among British pediatric anesthetists showed that while 80 percent believed infants less than one week old were capable of perceiving pain, 48 percent "never used" narcotic analgesics, and a further 41 percent "seldom" did so (Anonymous, 1987). This article pronounced verdict by saying, "It is clear that some newborn babies still receive no anesthetic [for surgery]. In 1987, this practice must be unacceptable, since there is overwhelming evidence that babies can feel pain." By 1992, there has been a dramatic decrease in neonatal surgery without anesthesia and a declining number of circumcisions, and this has been attributed in part to the greater recognition of the pain experienced by infants.

Flecknell (1985/6) cites documented failures to use adequate anesthetics to relieve post-operative pain in human children and adults. He says "the failure to use adequate pain relief in man has been attributed to a number of factors, including the lack of awareness of the problem by the medical staff concerned and a fear of the undesirable side effects, such as respiratory depression, which are associated with the use of opiates. It seems likely that similar factors are involved in the provision of pain relief in animals."

This perspective with human patients helps, I believe, to understand some of the problems faced by laboratory investigators studying animals. It is even harder to recognize pain in laboratory animals than in children, so the alleviation of pain can be delayed or overlooked. But changes are taking place and several factors contribute. Research has provided new insight into the recognition of pain in laboratory species; scientists are actively involved now in developing better anesthetics and analgesics specifically for lab species; training of laboratory personnel in both recognition of animal pain and in its relief is gradually improving. All told, the alleviation of pain in laboratory animals is being significantly improved.

Adverse mental states

We return now to the top of the phylogenetic scale to consider the adverse mental states of anxiety, fear, and suffering.

Anxiety and fear

The lesser adverse states of anxiety and fear appear to be present in some, if not all, vertebrate animals. J. A. Gray (1982), an authority on anxiety, has stated that "human anxiety, or something very like it, exists also in animals." In pain research on monkeys and rodents, one problem that can hamper the experiment is that after one or more exposures to the pain stimulus, the animals tend to "freeze" in anticipation of further painful stimuli. This is an indication of fear. It is reported that the sight of the experimental apparatus can induce this reaction and can confound the results. Also, when fish are faced with a dangerous situation, they can show evidence of increased arousal suggestive of anxiety and fear.

Various animal species have been successfully used to find and develop new drugs capable of relieving anxiety states in humans. The existence of specific binding sites for benzodiazepines (chemicals that apparently play a role in the pharmacology of anxiety in man) has been demonstrated in several species—rodents, carnivores, and artiodactyls (even-toed hooved animals such as pigs, llamas, giraffes, and sheep), three kinds of birds, a turtle, a lizard, a frog, a toad, and three bony fish (cod, plaice, and eel). Identical tests have failed to detect such sites in two lower chordates (hagfish and amphioxus), or in the following invertebrates: locust, lobster, woodlouse, squid, and earthworm (Nielsen et al., 1978). Rowan (1988) argues that the response of animals to the anxiety-relieving effects of the benzodiazepine drugs are relevant to the search for a dividing line for sentience. Certainly, it seems likely that if such a receptor exists, then the animal is capable of experiencing anxiety.

Anxiety, fear, and suffering are complex states, difficult to separate from one another. Patrick D. Wall, professor of anatomy at University College, London University and an authority on pain has commented on the "bizarre" relationship that exists between injury, pain, and suffering. He says, "in man, and I believe in animals, you can observe any form of coupling between these three. You can certainly have severe injury with no pain whatsoever, and you can have intense pain and suffering with no observable injury and all grades in between" (RSPCA Report, 1980, page 6).

Mental states can affect tolerance to pain. Tolerance varies significantly from individual to individual according to past experiences and to the current circumstances. The mental state can suppress or enhance the perception of pain. Soldiers in combat and participants in a sport who are in the midst of an important match may get seriously wounded without feeling much pain. The pain often comes when the combat or match is over. This phenomenon was vividly demonstrated by Henry Beecher (1959) of Harvard University in a study of Second World War victims. He found that there was a lack of pain in some wounded soldiers in dramatic contrast to similarly wounded civilians; this was attributed to the fact that for these soldiers, being wounded was a relief because it allowed them to escape from the front line.

Pain can also be enhanced by the situation. Controlled scientific studies have now demonstrated what was often thought to be the case, that the ambience of a dentist's office, for instance, can heighten the pain experienced (Dworkin and Chen, 1983). Anticipation and remembrance can enhance the experience of pain. Rollin (1981) points out that some animals as well as humans can remember, citing the example of a dog that fears the stick and trembles at the rage of his master's voice. On the other hand, he says, if animals cannot anticipate an end to pain, or remember a time without pain, as we can, then the "entire horizon of its universe is filled with pain, whereas we can see an end to suffering." Perhaps it is worse if you cannot see an end, he suggests.

Because human beings have more complex mental processes and richer cultural and social life, a reasonable presumption is that humans are capable of more fear, anxiety, and suffering than, say, a mouse. But it would be a rash person indeed who would suggest any exact cut-off point in the phylogenetic scale for these mental states. It is more a matter of degree.

Research into the mental states of animals is beset with problems but some approaches have proved useful. Dawkins describes how it is possible to probe the state of awareness of animals by means of ingenious experimental techniques (Dawkins, 1980a, pages 15–23). She claims that it is difficult "but not impossible" to design an experiment to show that an animal does have an abstract concept, such as that of number. An ability to distinguish between a small group of numbers has been demonstrated in jackdaws, for instance (Koehler, 1951).

Dawkins also describes experimental data that demonstrate how rats can identify what bodily position they are in, such as walking, rearing up, face-washing, or remaining still. Griffin (1976, 1978) has argued that evidence makes it very likely that many animals besides ourselves are conscious and have subjective feelings.

Dawkins says, "Many people may be inclined to change their attitudes to animals, for example, to killing them or inflicting pain, if they believe that those animals may be aware of what is happening to them, may have the capacity to form concepts and so on. The question "But they're not very intelligent, are they?" is one with which many people comfort themselves when drawn into arguments about animal welfare. . . . Some studies we have looked at may remove part of that comfort" (Dawkins, 1980a, pages 23–24).

To probe an animal's mind, Dawkins has emphasized experimental designs that allow animals to select for themselves between various options. The basic idea behind these experiments is to allow animals to "vote with their feet" and express some of what they are feeling by where they choose to go. "Giving animals the opportunity to *choose* for themselves which environments they prefer and to show what they find positively or negatively *reinforcing* is the closest we can come to being able to ask an animal what it is feeling" (Dawkins, 1980a, page 111).

Recently, a number of researchers and zoo personnel have tested what animals will select for themselves in the way of living conditions, such as light intensity, floor covering, space availability, temperature, and so on. In one such study mice chose lighting conditions comparable to moonlight. Self-selection experimental designs can provide important information for animal husbandry. Also, it is possible to test what adversities an animal will voluntarily undergo in order to achieve a certain choice of situation. For instance, hens will repeatedly choose to undergo the unpleasant experiences of having to squeeze through a narrow opening in order to reach a more spacious living area. This provides an idea of the relative importance of the reward to the animal.

It is worth mentioning that this type of experimental design can be a useful strategy in biomedical experiments to help ensure that the threshold of tolerance to pain or suffering is not exceeded (Dawkins, 1980a and b). By providing an option of escape from a painful stimulus, an animal can "vote with its feet" not to be subject to certain experimental procedures. This concept is indeed regularly used by some scientists and is part of the official policy of the International Association for the Study of Pain, which states "The animal should be able to control the effects of acute experimental pain (e.g., by escape or avoidance behavior)" (Zimmermann, 1980).

In our current state of knowledge it is impossible to know exactly what mental capabilities animals have. We do not know to what extent, if any, they have a sense of future. We do know that certain non-human primates can plan current strategies in order to obtain food in the future. But, other than human beings, do any species of terminally ill animals have a sense of impending death? We assume that animals, unlike humans, are not aware of certain things—such as the purpose of being in captivity or the purpose of what is being done to them in an experiment. Presumably non-human animals are limited in their ability to suppress or enhance the perception of pain based on a comprehension of the total

situation—they probably lack width of view of an event. There are more unanswered (or unanswerable) questions than answered questions about the mental
capacities of animals.

Suffering in both humans and animals finds expression in abnormal behaviors.
Human beings in deprived and overcrowded circumstances—in prisons for
instance—show withdrawal and increased aggression. Animals that have been
thwarted in the expression of their natural behavioral repertoire show peculiar
behaviors, including repeated pacing and other non-functional stereotypic movements, self-mutilation, and other behaviors collectively called vices. They may
also show excessive social withdrawal and aggression. Vices are typical of
agricultural animals kept in deprived or overcrowded living conditions. A wide
range of abnormal behaviors including vices is seen, especially in those captive
animals that have previously enjoyed freedom, such as wild-caught primates.

Grieving over a loss or death is a form of suffering. Anecdotal stories tell of
some pet dogs grieving over the death of their owner, and several wildlife
biologists have described the grieving of elephants over the death of one of their
social group. Sensitive primatologists recognize that grieving can exist under
laboratory conditions. In a situation where two primates have been housed together for a long time and one dies, the survivor may grieve. The new interest in
psychological well-being of primates has resulted in this topic's being addressed
at recent scientific meetings. Recommendations are made that laboratory personnel should take steps to relieve the grieving condition by providing extra attention
and other social outlets to the survivor.

Who can say whether an animal is suffering or not? To some extent, the
recognition of suffering depends on the sensitivity of the person observing it.
Indeed, suffering that is obvious to some may be denied by others. Some humans
fail to recognize or acknowledge the existence of suffering even in other human
beings whom they know well. This failure to acknowledge a mental state of
suffering is compounded when species lines are crossed.

People who are knowledgeable about animal behavior stand a better chance
than others of appreciating the mental state of an animal. But since animals do
not communicate in human words but have languages of their own, not all human
beings can comprehend the languages and signals given out by other species. It is
from people with exquisite understanding of animal life that we can learn most
about animal suffering.

Suffering in chimpanzees

One such person is Jane Goodall, world famous for her studies of chimpanzees at
the Gombe Stream Research Centre in Tanzania and author of many scholarly
works on the behavior and lives of these animals. She has keenly observed chimpanzees both in the wild in Africa and in captivity. In 1987, she visited SEMA,

an American laboratory under contract with NIH to conduct hepatitis research using chimpanzees. There had been public complaints about the welfare of these animals. She published her reactions during this visit in an article in the New York Times (Goodall, 1987). She graphically described the suffering of the chimps who were "far gone in depression and despair. . . . Young chimpanzees, 3 or 4 years old, were crammed, two together, into tiny cages measuring 22 inches by 22 inches and only 24 inches high. They could hardly turn around . . . there they will remain, living in conditions of severe sensory deprivation, for the next several years. During that time, they will become insane. . . . I shall be haunted forever by [this experience]." From such an authority as Goodall, surely it is reasonable to accept that chimpanzees suffer.

Several species of animals maintained in deprived sensory conditions have sometimes been used as a model of human depression and mental disorders. During the 1960s and 1970s, in particular, the use of laboratory animals to model human depression was popular (see Stephens' critical overview of these studies, 1986). Species used include rhesus, squirrel, pigtail, and other monkeys, dogs, cats, and rodents. Harlow and his colleagues conducted a long series of experiments that involved depriving monkeys of maternal care and social contact as well as extreme environmental deprivation. The aim was to determine which maternal characteristics underlie the infant's attachment to its mother. In some experiments, Harlow reared infant monkeys with cloth surrogate mothers whose bodies were made either of sandpaper, or included hidden spikes, catapults, or compressed air that could be made ice cold. Some newborns were reared in isolation chambers for up to 24 months. These animals showed signs of severe depression, and highly aberrant behavior, such as "whirling fits," crushing their own infants, and extreme withdrawal. Some died because they refused to eat. In one paper, the authors referred to the induced condition in rhesus monkeys as "psychological death" (Harlow and Novack, 1973). In another experiment, of nineteen infant monkeys used, seven died as a result of experimentally induced maternal deprivation (Spencer-Booth and Hinde, 1971).

The animal models of human depression are repeatedly criticized by the animal protection movement as inhumane. They are also criticized by some researchers as being invalid because the animals lack salient cognitive features of depression in humans such as negative thoughts about oneself, the world, and the future. But these experiments surely indicate that some species of animals suffer, and it is time that this condition is acknowledged in public policies.

Pain in cold-blooded vertebrates

Historically, England was exceptional in legally protecting cold-blooded vertebrates (fish, amphibia, and reptiles) as early as 1876, right from the start of their legislation on laboratory animals. Until the 1970s, general attitudes in the United

States were such that the use of cold-blooded vertebrates in injurious procedures fell outside the compass of humane concern. For instance, in 1965, the AVMA testified in Congress against inclusion of "all vertebrates" under the federal law on laboratory animals. They said, "This phrase [all vertebrates] is unrealistically broad" (Jones, 1965). Now, however, cold-blooded vertebrates are subject to protection in the United States under the 1985 PHS policy (but not under the AWA) and in several other countries.

Shortly after the newly revised 1978 version of the NIH (now PHS) policy on care and use of laboratory animals was issued, public attention was drawn to the need for coverage of cold-blooded vertebrates. The advisory council to the National Eye Institute (NEI) raised the question of whether or not the NIH policy covered cold-blooded vertebrates in addition to warm-blooded ones because the policy was not clear. The inclusion of cold-blooded animals was of significance to the vision research community because fish are used extensively. At the urging of council member Kenneth T. Brown, professor of neurophysiology at the University of California at San Francisco, the council adopted a policy in 1979 calling on all researchers financially supported by NEI not to inflict needless pain on cold-blooded vertebrates and to use effective procedures to minimize pain in these animals.

In an interview with *Science* magazine, Brown said that certain investigators do not take seriously the possibility that they may be inflicting pain. "For example," he said, "I have heard a first-hand account from a well-known investigator who systematically practiced removal of one eye from a live fish, which was then replaced into the tank, awaiting an experimental need for the second eye. . . . The investigator even joked about this in a group of experimenters in a social situation, which seems to indicate the generality with which such practices are accepted" (Carter, 1979). Brown said that the argument that these animals do not feel pain is "so strained that one wonders whether it would be advanced at all except in self-justification."

Among the reasons for using cold-blooded species in research is the belief of some investigators that no anesthetics are needed, thereby avoiding the undesirable effects (biochemical changes, etc.) of the anesthetics that are required in mammalian work. Also, nervous systems of cold-blooded vertebrates continue to function for long periods after procedures that would quickly kill mammalian nerve cells, a useful attribute for research on such cells; isolated tissues of reptile brain, for instance, remain viable for an hour or more in the absence of oxygen. Prolonged survival means, for example, that if a reptile, frog, or turtle is decapitated, the decapitated head may be capable of experiencing pain for several hours (see Cooper et al., 1986, and also UFAW, 1989). "In short," stated the NEI council report, "one of the main reasons for using cold-blooded vertebrates can also place these animals at particular risk of suffering." The council recommended that following decapitation, unless the experiment requires an intact brain, the brain should be destroyed immediately by pithing (destruction of the brain and spinal cord by thrusting an instrument into the cranium and spinal canal to destroy sensibility). This "should be done consistently, regardless of whether any further operative work is performed upon the head," said the report.

Fish caught from the seas for the commercial food industry enjoy no such consideration. They die by suffocation—presumably an unpleasant ending. But sports fishermen have been urged to set higher standards of humane death. For instance, Robert Schmidt, a wildlife biologist at the University of California Hopland Field Station, encourages anglers to kill their catch before scaling or filleting them rather than doing this while they are still alive (Schmidt and Bruner, 1981). Killing can be accomplished by a sharp blow to the head.

But do fish feel pain or are the behavioral responses to injury due to reflex actions? Are these concerns realistic? While fish have in their central nervous system neuropeptides that are similar to those found in mammals, it is not known whether they feel pain. Although fish demonstrate avoidance behaviors to aversive stimuli, they appear to behave quite normally when severely wounded. A cautious picture emerges and the jury is still out.

Little scientific work in this field bears on this question. Two studies—by the Royal Society for the Prevention of Cruelty to Animals in the U.K. and by a group of Dutch scientists—have come to the conclusion that fish do feel pain. The RSPCA set up a three-year panel of inquiry on angling and shooting under the chairmanship of Lord Medway, a distinguished zoologist. The panel heard many expert witnesses, and issued its report in 1980 (RSPCA Report of a Panel of Enquiry into Shooting and Angling, 1980, pages 7–10). This report states: "There is a difference between the detection of painful stimuli and the interpretation of those stimuli as being painful. The existence of an unusually rich innervation in certain parts of the body (e.g., the lips of fish) indicated that sensation in such areas is of great biological importance, but is not of itself evidence either that pain is or is not perceived. . . . The recognition of bradykinin and substance P and of the roles played by these chemicals in the perception of pain is of comparatively recent date. From the point of view of our Enquiry, these pharmacological discoveries provide an invaluable new tool, by which it is now possible to ascertain, with a higher degree of probability than hitherto, whether or not an animal possesses the capacity to experience pain." The panel invited two scientists to determine the presence of bradykinin and substance P in various parts of trout brain (olfactory tissue, forebrain, optic tectum, brain stem, spinal cord, and hypothalamus). The actual levels of these two substances are given in the report, and the conclusion is that "the recorded levels in the fish are of the same order as in a mammal." From these results, the conclusion is that "both substance P and enkephalins occur in all vertebrate classes from bony fishes to mammals. Their presence has not yet been sought in cartilaginous fishes or agnathes" (eel-shaped chordates such as lampreys and hagfishes).

The final conclusion of the RSPCA report is that "there may still be some people who will argue that we cannot prove beyond question that any vertebrate other than man, feels pain. We, however, conclude that if any do, then the evidence suggests that all vertebrates (including fish) through the mediation of similar neuro-pharmacological processes, experience similar sensations to a greater or lesser degree in response to noxious stimuli."

Another assessment of pain in fish comes from a team of researchers under the direction of Professor John Verheijen at the University of Utrecht in the Netherlands (Verheijen and Buwalda, 1988). They concluded that fish do feel pain and experience fear.

The Dutch researchers studied the behavior of thirty hooked carp, *Cyprinus carpio*. When caught by a hook and line, the fish darted, dived, shook their heads, and seemed to spit as if trying to expel unwanted food, responses that the researchers attributed to pain. When pressure was applied to the line, the carp displayed a type of behavior called "spitgas," prolonged spitting of gas from the swim bladder. These later responses could be produced in other ways, for example by adding to the water certain pheromones associated with distress. Since the pheromone-treated fish suffered no direct physical injury or pain, the researchers considered the "spitgas" and sinking responses to be due to fear.

Verheijen and co-workers believe that fish experience pain and fear not only from being hooked, but also as a result of the common angling practice of being maintained in a keep-net (holding fish captive for several hours in a confined net). The researchers rated the responses of carp on the category A to E pain scale (Table 6.1) and determined that holding fish in keep-nets "has some of the characteristics of Category D biomedical experiments" (significant pain) and that if the fish succumbs, the treatment should be rated as Category E (highly questionable or unacceptable).

By contrast, American ichthyologists who set national standards for field researchers stated that "capture of fishes by hooks . . . is an accepted practice of recreational fisherman . . .. many fishes are most efficiently captured" this way (Field Research Guidelines, 1987, number 3). Their approval of hooking is quite clear.

These official guidelines for fish and also those for amphibians and reptiles are a source of information about current thinking of scientists on the existence of pain in these animals. The wording is cautious. The word *pain* is used neither in reference to fish nor to amphibians and reptiles. The guidelines refer only to the existence of "distress" and "severe or chronic distress" in these cold-blooded vertebrates.

There is an anomaly in the guidelines for these cold-blooded vertebrates. Although pain is not ever mentioned, the use of anesthetics is recommended. The guidelines both for fish and for amphibians and reptiles use exactly the same wording. They state that "sedation, analgesia, or anesthesia" is required for procedures "that may cause more than momentary or slight distress" except where justified for scientific reasons by the investigator. I wonder if the word *distress* is not being used here when *pain* would be a more accurate choice? Distress is not a condition in which one would use anesthetics; pain is.

Not quite such a cautious approach is seen in either the British or Australian policies, which seem to assume that cold-blooded vertebrates *are* capable of pain. In commenting on the 1990 Australian Code, two Australian scientists have stated, "In the absence of any contrary information, it must be assumed that painful stimuli are felt [by cold-blooded species], and that humane restraint, analgesia and anesthesia should be adopted whenever necessary" (Arena and Richardson, 1990). Also, the recommendation to use anesthetics for fish is made by a recent Committee Report on Pain and Distress in Laboratory Animals convened by the National Research Council, National Academy of Sciences (1991).

The American field research guidelines require that fish, amphibia, and reptiles that would otherwise experience "severe or chronic distress" that cannot be relieved shall be euthanized at the end of the procedure, or, if appropriate, during the procedure. This is a useful directive, but the question then arises just what methods of killing are acceptable? The fish guidelines state that anesthetic overdose is acceptable, as is destruction of the brain, but they are not strict about killing methods. As we have seen, hooking fish on a line with subsequent suffocation is approved. Both the fish and the amphibian and reptile guidelines approve immersion in formalin for certain species. Formalin, a solution of the powerful disinfectant gas formaldehyde, serves as a fixative and preservative and is commonly used by field researchers to retain details of morphology for scientific study. It is also used by pain researchers as a method of simulating chronic pain in mammals. The rapidity of death by immersion in formalin depends on how quickly this toxic substance is absorbed through the skin and gills, and therefore on the size of the animal. For stickleback fish, death occurs in a few seconds (considered acceptable by the guidelines); in sharks, which have a thick integument, death is protracted (considered unacceptable unless the animal has been previously anesthetized). Inasmuch as formalin is an extremely irritant substance, and its use in conscious animals condemned by many, a more clearly humane method of death for all species of fish is an overdose of anesthetic agent added to the water followed by destruction of the brain.

When large numbers of animals are killed for commercial trading, the least costly methods of killing are frequently selected, and these can easily trump humaneness. Formalin is sometimes used as a killing method in biological supply houses, which receive sacks of wild-caught live frogs or crabs and sell the dead animals to schools for dissection. Veterinarian John E. Cooper, who has authored a number of articles on recommended killing methods for lower organisms, has said, "Personally I would be cautious about using formalin to kill anything except a single-celled organism or perhaps, a very small metazoan, e.g., a sponge" (John E. Cooper personal communication, September 3, 1990).

According to the amphibian and reptilian field guidelines "killing unanesthetized specimens by immersion in a formalin solution is unacceptable, unless justified for scientific reasons." This is qualified, however, by the statement that formalin may be the only way to fix certain details of morphology critical to the success of the work, and therefore, in these cases, formalin immersion of unanesthetized animals is sanctioned. It is advised that prior light anesthetization be used.

In the culinary frog leg trade, the legs are severed from the body while the animal is still alive (Watkins, 1990). Concern over these issues in Britain led to the preparation of a report on acceptable methods of killing amphibians and reptiles prepared by Universities Federation for Animal Welfare and the World Society for the Protection of Animals (Euthanasia, 1989). Reporting for the working party, Cooper provides detailed information on acceptable and unacceptable methods of killing, and this much-needed report is essential reading for any scientist whose work may involve killing these species. The World Society for the Protection of Animals is currently trying to persuade the frog leg tradespeople to kill by electrocution.

Pain in mollusks

Mollusks comprise several classes, the most commonly known being the bivalved organisms such as oysters and clams, and the gastropods (snails). Another class, the cephalopods, includes the octopus and squid, whose nervous systems are quite complex and unequalled among other mollusks.

Traditionally, mollusks have not been subjects of humane concern. In the United States, as is typical for most countries, invertebrate animals are not currently protected in the public policy, but this appears to be changing.

Octopus and squid have been used for several purposes in biomedical research, including studies of learning and behavior by neuroscientists. George Wald won his Nobel Prize for studies of visual perception that utilized, among other organisms, the octopus. The reviewer of a new book *Squid as Experimental Animals* writes that "Few life scientists, including squid specialists, however, are likely to appreciate the range and number of basic discoveries that also have stemmed from research on squid and its cephalopod cousins, the octopus and the cuttlefish. Much of this work has utilized the giant axon system to provide insights into active transport of ions and metabolites across cell membranes, microtubule-based organelle transport, and synaptic transmission, but there have been numerous contributions in other areas as well, such as hemo-cyanin-based oxygen transport" (Gilly, 1991). The "giant axon" of the squid is a much-used system because of its large size and therefore relative ease of manipulation for determining the nature of neural activity.

Octopuses are poikilotherms (their bodily temperature is dependent upon environmental temperature), but they respond to pain in ways similar to higher animals. Researchers such as Pieron in 1930 and Buytandijk in 1943 and 1953 concluded that the octopus does feel pain (quoted by Fiorito, 1986).

Other classes of mollusk, such as snails, do not possess such complex nervous systems as cephalopods, but they too have utility in biomedical research. For instance, Martin Kavaliers of the University of Alberta and co-workers have developed a sensitive system of testing anesthetics by using gastropod land snails (Kavaliers et al., 1983). This pioneering work establishes a useful invertebrate model for research on the analgesic qualities of various drugs where formerly only mammalian animals were used. When placed on a surface warmed to 40°C, within a few seconds a land snail demonstrates the aversive nature of this temperature by lifting the anterior portion of its extended foot. "This response," says Kavaliers, "is comparable to that occurring in rodents placed on a warmed surface (50–55°C) where the animals quickly lift their feet or attempt to escape from the heated surface." Under the influence of anesthetic drugs, this response is suppressed.

Canada is exceptional in including certain invertebrates in its national policy—protocols involving these animals must be approved by institutional oversight committees. According to CCAC policy, "Cephalopods and some other higher invertebrates have nervous systems as well developed as in some vertebrates, and may warrant inclusion in [pain] Category B, C, D, or E." Thus, some invertebrate procedures may fall in the highest pain categories of severe distress (Category D), and unacceptable (Category E).

In the United States, some voluntary recommendations for student use of animals include mention of humane treatment of cephalopods (Institute of Laboratory Animal Resources, 1989). This is probably the first policy in the United States to mention these creatures.

Pain in insects

Although concern about pain existing below the level of mollusks is rare, some entomologists do raise the issue of pain in insects. It is an intriguing question, and a mixed picture emerges.

Several entomologists have stated that they believe that insects feel pain. For instance, the eminent entomologist V. B. Wigglesworth (1980) of Cambridge University has said, "I have no doubt the *Rhodnius* [a vector of Chagas' disease] feels pain when a red hot poker, in the form of a heated needle, is brought close to the antennae; it reacts violently; and if the treatment is repeated it becomes wildly excited and endeavours to escape. . . . I am sure that insects can feel pain if the right stimulus is given. . . . For practical purposes why not assume that that is so? Most operations on insects are actually facilitated if the insect is narcotized." Lockwood (1987, 1988), an entomologist from the University of

Wyoming, believes it is "ethically mandatory" to anesthetize insects prior to dissection or other potentially painful treatment in the laboratory.

Not all entomologists go along with this. Eisenmann and co-workers (1984) believe that insects react to painful stimuli in a reflex fashion. This might be rather as a quadriplegic human being might withdraw a foot from a heat source due to the action of the spinal reflex system. Along with programmed avoidance and escape behavior, this would suffice to explain an insect's response to a painful stimulus. The matter is unresolved, but the recommendation is usually made to use anesthetics to be on the safe side.

Below the insects, nociception appears to provide a full enough explanation of events. Even so, humane methods for handling and killing earthworms and other lowly creatures in the laboratory or classroom have been recommended (Orlans, 1977).

Conclusion

There is a decreasing level of certainty about capacity of a species to experience pain as one descends the phylogenetic scale. Pain exists among warm-blooded vertebrates, among some, if not all, cold-blooded vertebrates, and among some cephalopods. Pain may *perhaps* exist down to the insect level—anesthetics appear to be effective right down to this level. Much uncertainty exists. Suffering exists at least in the higher vertebrates. The current trend is that policies to protect animals from adverse states are being extended to include additional species lower on the phylogenetic scale, and this trend appears likely to continue.

10

Testing

Products such as cosmetics, toiletries, drugs, and pesticides have been routinely tested on animals to check for safety before they are marketed. The rationale is that what is harmful to animals is likely to be harmful to humans. Two widely-used tests—the Draize and the LD50—have been the focus of a largely successful campaign to make animal testing more humane. The Draize, as used in the past, could cause blindness in rabbits, and the LD50, used on rodents and dogs, causes slow painful death.

The industry most exposed to criticism has been the cosmetic industry—the makers of beautifying products, shampoos, antiperspirants, etc. Many ask why animals should suffer for the nonessential purposes of developing a new eye shadow or lipstick. The search for alternatives and the reduction in the use of animals used in testing since 1980 is described below.

Many facilities where animal tests are conducted fall outside the laws protecting laboratory animals. Neither the Public Health Service nor the Animal Welfare Act policies necessarily apply. The PHS policy does not apply because overwhelmingly these are commercial enterprises that receive no PHS funds. Also, the facility can fall outside the purview of the AWA if only rats and mice are used. What oversight does exist often stems largely from in-house quality control established by the company itself.

Nationwide, the number of testing facilities that are not subject to any animal protective law is unknown. To my knowledge, the only data on this matter is from the city of Cambridge, Massáchusetts, where in 1991 there were a total of twenty-three facilities that conduct animal experiments; of these, thirteen (or 57 percent) fell outside the laws of PHS and AWA.

The Draize and LD50 tests

Both the Draize and LD50 tests are notable for the pain they inflict, for wastage of animal life, and, at least in the past, for widespread use. In the Draize test, first introduced in the 1940s, potentially irritant and toxic substances are applied directly to the eyes of conscious rabbits. The eyes are chosen because of their great sensitivity, the rationale being that this provides a margin of safety with regard to human exposure. The animals are sometimes restrained in a holding device with only their head protruding to prevent them from scratching or rubbing their eyes. The test substance is applied and the eye held closed. Sometimes the application is repeated. The rabbits' eyes are then observed many days for signs of tissue damage—ulceration or opacity of the cornea, iris inflammation, and conjunctival inflammation—and this is rated on a scale. The score is used to indicate the irritancy potential of the substance. In the past these tests were used for such substances as bleach and concentrated shampoo, but these practices have stopped. The test has been repeatedly criticized as crude and unreliable, but it continues to be used albeit far less widely and often in a modified, far more humane manner.

The LD50 test (median lethal dose) is the dose of a test substance that causes death in 50 percent of the treated animals in a specified time period. To conduct this test, various doses of a drug or other substance are administered to groups of animals to determine the lethal dose at which half the number of animals die. With relatively toxic substances, this death rate is achieved with relatively small volumes of the test substance; but large volumes are needed for some non-edible or relatively non-toxic substances. Reports from the past show that LD50s were determined for substances like paper, lipstick, and distilled water. The animals were virtually blown up with excessive volumes forced down tubes into the stomach. These practices have now stopped.

In the classical LD50 test, from forty to a hundred animals are used per substance to be tested. The deaths are often protracted, taking days, weeks, or even months. During this time, the animals may exhibit typical symptoms of poisoning such as vomiting, diarrhea, paralysis, convulsions, and internal bleeding. Since death is the required endpoint, dying animals are not put out of their misery by euthanasia.

The test was developed in the 1920s and gained popularity in part because different lethal substances have different effects, and death is the only one common to them all. A test that uses death as an endpoint provides a notion of uniform testing. Indeed, the LD50 dose level for a substance has come to be treated as if it were a biological constant (like a molecular weight) although this is far from true. The test is easy to perform even by the unskilled, and this probably added to its popularity. Practically all government guidelines that regulate toxicological testing of chemicals have at one time required this test.

It is notable that criticisms of these two tests came first from scientists, not from the animal activists. An early critic was physiologist David H. Smyth (1978) of the University of Sheffield, U.K., and then chairperson of the Research Defense Society. In his book *Alternatives to Animal Experiments* he questioned whether the Draize test was necessary at all, and if so whether it needs to be carried to the extent of causing severe eye damage. He attacked the LD50 because it is unreliable; the lethal dose depends upon numerous factors, he wrote, including species, strain, sex, age, ambient condition, nutritional status, and route of administration, and it can vary from time to time within the same laboratory and between laboratories. It was Smyth, says the New York animal activist Henry Spira, who inspired him in 1988 to start the campaign to ban the Draize and LD50 tests.

Other scientists, too, have been strongly critical of the LD50. Notable among them is Gerhard Zbinden (1973), a world-renowned toxicologist at the University of Zurich who has done much to promote animal welfare. He called the LD50 test "a ritual mass execution of animals" (Zbinden, 1973). In 1981, he and Dr. M. Flury-Roversi published a review of the LD50 test, concluding that it is unreliable and inconsistent. They found the test poorly suited for the evaluation of human risk from toxic compounds.

Evidence on lack of reproducibility of the LD50 test was particularly damning. For example, Zbinden and Flury-Roversi presented information from a large study that was conducted in Europe in 1977 by Hunter and colleagues. This involved 65 toxicological laboratories in eight countries that used their own standard procedures and tested five substances. The numerical values for the LD50 of the five substances showed considerable differences from lab to lab: for PCP it ranged from 44 to 523 mg/kg, and for sodium salicylate from 800 to 4,150 mg/kg. For the five substances, there were 3.7- to 11.9-fold differences between the various labs.

Then a second inter-lab trial was conducted with the same substances but with stricter controls on testing procedures. Even so, the results were still widely variable. The range of maximal to minimal values among the substances was from 2.5 to 8.4 mg/kg—still over a 3-fold difference. At the conclusion of their review, Zbinden and Flury-Roversi recommended that the LD50 test should be replaced by a more comprehensive short-term test that can be done with small numbers of animals.

With this lead from the scientific community, the animal rights activists picked up the challenge to eliminate the LD50 and the Draize tests.

The movement for reform

Henry Spira, a former high school English teacher and civil rights activist in New York City, had already made his mark as an animal activist by organizing successful public protests against sex experiments on cats at the American Museum of Natural History that were stopped in 1976. In 1978 and 1979, he put together a coalition of more than 400 American humane societies to ban inhumane animal tests. The goal was not to stop consumer product testing but to stop cruel animal tests. They started with the Draize test (the LD50 campaign came soon after) because it is easy for the public to relate to the pain of having something toxic in your eye.

In early 1980, this coalition approached a major cosmetic company, Revlon, to suggest (a) that Revlon should approach the Cosmetic, Toiletry and Fragrance Association (the trade association) with a proposal that the CTFA coordinate a collaborative effort by industry to seek an alternative to the Draize test; and (b) that Revlon should commit $170,000 (0.01 percent of their gross income) to the project (Rowan, 1984, p. 223). A key to Spira's success in this and the several other campaigns he has run is that he defines the targets and goals to ensure that the self-interest of the manufacturing firm (or other adversary) is clearly served by going along.

Revlon responded in a letter dated February 13, 1980, saying that the proposal had been turned over to a relevant committee of the CTFA and that "neither Revlon, or any other single company, can give any assurances as to what action, if any, this committee or any other committee of the CTFA, may take except to say that it will receive consideration." But this was not satisfactory to the coalition. On April 15, 1980, a full-page ad appeared in the *New York Times,* paid for by The Millennium Guild in New York City, with Revlon as the target. The ad said, "How many rabbits does Revlon blind for beauty's sake?" This ad sent shock waves through the cosmetic industry. By the year's end, Revlon announced it was making a three-year grant of $750,000 to Rockefeller University to research possible alternatives. (In 1988, Revlon announced a moratorium on animal tests conducted in their own facilities).

Over the next decade, the impact of Spira's campaign spread in several directions. Revlon's grant opened a new source of funding for alternatives in the United States (see Appendix B for chronology on funding for alternatives). Alternatives were soon sought for other animal tests that caused pain or death— not only the LD50, but skin irritancy and inhalation toxicity tests. The campaign extended throughout the cosmetic, toiletry, and pharmaceutical industries. Various types of public protest were used to urge firms to use alternatives to the Draize and LD50. Pressures were placed on the regulatory agencies (the FDA and others) and on Congress to ban these tests. Legislation at the city, state, and federal level was also introduced to ban them.

The campaign was not confined to the United States but had international dimensions. In the U.K. a group called FRAME (Fund for the Replacement of Animals in Medical Experiments) has issued recommendations and publications and has organized scientific meetings to stimulate the search for alternatives and changes in public policy throughout Europe.

In the United States, the campaign has achieved successes in several areas: (1) the development of alternatives to the LD50 and Draize tests, (2) the reduction in animal use by industry, (3) changes in the policies of the regulatory agencies, (4) legislative efforts to ban the Draize and LD50 tests, and (5) a new focus on corporate conscience.

Alternatives: general comments

Apart from the humane advantages of using alternatives in toxicity testing, there are scientific benefits also. One is the encouragement given to improving the technology of toxicity testing. *In vitro* tests have brought a new emphasis on the molecular level. Often nowadays a battery of tests is used instead of a single one like the Draize (an *in vivo* test), and this provides a broader spectrum of scientifically significant information. Some of the new tests use human cells and thus avoid the problems of species variation and non-applicability to the human condition. However, problems still remain in extrapolating from a single cell to a multi-cellular situation.

Furthermore, *in vitro* tests are less time-consuming and sometimes less costly than using live animals. As an example, it is claimed that the agarose diffusion test takes only 24 hours to complete and costs $50 to $100, compared with up to three weeks and $500 to $700 for the Draize.

Many alternatives to the LD50 and Draize tests have now been developed as shown in the sampling given below.

Alternatives to the LD50 test

FIXED DOSE PROCEDURE (FDP). One of the most important alternatives is the FDP, developed by the British Toxicology Society, whose aim was to reduce the amount of pain and stress to the animals. The FDP involves administering the highest toxic dose not producing lethality to a small group of animals. The fixed doses chosen are keyed to the cut-off points for acute oral toxicity in the hazard classification system used by the European Economic Community (EEC). A dose causing moderate toxicity is then used to project a dose range in the EEC classification that would produce lethality. The validation trial of the FDP conducted by van den Heuvel et al. (1990) showed that laboratories could obtain much more uniform results by using signs of toxicity such as recognizing the presence of pain.

The FDP was recently endorsed by the Organization for Economic Cooperation and Development (OECD). Members of the OECD include individual European countries, the United States, and Japan. In late 1991, they agreed on mutual acceptability of FDP data, thus avoiding duplication of animal tests. This agreement is similar to a treaty obligation on the part of the participating countries, so the U.S. regulatory agencies now have agreed to accept FDP data.

THE LIMIT TEST.   About five rats or mice are given a single high dose of the test substance to assess acute toxicity. If no animal dies, the substance is considered non-toxic and no more tests are run, and a further search for a precise LD50 is abandoned. By 1985, the numbers of animals used by cosmetic companies reportedly dropped 75 to 90 percent because of adoption of the Limit Test (Welsh, 1990, page 69).

THE UP-AND-DOWN TEST.   Each animal receives a single dose, which is lowered after signs of severe toxicity develop or is raised after an animal survives one week without such signs. The resulting information is evaluated in a commonly available computer program and provides an estimated LD50 value. This method reduces the use of animals from 40 to 60 in the classical LD50 test to 6 to 10 per test.

TIER TESTING.   This approach includes the use of data from structurally related chemicals, the use of the Limit Test, and a three-dose multiple endpoint evaluation. The resultant reduction in animal use is substantial.

Alternatives to the Draize test

THE CAM ASSAY.   In this assay system, a small piece of egg shell is removed from a chick egg, leaving the heavily vascularized, underlying chorioallontoic membrane (CAM) intact. The membrane has no nerve cells, so no pain is perceived. It is a complete tissue that responds to injury with classical inflammatory reactions. A few drops of suspected toxin, dissolved in saline, are placed on the exposed membrane and the amount of blood vessel breakdown is taken as a measure of toxicity. The CAM test was developed by Joseph Leighton, Ph.D. of the Medical College of Pennsylvania. It is used by Colgate Palmolive for prescreening of new formulas and new ingredients.

THE LOW-VOLUME EYE TEST.   Griffith et al. (1980) of Proctor and Gamble found that the use of 0.1 ml of test material (the standard volume used at that time) into the rabbit eye leads to an overestimation of human hazard. From their research of comparing rabbit eye responses when tested with 21 chemicals which included surfactants, acids, and alkalies, they concluded that a dose volume of

0.01 ml was a more accurate predictor. The low-volume test that uses one-tenth of the previous dose volume is more humane and is now widely used.

TESTSKIN.   An artificial skin, developed by Organogenesis, of Cambridge, Massachusetts, consists of skin cells grown on sheets to produce a tissue resembling human skin. It has several layers of differentiated cells, just as human skin does, and it is supported by its own synthetic skeleton and circulatory system. The artificial skin is used to determine the safety of household and other consumer chemicals by direct application and assessment of resultant damage. This method has been adopted by several major companies including Avon and Revlon.

EYTEX™.   A large number of test materials have been evaluated in this assay based on a reagent (containing a protein derived from the jack bean) that becomes opaque when test materials are added. The degree of opacity induced in the reagent by a test material is reported to be proportional to the Draize eye irritation test score of the substance evaluated. The measurement of opacity is done in a simple spectrophotometer.

AGAROSE DIFFUSION METHOD.   This test has been widely used to establish the safety of plastics in medical devices implanted in the human body. Noxell Corporation, which makes cosmetics, developed the test for use with liquids, creams, powders, and pastes, and adopted it for testing their products in 1989. Substances being tested seep through an overlay that protects the culture from direct contact. This test uses cell cultures from mice that are now available in immortal cell lines, so no more animals are required.

USE OF COMPUTERS.   Predictions of toxicity are based on computer analyses of the substance's structure and properties. Such models are widely used by scientists in conjunction with other tests and many systems have been developed. Some help predict toxicity by comparing the molecular structure of known substances of known toxicity with new chemicals. Some work by producing intricate and accurate three-dimensional color pictures of enzymes responsible either for inactivating poisonous chemicals or activating them to a toxic form. A number of novel chemicals, predicted by this computer system to be toxic, have already been withdrawn from development, saving animals from painful tests.

Validation programs

Several large-scale programs to validate these tests are in progress now. The purpose is to select which tests, or combination of tests, is the most useful for predicting human toxicity. For instance, a program to validate alternatives to rodent LD50 tests has been organized by Björn Ekwall of Uppsala University. This program—involving forty-five laboratories worldwide—is designed to test a large number of varied chemicals by several different assay systems. The results should help identify those tests that are most useful for general application.

The Cosmetic, Toiletries and Fragrance Association has organized a multi-year "Evaluation of Alternatives Program" to study about twenty-five potential alternatives to the Draize test (see Gettings and McEwen, 1990). Research so far conducted suggests that a battery of tests is needed to replace the Draize test, and that different batteries of tests will probably be needed, depending upon product type.

Will the Draize test be eliminated? According to one commentator, its use had already been reduced by more than 50 percent by 1988 (Holden, 1988). In 1991, Sidney Green, director of the Division of Toxicological Studies at FDA, said that the validation of alternative test methods will take many more years of research before sufficient data are available to determine whether or not the Draize test can be discontinued. The trends appear to be that use of the Draize test will continue to decline, and some predict that by the turn of the century it will be eliminated.

Industry and the federal regulatory agencies

Industry's recognition of the non-essential nature of some animal testing has led to major reductions in animal use. Testing will continue, but it will be less and less dependent upon use of animals. In 1988, Avon Products became the first major U.S. company to announce an end to the use of animals for product safety testing. This was the culmination of many years of planning. Avon's use of animals had been steadily declining since 1981 (see Table 10.1). In 1986, the company opened an in-house cell culture laboratory where their toxicologists have worked on validating the Eytex method and, according to a press release, have established that it is "in total agreement with the Draize eye irritation tests for eye-liner, mascaras, hair tonics, skin moisturizers and non-tear shampoos. . . . [It] slightly overestimated the irritation for eye shadows, colognes, perfumes, hair shampoo and skin creams . . . but this is acceptable because the margin of difference is on the side of safety." Nowadays, the methods used by Avon for skin irritancy are a combination of alternative methods using the company's computer data base and human volunteers to confirm the mildness of the product.

In November 1988, some months after Avon's announcement that it would end animal testing, Benetton Cosmetics Corporation—the target of an international "compassion campaign" by PETA and others—announced that they too had stopped all animal testing. Within short order, similar announcements of mor-

TABLE 10.1 Decline in animal use at five major U.S. companies

Year	Avon Products	Proctor & Gamble	Colgate Palmolive	Hoffmann-La Roche	American Home Products*
1979				948,517,000	
1980				NA	
1981	14,550			NA	
1982	7,320		4,270	NA	
1983	9,420		11,840	NA	
1984	7,010	10,781	3,750	NA	348,800
1985	5,050	6,940	3,120	NA	NA
1986	4,720	6,860	2,740	NA	NA
1987	4,060	4,800	1,720	NA	NA
1988	2,240	4,710	1,430	238,012,000	NA
1989	0	NA	1,670	200,000,000	319,298
1990	0	NA	NA	226,000,000	269,105

This table shows how five major companies have decreased the numbers of animals used in testing. If the first year for which data for any one company is taken to be 100 percent, then the percentage reductions in animal use over the period of time shown for that company are: Avon Products (cosmetic manufacturers) reduced by 100 percent; Proctor and Gamble (household products) reduced by 56 percent; Colgate Palmolive (toiletries and household products) reduced by 61 percent; Hoffmann-La Roche (pharmaceuticals) reduced by 75 percent; and American Home Products (pharmaceuticals) reduced by 23 percent.

All figures are rounded to the nearest ten. NA = not available.

*Comprises five divisions that use animals; Ayerst, Fort Dodge Laboratories, Sherwood Medical, Wyeth, and Wyeth-Ayerst, and includes test animals used in outside contracts as well as those used in-house.

Sources:

Avon and Proctor and Gamble: from Welsh, 1990, pages 94 and 122 respectively. This information was compiled by IRRC from data from USDA and the companies. The Proctor and Gamble data covers P & G's main laboratory and leased facility in Cincinnati.

Colgate Palmolive: from Colgate Palmolive Company 1989 Report of Laboratory research with animals, February 1990, 11 pages, New York. The numbers represent the totals if animals used both in-house and by outside contractors.

Hoffmann-La Roche: Personal communication Martin Hirsch, Senior Manager, Public Relations, Hoffmann-La Roche, May 29, 1990. The figures for 1989 and 1990 are approximate. The rise in numbers of animals used in 1990 is due to use of mice in research in new techniques.

American Home Products: Personal communication May 30, 1991 from Nancy Barrett, Department of Public Issues, American Home Products.

atoriums were made by a dozen other big-name companies including Noxell, Amway, Mary Kay Cosmetics, Revlon, Charles of the Ritz, Elizabeth Arden, Fabergé, Germaine Monteil, Shaklee, and Estée Lauder. By 1990, Revlon was running full-page ads in women's magazines publicizing its "Pure Skin Care" line with a "100% nonanimal tested formula." According to PETA, over 350 companies have now stopped testing products on animals.

A few companies have announced the actual numbers of animals used so that reduction trends are documented. Table 10.1 provides data on Avon, Proctor and Gamble, Colgate Palmolive, Hoffmann-La Roche, and American Home Products. These companies are not comparable for animal use reductions because the range and number of products that each produces are very different. Other companies show similar trends. All told, the corporate response has been highly effective in reducing animal use.

This response of industry has been ahead of what was required by the federal regulatory agencies. Indeed policies of the federal agencies on animal testing have often been unclear and contradictory. But recently the agencies have been edging toward accepting alternatives and issuing statements discouraging use of the classical LD50 and Draize tests.

Three government regulatory agencies are primarily concerned with animal testing of consumer products that are not medically related—the Food and Drug Administration (FDA), which has received the most attention because of its authority over cosmetics, the Consumer Product Safety Commission (CPSC), and, to a lesser extent, the Environmental Protection Agency (EPA).

The purview of these three regulatory agencies is as follows. Since 1938, the FDA has administered the Federal Food, Drug, and Cosmetic Act. The incident that led to passage of this law was the 1933 blinding and disfigurement of a woman who had dyed her eyelashes with a coal-tar product called "Lash-Lure." The AMA documented seventeen similar cases, some resulting in death. Lash-Lure remained on the market for five more years because, until the Act passed, the federal government did not have authority to seize such products. The law has been tightened up over the years to keep pace with increasing consumer demands that what is in the marketplace must be safe.

The law currently requires that cosmetics be free from deleterious or poisonous substances; it prohibits the distribution of adulterated or misbranded cosmetic products. Under the Act, the FDA has issued a regulatory requirement that either the safety of each cosmetic ingredient and each finished cosmetic product be adequately substantiated before it is marketed, or that the product be labeled with a warning that its safety has not been determined. The law does not specifically *require* animal testing, but historically the FDA has relied on animal toxicity data to assess consumer safety. Nowadays, the production of new varieties of eye shadows and lipsticks generally requires minor formulation changes for which safety testing is often unnecessary. However, animal tests are used in the development of new products such as sunscreens, fluoride toothpaste, and many others.

The CPSC administers the Federal Hazardous Substances Act, which provides for proper labeling of hazardous products. This Act covers most household products other than foods, drugs, and cosmetics that are regulated by the FDA, and pesticides that are regulated by the EPA. Typical of the products monitored by CPSC are drain cleaners, anti-freeze, and furniture polish.

The EPA has jurisdiction over pesticides, industrial chemicals, air and water pollutants, hazardous wastes, and some radiation hazards.

The federal agencies have not agreed on which animal tests are required and which alternatives to the classical LD50 and Draize are acceptable. Some agency statements have been so ambiguous that they could be interpreted as both accepting and rejecting the same test. These ambiguities have been a source of confusion and irritation to some, especially the reformers.

The FDA was pressured to make a clear statement in 1986. Twenty humane societies including the ASPCA filed a petition requesting clarification of the FDA policy on the classical LD50 test. The FDA finally responded with an announcement in the Federal Register on October 11, 1988. "FDA has adopted a policy that the 'classical' LD50 test is not a required toxicity study. The agency supports efforts to eliminate continued conduct of the 'classical' LD50 test and to reduce the numbers of animals used." FDA further stated that it will not refuse to accept data from classical LD50 tests "if they are relevant to a decision FDA must make." Commenting on this statement, an ASPCA report stated, "Rather than clarifying the agency position, it has perpetuated the confusion." Keeping well-seated on the fence, the FDA later said it "supports efforts to eliminate continued conduct" of the classical LD50 test, but many of the FDA's guideline protocols and regulations referred to the LD50 test and how it should be conducted.

The EPA was rather more forthright. A revised policy of September 22, 1988, announced that the EPA will only accept data from tests using fewer numbers of animal subjects than those used in the classical LD50 test. They recommended use of the limit test, and stated that no further testing is necessary in the absence of lethality at a 2 g/kg dose. They emphasize the use of a tiered approach and the need to collect data on behavioral effects and gross pathology as well as lethality.

The critical event in late 1991 was the mutual agreement of the OECD countries to accept the Fixed Dose Procedure. This effectively means that the U.S. regulatory agencies have moved significantly forward with respect to replacing the classical LD50 test.

Recently, some representatives from industry and the three key U.S. regulatory bodies have worked informally toward a consensus about eye irritancy tests. In September 1991, they cooperated in a workshop on alternatives (mainly refinement and reduction) to eye irritation tests in Washington, D.C. Its purpose was to promote standardization and harmonization of testing guidelines and to discuss possible modifications. The proceedings were reported by Andrew N. Rowan of Tufts University in *The Alternatives Report,* of which he is editor (September-December, 1991 issue). Dr. Robert Scala of Exxon Corporation closed this two-day session voicing strong praise for the courage of the government scientists who took the initiative on the issue of alternatives in the absence of any policy guidelines. According to Rowan, Scala "urged the government agencies to pull for data on refinement and *in vitro* systems, so that industry can push its management to provide the funds for changes."

Despite this progressive move, David A. Kessler, the new FDA Commissioner, issued a clear statement on April 18, 1991, in favor of the Draize test and opposition to the proposed California state ban on it (Kessler, 1991). He wrote, "The Draize eye irritancy test is currently the most valuable and reliable method for evaluating the hazard or safety of a substance introduced into or around the human eye. . . . There are presently no non-animal tests available to completely replace the Draize." Reaching a consensus on this test will take time.

Legislative efforts

Historically, there have been two major thrusts in the legislatures: one to ban the LD50 and Draize tests and the other to require labeling about use of animal tests.

Two cities, known as bellwethers on many issues, have banned some toxicity tests: Cambridge, Massachusetts, and Berkeley, California. On March 4, 1991, the Cambridge City Council established a policy that the LD50 and Draize tests "shall only be used after all other alternatives are exhausted." In 1991, in another unanimous vote, the Berkeley City Council passed legislation which states: "Except as specifically required by State or Federal law, no person shall perform either the Draize eye irritancy test or the skin irritancy test for any purpose within the city of Berkeley. Any Berkeley resident may enforce the provisions of this chapter by means of a civil action for injunctive relief."

Efforts to enact state laws to either ban or limit animal testing have generated considerable controversy and so far have failed. In these legislative efforts, strong campaigns were launched on both sides along familiar lines. The animal rights and animal welfare groups were on one side, and the Foundation for Biomedical Research (FBR), medical researchers, the CTFA, and certain segments of industry on the other. A common thread in testimony against these bills that target only consumer products is that even the most modest animal test prohibitions will adversely affect medical research as a whole.

This strategy of opposition was successful in California where a bill to ban the Draize only for cosmetic and household cleansers—no more—successfully passed the state legislature twice but was vetoed by the governor. Typical of the position taken by opponents of these bills is the statement in a booklet issued in 1988 by the Foundation for Biomedical Research that referred to the LD50 as "still absolutely necessary in the development of certain new pharmaceutical products" (FBR, 1988). According to an FBR newsletter, in a press conference held April 29, 1990, in Washington, D.C., former U.S. Surgeon General C. Everett Koop, an FBR board member, maintained that there is no substitute for animal testing if Americans want to ensure the safety of consumer products. He said, "If the California legislature does not act responsibly and oppose this legislation, other states might take their cue from California and fall prey to extremist pressures." He further stated, "I care about animals. But I care about people more. . . . I have seen children brought to emergency rooms because of accidental poisonings and have seen children born HIV positive. Obviously, the animal rights extremists have not, or they would never be so inhumane as to be making the inane remarks that they do."

In the first veto message, California Governor George Deukmejian said on June 25, 1990, "I am concerned that this bill would preclude a viable testing option that may be necessary to ensure that cosmetic and household products are not harmful to the health of consumers. Although I am supportive of efforts to find alternatives to animal testing, the U.S. Environmental Protection Agency, the U.S. Food and Drug Administration, and the U.S. Consumer Product Safety Commission all agree that these particular tests remain the most valuable and reliable method in determining the safety of new and reformulated products that may come in contact with the eyes or skin of consumers."

The California bill was re-introduced in the next session and passed both the Assembly and Senate. The CTFA allocated one million dollars to defeat this and similar bills. The bill was vetoed by the new governor, Pete Wilson, on September 9, 1991.

At the federal level, on November 25, 1991, Representative Barbara Boxer (D–Cal.) introduced legislation, the Consumer Products Safe Testing Act in the 102nd Congress. This bill (H.R. 3918) calls on the federal agencies to say which alternatives to the LD50 and Draize tests should be used at the present time. This bill had been co-sponsored by over 130 Representatives in the previous 101st Congress. The 1991 version has been now modified to take into consideration comments presented by the medical research community and federal agencies and now specifically exempts medical research. The bill instructs federal agencies to review and rewrite regulations with acute toxicity testing, including the Draize test, to reflect human reactions to products more adequately and therefore to better protect human health. The bill would ensure that alternative testing procedures that are of equal value as indicators of toxicity levels and that are less costly in terms of dollars and animal lives are encouraged by the federal government. Alternative tests such as the Eytex system, cloned human skin cells, and computer models have been developed and more are on the way, says a 1991 statement from Representative Boxer.

The bill's proponents argue that the federal agencies are not making decisive moves to encourage alternatives. "It seems the regulatory environment is not receptive to alternatives. I think the Congress can break this inertia," said Representative Boxer at earlier Congressional hearings. However, opposition has been strong. This bill had not yet been voted out of committee by mid 1992.

At the state level, a new approach aimed at increasing consumer awareness about animal tests was made in California during the 1989 legislative sessions. The "Humane Product Testing Law" (SB 60) prepared by State Senator Robbins would require those household products and cosmetics that used live animals in their consumer-safety tests to say so conspicuously on their labels or packages. Household products would include cleansers, paints, solvents, and polishes, and cosmetics would include soaps and beautifying articles applied to the human body. Products intended for human consumption would not be included. By mid-1992, no such measures had been adopted in California or elsewhere.

Some products are already advertised as "cruelty free." For instance, a line of cosmetics called "Beauty Without Cruelty," prominently labeled as having been produced without any animal testing, has been successfully marketed for several years. But the term "cruelty free" is misleading because it would be difficult to identify ingredients that have not been tested on animals at some time.

The animal rights groups have fostered the notion of "cruelty free" throughout a wide range of products—one English group even tells you where to obtain "cruelty free" bagpipes, traditionally made from a sheep skin or hide, but now available in Gore-Tex fabric! In the U.K. in 1991, there were proposals in the House of Commons to require labeling of fur products according to whether they are "cruelty free." Presumably anything that involved real animal fur would be considered "cruel," with no distinction made between the methods of trapping or killing used.

These labeling proposals have problems. FRAME opposes proposals to require a label "tested on animals" if the products or ingredients they contained had been tested on animals within the preceding five years. This group argues that such a requirement would cause a "nightmare of confusion" because manufacturers could not be expected to know whether or not their products had been tested on animals—it is unrealistic. FRAME points out with justice that since there is no law requiring that the results of tests be made publicly available, it would be impossible to tell whether the absence of a "tested on animals" label was legitimate or was a dishonest marketing ploy.

Corporate conscience

A book that might have passed unnoticed a few years ago—*Rating America's Corporate Conscience* by S. Lydenberg—generated attention as the first book to use animal protection as a measure of corporate responsibility. It was published in 1987 by a watchdog organization, the Council on Economic Priorities, in New York.

The Council on Economic Priorities also initiated an Animal Rights Corporate Conscience award. The first recipient was Proctor and Gamble, cited in February 1988 as "a leader in seeking alternatives to using animals in tests, and for prodding Federal agencies to look at these alternatives." In their 1991 shopper's guide to socially responsible supermarket shopping, the Council rates companies according to their activities on animal testing. The criteria are whether or not the company has given up animal tests, has reduced animal tests more than 40 percent over the last five years or less, and has given $250,000 or more annually to alternative research through in-house or independent labs. Among the large companies that have received top rating are American Home Products, Bristol-Meyers Squibb, Colgate Palmolive, Johnson and Johnson, Kellogg, Proctor and Gamble, and Ralston Purina.

In line with this new trend, the business sections of newspapers like the *Wall Street Journal* and the *New York Times* have begun running occasional articles about *in vitro* toxicity testing and other ways to reduce animal testing. A typical one is entitled "Beyond White Rats and Rabbits" (*NYT,* Feb. 28, 1988).

Another group, Investor Responsibility Research Center of Washington, D.C., compiles and analyzes information on the activities of business in society, on the activities of institutional investors, on efforts to influence such activities, and on related public policy. Their 1990 book on animal testing authored by H. J. Welsh relates how some animal rights groups have recently started using a tactic that is squarely within the tradition of moderate activists—shareholder resolutions (page 20). PETA has bought stock in Avon, Bristol-Myers, Gillette, and Proctor and Gamble so that it could act as a shareholder proponent. PETA has also solicited its members who hold stock in consumer product companies to submit shareholder resolutions for disclosure of animal use figures.

In 1987, the first year, three companies were affected. A PETA resolution asked Greyhound (of which Armour-Dial of Dial soap is part) to halt animal testing not required by law and to begin to phase out products that cannot be marketable without animal tests (6.7 percent voted in favor of this resolution). Less favorable votes were obtained at two other companies; a resolution asking for a halt to animal tests not required by law received only a 2.2 percent vote at Proctor and Gamble; a proposal asking IBM to donate $200,000 for research on alternatives to animal testing got 1.7 percent of the vote.

In subsequent years, similar actions have been taken. For instance, the ASPCA has submitted proposals on factory farming to McDonald's and to Pepsico; several groups have proposed resolutions to U.S. Surgical on the company's use of dogs for training their marketing personnel in the use of surgical staples; and PETA has submitted a resolution on selling fur coats to American Express.

This campaign has had some impact in increasing the awareness of the animal issues. Also, as a result of these resolutions, several companies have released more accurate data about the numbers and species of animals used in experiments at their facilities (see Table 10.1.) It is likely that shareholder scrutiny will continue to influence voluntary reporting of animal data and will make companies take the animal protection movement more seriously.

Current trends

The campaign for more humane toxicity testing methods has not run its full course. Vetoes and legislative opposition to bans on the LD50 and Draize tests have not stopped progress. To varying degrees the attention of the public has been captured, leading firms are listening, and federal agencies are taking useful steps. One indication of progress is that the rise in scientific publications about *in vitro* toxicity testing has been dramatic. There are now many journals and several newsletters devoted to alternatives in testing. Some of the journals and the year in which they were launched are *Alternatives to Laboratory Animals* (published by FRAME, 1972), *Cell Biology and Toxicology* (1984), In vitro *Toxicology* (1986), *Alternative Methods in Toxicology* (1987), *Molecular Toxicology* (1987), *Toxicology* in vitro (1987), and *Toxicology and Industrial Health* (1985). Among the newsletters are the *Newsletter of the Johns Hopkins Center for Alternatives to Animal Testing* (CAAT, 1983), *Frame News* in the U.K. (1984), and Tufts University's *Alternatives Report* (1989). In 1991, Proctor and Gamble started issuing a quarterly newsletter called *Alternatives Alert* for company employees who are engaged in product research. These publications, many of which reach scientists and the public, contribute to the increasing awareness of alternatives in animal testing.

A future increase in political support is also a real possibility. Vice President Albert Gore, Jr., in addition to being an outspoken advocate on environmental issues, has also expressed his opinion on the LD50 and Draize tests; "I believe both these tests should be eliminated" (Letter to a Tennessee constituent, Don Elroy, from the then U.S. Senator Gore, April 22, 1992).

11

From Sunshine Laws and Civil Disobedience to Raids

Over the years, methods used by watchdog organizations to voice their concerns about animal experiments have become increasingly forceful. Early methods used by the antivivisectionists and animal welfarists had been mild—searching the literature and the like. Another strategy has been to invoke "sunshine" laws, intended to bring the activities of government into the open, to legally obtain information about government-funded research and the activities of Institutional Animal Care and Use Committees. Starting in the mid-1970s, civil disobedience tactics began to be adopted. First, street demonstrations and later sit-ins and other peaceful methods of protest were used. The laboratory raids, which started in 1981, appreciably escalated the level of aggressiveness. They involve infiltration, illegal entry, and theft; and at least during the 1980s increasingly arson and bombs have been used. In 1992, the American wing of the clandestine Animal Liberation Front, the group primarily responsible for the raids, was listed by the Federal Bureau of Investigation as one of the ten most dangerous terrorist organizations.

In reviewing these progressively aggressive tactics, it is important to keep in mind who approves what method of protest. The raids are perpetrated by the most extreme groups. Support for raids is found among animal rightists. (However, to some extent, support depends on the particular circumstances surrounding each individual raid). The animal welfarists (humane societies and the like) tend to disassociate themselves from the raids and to choose peaceful and legal means of pursuing their goals.

169

As the laboratory raids have progressed, their objective changed from information gathering to economic sabotage and personal harassment. This shift in objective has caused something of a backlash and public sympathy has turned, to some extent, in favor of the beleaguered researchers. This chapter relates this history and analyzes the issues involved.

Access to information

Before the raids, three methods to gain access to information were used: literature search, conducted tours, and inspection of government records.

To this day, the most common way of obtaining information about the treatment of laboratory animals has been to search the scientific literature. Based on this information, various campaigns of protest have been launched.

Before the raids, antivivisectionist and, less frequently, humane organizations compiled extracts from published accounts of experiments and used them to persuade the public that animals had been abused. Highly invasive experimental methods were cited such as deprivation of sight, intentional fracture of bones, administration of lethal substances, or exposure to lethal infections. Typically, the harms to the animals were described but no information on the purpose of the experiments was provided. Much-favored for quotation were articles in which the investigators had reported that the results were inconclusive or that more research was needed along similar lines. Since the purpose of the protesters was to embarrass the investigators and to discredit animal experimentation as a whole, no effort was made to achieve a balanced presentation.

This approach nourished the antivivisectionists but had little or no effect on the scientific community or general public. Skeptical and unsympathetic readers were put off by the one-sided presentations. Animal researchers rarely saw these write-ups, and when they did, dismissed them. On the whole, the protest organizations achieved little or nothing. The scientists were not listening, the media ignored the issues, and the public was not persuaded to bring any pressure for change.

Nowadays a broader range of people publicly comment on the humaneness of certain experiments. Starting roughly in the early 1980s, reform-minded physicians, veterinarians, and animal researchers began to publicly report their reviews of proposed or ongoing animal experiments. Typically, their assessments present the reasons for conducting the experiments, identify omissions and commissions in experimental procedures, and suggest ways in which animal suffering could have been minimized or abolished. Their criticisms of the animal experiments are intended to be taken seriously by the scientific community. Good published examples are found in Smith and Boyd, 1991. In line with this trend are the open discussions of real cases of questionable animal procedures that have occurred at conferences organized by the Canadian Council on Animal Care. The latest such conference was in February 1992, and was attended by over 200 persons, both scientists and non-scientists.

In the past, a second method of obtaining information about laboratory conditions was the conducted tour of research facilities. Tours were sometimes part of a community outreach program sponsored by research facilities; occasionally they were conducted on request. Very few requests for such visits were made and not all of them were granted. Since visits were tightly controlled, they did not turn up much interesting information for reformers and, on the whole, neither the public nor the media was interested. One exception was the Animal Welfare Institute (AWI), which sought a number of conducted tours in the 1950s and 1960s. This organization's trained observers were able to obtain useful information on conditions of animal housing and to report publicly both the favorable and unfavorable evidence. Since the start of the raids, research facilities have been less inclined than before to permit such tours.

Ever since the AWA was enacted in 1966, reports of USDA inspections of animal holding facilities have been made public. On the whole, the humane movement did not avail itself of much of this information, but AWI representatives made a point of keeping up with it. They regularly reported to the public deficiencies of animal transport and holding facilities that the USDA inspectors had encountered and how long it took to get the problems corrected, if ever.

All three sources of information (articles, tours, and records) were limited in their range and frankness. Watchdog organizations constantly complained that the laboratory door was shut and the public was not allowed to see behind it. Until the 1980s, this was largely true and the public had little knowledge of what was going on in animal labs, either good or bad.

Freedom of Information Act

Since the passage of the Freedom of Information Act (FOIA), the public has succeeded in gaining access to much more valuable information. The FOIA, amended by Public Law 90-23 in 1967, requires most federal agencies to release information to interested persons unless it is classified or meets other exceptions. The burden is on the government to show why information should be withheld.

Certain exemptions apply to what is available from both USDA and NIH. For instance, most reasonably, the public is denied access to information on the progress of PHS-funded research that has not yet been published unless the scientist wishes to release it voluntarily. Arguably with less reason, the public cannot find out how requirements of providing for the psychological well-being of primates and the exercise of dogs are being carried out because the research institutions' plans to fulfill these requirements do not have to be submitted to USDA. If they were provided to USDA, they would be subject to public access.

Requests to government agencies under the FOIA have steadily increased over the years. The USDA, NIH, and the Department of Defense (and indeed all other government agencies) are subject to the Act's provisions. For instance, over a recent four-year period, requests to the USDA have more than doubled—from

303 received in 1986 to 665 in 1990. Documents most often requested are copies of inspection reports, reporting forms, records, and forms used to apply for licenses or registrations. In 1986, the Office of Technology Assessment noted that the AWI made more requests for USDA information than any other organization.

NIH is most frequently asked to provide descriptions of animal research involving highly invasive procedures, and PETA makes the most requests. Information made public includes the experimental rationale, the number and species of animals, the total amount of public funding, and the projected life of the study.

Instead of having to wait until the research is published, by use of the FOIA the public can find out about proposed animal research projects at the start of federal funding. This opens up the possibility of raising public concern about certain experiments early in the project.

Information obtained under the FOIA has formed the basis of many protests about animal experiments. The first was made in 1975 when Spira obtained information about some cat sex experiments conducted at the American Museum of Natural History. After 18 months of street demonstrations every weekend and a sympathetic write-up about the case by Nicholas Wade in *Science* (1976), the experiments were finally halted.

A more recent case involved studies at Cornell University of barbiturate drug addiction in cats. The drugs were withdrawn abruptly, causing severe withdrawal effects that included convulsions and death. This work, which had received approximately $250,000 per year from NIH for 13 years, was considered of high merit by scientists because it provided information on the mechanisms of drug addiction. In August 1987, after some months of almost daily street protests by animal advocates, a group called Trans-Species Unlimited obtained an agreement from Cornell officials to end the cat experiments. Then, Trans-Species found out through a FOIA request that the university had signed a new grant application to the National Institute on Drug Abuse specifying use of thirty more cats for similar research. This grant was approved for funding in 1988. This inconsistency caused embarrassment to Cornell and, at the investigator's request, Cornell handed back the investigator's NIH grant renewal worth $600,000—an unprecedented event. Some members of the biomedical community were outraged at Cornell for "caving in" to the animal rights groups.

Requests for information under the FOIA have not always gone smoothly. Starting in 1989, a radical group, In Defense of Animals (IDA), has filed a series of FOIA requests with the Department of Defense, seeking information on the use of primates and other species in weapons testing. According to Michael Budkie, an IDA spokesperson, the information released omitted mention of five military establishments that conduct animal experiments. Furthermore, IDA's president Dr. Eliot Katz charged that FOIA requests for research protocols involving primates at Wright Patterson Air Force Base in Dayton, Ohio, for the years 1989 and 1989 were denied by the Air Force on the basis that no records existed for research protocols during those years. Yet documents filed voluntarily during the years in question with the USDA show that 110 primates were used in research during these years. These charges were made in testimony of Katz before the Research and Development Subcommittee of the U.S. House of Representatives Armed Services Committee on April 7, 1992, in hearings where a number of public concerns over military use of animals were aired. As a result of the hearings, an amendment to the Defense Appropriations Bill was approved by the committee calling for a detailed annual report by the Department of Defense to Congress on animal experimentation, and the establishment of programs to develop alternatives to animal research. In its strongly-worded report, the committee directs DOD facilities to appoint "animal advocates" to their IACUCs.

Sunshine laws

The FOIA is but one example of a "sunshine law"; there are many others. These include both federal and state laws that require public access not only to certain records, but also to certain meetings. State laws vary in their wording, but all fifty states have open meeting laws, and in addition, many mandate public access to certain records. At issue has been whether or not the state sunshine laws pertain to IACUC meetings and IACUC records. These battles have often been fought in court.

To the animal rights movement, state sunshine laws offer significant advantages over the federal law. Under the state laws, information can be obtained from state-funded institutions at an earlier time, and from a wider range of funding sources. In contrast, the federal law applies only *after* funding has been approved, and excludes commercial funding. Also, animal rights groups claim that their presence at IACUC meetings will influence researchers to pay more attention to the ethical implications of their research.

The right of the public to attend IACUC meetings under the open meeting laws has been highly controversial. The universities have given several reasons for resisting the open meeting laws: having animal rights sympathizers in the buildings to attend IACUC meetings involves a possible security risk—this would be especially true if the public were allowed to go on inspection tours of the animal facilities, a legally required activity of the committee; providing names of IACUC members could result in harassment or litigation against the members; making IACUC discussions or records public provides information on ongoing research, which could stifle the review process and make IACUC members more guarded in their comments, result in public protest and possible stoppage of certain experiments, and be unjust to individual investigators because science is a competitive endeavor and creative ideas should not be usurped by premature disclosure. The universities argue that the mandated review by IACUCs is confidential; indeed the AWA prohibits IACUC members from releasing any "confidential information of the research facility." This provision, they argue, makes confidential any discussion of experiments. Another argument against open meetings is the fear that animal rights sympathizers might distort what they hear and unfairly smear the reputation of researchers.

The case for opening IACUC meetings to the public has been stated by Elinor Molbegott, counsel for the American Society for the Protection of Cruelty to Animals. At a 1987 conference for scientists held at Rockefeller University, she said, "True, the information learned at meetings may be distorted by some [members of the public] but few would argue that our press should be censored, or freedom of speech denied because some people in the media distort the truth now and then. The same reasoning should apply here. Furthermore, in the event this does occur, there are laws regarding defamation and harassment. It's unfortunate that some [IACUC] members may choose to be more guarded at the meetings, but the overall benefit of having public access to meetings surely exceeds the possible detriment of denying access. . . . One can argue that to deny information merely gives the interested public few options, one being to break in and actually see what is going on. To deny access . . . could encourage the unlawful behavior that many scientists and administrators at research institutions are so concerned about."

A few universities have agreed to open IACUC meetings to the public. For example, meetings at the University of Florida in Gainesville have been open since 1985. After national protests led to the discontinuance of two research projects, the university hired a veterinarian, Farol N. Tomson, to oversee the animal facility, and no further public protests have taken place. In a 1991 interview, Tomson, who chairs the IACUC, told me "It is only right and proper these guests should be there. It is the best way to tell our story." The IACUC meetings are advertised in the local newspaper and typically five to ten animal rights persons or press members come to each meeting. Visitors are given the minutes of the last meeting and may comment halfway through and at the end of each meeting. This system, says Tomson, has worked well.

Nationwide, the denial of requests to attend IACUC meetings have often led to legal suits brought by individual animal advocates and such groups as the ASPCA, the New England Anti-Vivisection Society, and the Progressive Animal Welfare Society. Decisions have gone both ways—in six states meetings are open, and in five states plus the province of Ontario they are closed (see details in Appendix C, page 281). No information is available on what proportion of institutions nationwide hold open meetings.

Civil disobedience

Many leaders in the animal rights movement pay tribute to the pioneers of the civil rights movement. Peter Singer, Tom Regan, Ingrid Newkirk, Henry Spira,

Joyce Tischler, and others say they have drawn inspiration and learned strategies for effecting social change from Mahatma Ghandi and Martin Luther King. Civil disobedience tactics are now widely used within the animal rights movement. These include street demonstrations, boycotts, and hunger strikes. By definition, civil disobedience is characterized by *nonviolent* actions.

Civil disobedience has been used to correct injustices where other traditional methods of social change—through the courts or through legislation—would not have brought results, or at least not so quickly. Henry David Thoreau protested slavery by refusing to pay his taxes and explained his position in his famous 1848 essay on civil disobedience. In this century, Gandhi led a movement of passive resistance in both South Africa and India to protest unjust racial laws. Similarly Martin Luther King, much influenced by Gandhi, led the fight against racial injustice in the United States. The strategies involved not only passive resistance but also invading the territory of whites, as when Afro-Americans sat in the front section of the bus or at lunch counters traditionally reserved for whites only. In a number of instances, these actions were illegal. The laws were unjust and had to be changed. Illegality does not necessarily make an act unjustified.

The animal rights movement claims that several of their tactics are in this honorable tradition (see Jackson, 1989, and Siegel, 1989). Several members of the animal rights movement advise their constituency that methods such as raids should not be utilized as a method of coercion until virtually all legal methods have been tried and have failed. For instance, an Animal Liberation Front member reported by Jackson says, "When repeated and widespread legal actions fail to yield results, pessimism, bordering on despair, can grow into a controlled and thoughtful rage, inciting people to actions they would not do in less drastic circumstances" (Jackson, 1989).

Raids have been variously called acts of civil disobedience or crimes. For instance, Holly Jensen of the ALF and Ingrid Newkirk, National Director of PETA, consider that the 1984 raid on the NIH-funded University of Pennsylvania baboon head injury labs was an act of civil disobedience (Fox, 1984). On the other hand, James B. Wyngaarden, as the government spokesperson for NIH, said, "I think there's a limit to what can be tolerated as civil disobedience. I personally believe [the Gennarelli] break-in is a crime" (Fox, 1984).

Those who participate in acts of civil disobedience pay a price for asserting their convictions. Arrests, fines, and prison sentences can result from such acts, and worldwide several animal rights sympathizers have suffered these penalties. In planning an event of civil disobedience, the level of likely self-sacrifice demanded of participants is taken into consideration. One particular protest— over use of nuclear weapons—serves to illustrate the stringent tests sometimes used by protesters. I heard a talk by a religious leader who had helped to organize a nuclear weapons protest. She was prepared to give her life for this cause. She had just emerged from several months in prison for illegal entry into a military base. She said that her protest group took months to plan an act of civil disobedience. The target was carefully selected to be relevant to their mission and the action of protesters had to have symbolic meaning. The selection of participants was critical; great care was needed to ensure that no infiltrators could bring disrepute to the group. Strict rules on nonviolence were established and all were instructed not to resist arrest. All knew beforehand that their illegal action would make jail inevitable. Adding up the sentences of those who participated, the total toll was 25 years in prison against 15 minutes of hammering a nuclear missile with kitchen hammers. In the planning, they had assessed the cost in terms of the level of self-sacrifice required against the costs to the military in terms of damage done to the missile. A criterion for proceeding with any action was that the level of self-sacrifice had to far outweigh any damage.

To use civil disobedience effectively involves maintaining what is sometimes a delicate balance between garnering public support because of the injustices that are protested and incurring public condemnation for the illegality and other events surrounding the event. According to Paul Hardin (1988), Chancellor of the University of North Carolina, public tolerance depends on (a) the gravity of the wrong protested or importance of the cause advanced, (b) the relevancy of the legal violation to the alleged wrong or cause, (c) the severity of the harm flowing to others in consequence of the act of civil disobedience, and (d) the relationship of those inconvenienced by the act of civil disobedience to the alleged wrong. Hardin describes civil disobedience as a well-calculated violation of the law. "In my view public agencies, including states, towns, and state universities, cannot by their nature *approve* civil disobedience. The essence of civil disobedience is the absence of permission. It is an individual's decision to violate the law with a full realization that the act is illegal and a willingness to accept the legal consequences of the unlawful act, as a means of dramatizing the importance to the actor of the cause being advanced or the injustice being protested." Applying Hardin's criteria provides a test of one's opinions about the animal reform movement.

The start of the American raids

The first laboratory raid in the United States was conducted by police on the laboratory of Edward Taub, Administrative Director of the Behavioral Biology Center at the Institute for Behavioral Research (IBR), in Silver Spring, Maryland. On September 11, 1981, the police confiscated seventeen monkeys (thereafter known as the Silver Spring monkeys) acting on evidence provided by a worker at the facility, Alex Pacheco, and testimony of five scientists (a primatologist, a veterinarian, a physician, and others who had been secretly let in at night by Pacheco) that conditions in the NIH-funded lab violated Maryland state anti-cruelty laws. The raid took place in view of prearranged television crews so that maximum publicity was obtained by the animal rights movement. Within weeks of the raid, NIH cut off funding to the lab—an unprecedented action. The case was also tried in a state court. It won widespread media attention and public sympathy for the animal protection movement.

A second raid was made in 1984 by members of the Animal Liberation Front (ALF), who illegally entered the University of Pennsylvania's baboon head injury laboratory. The raiders stole tapes that the NIH-funded investigators had made of their studies. The evidence was self-incriminating. Again NIH cut off funding, but only after a year-long delay, a sit-in demonstration at NIH by animal advocates, and substantial public pressure.

These first two raids stand apart from the many others that followed because they were better planned and more effective. Both succeeded in publicly embarrassing the animal research community and NIH and in stopping the research. Evidence from the raids played an important role in the passage of the 1985 strengthening amendments to the AWA. It is worth recounting these two cases here because they have been influential, and because memories about abuses are short and because stout defenders of both projects have sought to exonerate the laboratory personnel involved.

I was working at NIH at the time of the first raid, and I followed these events closely as they happened. I was not involved in any of the staff work on this case, but I was surrounded by colleagues who reflected the perspective of the funding agency.

The Silver Spring monkey case

The Silver Spring monkey case was orchestrated by Pacheco, aged 23, who was employed at this laboratory as a temporary summer employee. He was also a part-time undergraduate student at George Washington University. He had previously been involved with Sea Shepherd, the environmentalist activist group, and later went on to become the chairperson of PETA.

Taub's laboratory monkeys—sixteen crab-eating macaques and one rhesus macaque—were being used in research related to the rehabilitation of stroke victims. Twelve had undergone dorsal rhizotomies resulting in total denervation of a forelimb. The research was intended through behavioral and anatomical studies to define quantitatively the deficit in movement following forelimb deafferentation. The behavioral aspect of the study was intended to investigate adaptive behavior in monkeys forced to use forelimbs in which sensation had been abolished. The anatomical aspect included regeneration studies of axonal sprouting. Deafferented monkeys are notoriously difficult to take care of because they treat the deafferented limb as a foreign object, and frequently chew off fingers. Many deafferented monkeys have continuous sores in various stages of healing.

The monkeys confiscated by the police showed evidence of improper treat-

ment, purulent lesions on some of them, untreated wounds, and filthy laboratory
conditions. The bad conditions appeared to be of long standing. Among the
group of twelve deafferented monkeys, thirty-nine digits were missing or deformed because of self-mutilation. Photographs of the animals' deformed hands
raised strong public emotions.

Funding from NIH for Taub's research was in its ninth year and in 1981
amounted to approximately $144,000. Immediately after the police raid, NIH
carried out its own investigation, which included a site visit and a review of 117
photographs taken by the police and of other relevant evidence. Its purpose was
not to judge the scientific merit of Taub's work, but to ascertain whether or not
the Institute for Behavioral Research had complied with the PHS Animal Welfare
Policy and the NIH Guide for the Care and Use of Laboratory Animals.

The conclusions of the NIH's careful report, dated October 7, 1981, were that
adequate veterinary care had not been provided, the Animal Care Committee was
not properly constituted and had failed to provide adequate oversight of the
facilities, the physical facilities for housing the monkeys were inadequate, the
occupational health programs for IBR staff were inadequate, and the condition of
the laboratory at the time of the police raid was "grossly unsanitary." As a result,
after review of this report by senior NIH officials, NIH determined that IBR had
failed in significant ways to comply with PHS policy and withdrew its funding.

Such a decision by NIH was not made lightly. Indeed, it was well-recognized
by Thomas E. Malone, Acting Director, and by other senior NIH officials that to
stop funding a project because of animal welfare concerns would cause bad
feeling, even ire, within the biomedical community. However, they believed it
would have been impossible for NIH to maintain credibility with the public and
Congress without this action.

Some segments of the research community came to Taub's defense. Neuroscientists in particular praised the value of Taub's research and the applicability
of his findings to human neurological disorders. A group of scientists from New
York University, Johns Hopkins, the University of Pennsylvania, and elsewhere
established a legal defense fund to help with his court expenses; the American
Psychological Association made a contribution from its organizational funds;
members of the Society for Neuroscience were urged by their president to send
checks. Taub garnered sympathy by presenting himself as a modern-day Galileo,
victimized as he said by "forces of ignorance and zealotry." In his court testimony, Taub said, "What has happened to my work harks back to the middle ages,
and to the period of religious inquisition, when scientists were burned at the
stake."

Court action proceeded and Taub was initially convicted on six counts. These
were later reduced to one, and later still in 1983 the conviction was reversed on
appeal on a technicality (the Maryland Court of Appeals ruled that the general
provisions of the state anti-cruelty statute do not apply to federally supported
scientific research). Taub and some members of the research community used

this decision to claim his vindication although nothing in the ruling contradicted the previous findings. The decision related only to the jurisdictional question. NIH held firm, and in 1982, the NIH director James B. Wyngaarden informed IBR that NIH reaffirmed its previous findings that IBR had failed to provide adequate veterinary care. IBR subsequently changed its name from Institute for Behavioral Research to Institutes for Behavioral Resources, which operates foster care facilities for young people and the mentally retarded in Washington, D.C.

Taub received a prestigious Guggenheim Fellowship in 1983, and in 1986 he was elected a Fellow of the American Association for the Advancement of Science at its Philadelphia conference. He has been hired as a professor of psychology at the University of Alabama, Birmingham, but has stopped conducting animal research.

Litigation has continued for several years over such questions as where the Silver Spring monkeys should be housed, whether any further experimentation should be conducted on them, and if and when individual animals should be killed. In mid-1992, some litigation was still not resolved.

University of Pennsylvania's head injury lab

The second raid came on May 28, 1984, when self-professed members of the ALF stole videotapes that recorded day-to-day experiments of Thomas A. Gennarelli, associate professor of Neurosurgery at the University of Pennsylvania and clinical director of the Regional Head Injury Center, in which baboons had been inflicted with serious head injuries. Also involved was Thomas W. Langfitt, chairperson of Neurosurgery and overseer of the work; he was the principal investigator on the Head Trauma Program Project grant from NIH of which Gennarelli's project was part.

The purpose of Gennarelli's research was to develop an animal model to study the functional and anatomical effects of head injury, such as that which occurs in car accidents, and thus provide insight into human head injuries. The experimental procedures involved securely cementing the head of each baboon in a helmet and subjecting the head to a sudden jerking movement delivered by a specially designed piston. The head jerks sharply back at an angle of about 60 degrees, and the body responds violently at the thrust. The neurological damage that results is proportional to the severity of impact and resultant coma.

These studies had received NIH funding for 15 years; in the year 1984, Gennarelli received about $330,000 for these studies. PETA and other animal rights groups repeatedly misrepresented the amount of money involved in the studies by citing the total composite grant to Langfitt—on the order of one million dollars a year—which covered not only the baboon studies (which amounted to a small fraction) but human studies of head injury.

The raiders stole videotapes and sabotaged a computer and other equipment, causing damage of approximately $20,000. ALF members handed over copies of the videotapes to PETA, and thereafter PETA acted as the front-persons and negotiators. In subsequent raids, PETA has continued to play this role.

PETA gave a copy of the 60-hour-long tapes to NIH. In addition, the group produced a half-hour of excerpts, which were widely shown both in the United States and abroad. This film was called *Unnecessary Fuss,* picking up on Gennarelli's words to the *Toronto Globe and Mail* when he had said he was "not willing to go on record to discuss the laboratory studies because it has the potential to stir up all sorts of unnecessary fuss among those who are sensitive to those kinds of things."

The tapes showed violations of the AWA, such as inadequate levels of anesthesia and non-sterile surgery on the baboons. A reporter for *Science* described the tapes as ranging from "embarrassing to disastrous" (Fox, 1984). The hallucinogenic drug phencyclidine, also known as "PCP" or "angel dust," was given to the primates to restrain them, but this is not an anesthetic. In one sequence of the film, a researcher can be heard to say, "the animal is off anesthesia" just before infliction of the brain injury. During the procedure of administering the head injury, the animals could be seen writhing on the operating table. The laboratory personnel mocked the injured animals.

Excerpts from the video "Unnecessary Fuss" were shown on NBC's "Nightly News" and "Today Show" and Cable News Network. Newspapers and radio stations were also quick to recount events and media attention reached international proportions. The film was an important mover in changing public and official opinion. It moved James J. Kilpatrick (who is no radical) to write a column entitled "Brutality and Laughter in the Lab," which ran in papers across the country. Kilpatrick (1985) wrote, "I watched [the video] a few days ago, and although I am no anti-vivisectionist, I found it appalling . . . Well, it was high time for someone to rescue these baboons." This video also affected the opinion of lawmakers in Congress, who later that year added significant strengthening amendments to the Animal Welfare Act.

By September, four months after the raid, congressional hearings were held about the use of federal funds for this research. PETA had planned to show *Unnecessary Fuss* at the hearings, but NIH and USDA officials threatened not to attend if the stolen tapes were shown. So PETA arranged showings at a nearby church during the lunch break, and I was among the many people who first saw the film there. The laboratory conditions depicted were such that it was hard going for many to watch. Respected newspaper columnist Henry Mitchell reported on September 21 in the *Washington Post* that seeing the film made him feel ill.

But defenders quickly came forward. Within weeks of the raid, NIH director Wyngaarden made a public statement describing Gennarelli's lab as "one of the best in the world." University of Pennsylvania officials said accurately that Gennarelli's experiments had, in the past, been reviewed repeatedly and found to conform to NIH guidelines. According to a report prepared by an investigating committee from the Society for Neuroscience chaired by Robert E. Burke, "the University's own animal care committee was particularly thorough and detailed" in its review of these baboon experiments which have "been conducted in accord with accepted standards of humane care. . . . Dr. Gennarelli made a convincing case that the . . . procedures represent an ethical and humane way to produce an animal model of human head trauma. This goal has been judged to be scientifically valid" (Society for Neuroscience, 1984). Langfitt argued that primates are the only useful subjects available for discovering what happens to the brain upon the moment of injury. He claimed that as a result of the studies from the University of Pennsylvania, researchers were on the threshold of discovering major improvements in the treatment of human head injuries caused by severe falls or automobile accidents. *The Bulletin of the American Association for Laboratory Animal Science* raised the "likelihood that animals in the [videotape] sequences were either anesthetized or already dead" (Anonymous, 1984)— suggestions not born out by the facts.

In contrast to the Silver Spring monkey case, NIH did not act promptly to cut off funding, but instead initiated an investigation. Each side blamed the other for the protracted nature of this inquiry. Twelve months after the raid, at its May 1985 meeting, the advisory council to the National Institute of Neurological and Communicative Disorders and Stroke (NINCDS) approved a recommendation from an NIH Study Section to renew Langfitt's grant (which included that of Gennarelli) for a further five years starting on August 1, 1985. The NIH Study Section had given a high priority score to this grant, in the 120s (on a scale of 100 to 500, with 100 being the best score). Everything was set for a renewal of Gennarelli's grant.

Opposed to a renewal of funding, members of the animal rights movement urged members of Congress to take action. In May, some sixty members of Congress petitioned Health and Human Services Secretary Margaret M. Heckler (who had authority over NIH) to stop the funding of this lab until the NIH investigation was complete. But Heckler did not act immediately.

As a result of the delays, the animal advocates undertook a major campaign of peaceful civil disobedience to press their case to stop this research. On July 15, 1985, some fourteen months after the initial raid, a sit-in started at NIH, organized by PETA. Over 100 advocates from across the country walked into the office suite of Murray Goldstein, director of NINCDS. According to a report in *The Animals' Agenda,* this was done "because professional backscratching and conflicts of interest have blocked every legal path." Many well-known animal rights proponents were among those who barricaded themselves in, including Alex Pacheco, Tom Regan, and Elliot Katz. Demonstrators draped a banner proclaiming "Cruelty and Deceit" from the outer windows; they had food delivered; they sang and chanted. As originally planned, the action was to have lasted only a few hours, not four days.

In an attempt to keep the protest at low profile, the police and NIH officials made no arrests. But media coverage mounted each day. As the sit-in went into its fourth day, Secretary Heckler announced, on July 18, that "until all questions about the use of primates in these head injury experiments have been satisfactorily resoled, I have instructed NIH to suspend the use of federal funds." NIH announced the same day that it had put the five-year renewal for Gennarelli's grant on hold (the other parts of Langfitt's grant were not affected). This suspension was done with a grace period though, and Gennarelli's existing grant was extended at the current level of funding for an additional six months, through January 1986. NIH required that the university negotiate a new "assurance" of compliance with PHS policy.

Penalties to the University of Pennsylvania finally came some 16 months after the raid. In August, USDA imposed a $4,000 fine for violations of the AWA in the university's baboon head injury lab. In September, Wyngaarden extended the suspension of the five-year grant renewal (although the grace-period funding was not affected). After reviewing the NIH committee's final report, Wyngaarden concluded that the university had "failed materially" to comply with conditions of the grant with respect to the care and use of non-human primates. In a September 23 letter to the university's medical school, Wyngaarden cited five areas of noncompliance and spelled out conditions the school must meet if funding were to be resumed. Among other problems, the deficiencies concerned management of anesthesia for the baboons, adequacy of techniques to achieve a sterile environment, and adequacy of the laboratory environment.

On the same date, a press release from the University of Pennsylvania announced that the university "has indefinitely suspended all research using primates in the Head Injury Clinical Research Laboratory at its Medical School and has reprimanded the researchers who were responsible for supervising the experiments." A letter of reprimand was sent from the university's president, Sheldon Hackney, and provost, Thomas Ehrlich, to Gennarelli and Langfitt. It stated, in part, "We conclude that there has been less than satisfactory discharge of the responsibility expected of research faculty at the university." The university officials noted, however, that the primate research is highly regarded by peers and is of great importance to human welfare. In a published response, Gennarelli and Langfitt expressed regret about some of the deficiencies (Gennarelli and Langfitt, 1985).

What has happened since then? Gennarelli has continued his research without using primates. In a new NIH award to run from 1991 to 1996, Gennarelli will use the same head injury device that was the subject of the raid not on primates, but on minipigs.

Some members of the biomedical community at first spurned the film *Unnecessary Fuss,* refusing to view it or to purchase it from PETA. However, after training programs for laboratory personnel were mandated by Congress in 1985, NIH was among the first to start using this as a training film for investigators. A number of labs now use this film in a similar way.

The Animal Liberation Front

The University of Pennsylvania raid marked the presence of the Animal Libera-tion Front, an international underground movement, in the United States. It originated in the 1970s in England, evolving from a group called the Band of Mercy whose members sabotaged the vehicles of hunters and destroyed guns used in bird shoots. In 1973, members of the Band of Mercy decided that their campaign should expand to include all forms of animal exploitation. Not only were laboratories targeted for infiltration and raids, but also biological supply houses, abattoirs, chicken farms, butchers' shops, fur salons, hunting events, live pigeon shoots, and other activities that involve harming and killing animals. The ALF views animal research as the most powerful symbol of human domin-ion over and exploitation of animals, and it devotes much of its energies to this issue. Active ALF chapters are believed to exist now in forty-five countries including several in Europe, Australia, New Zealand, Africa, and Canada, as well as the United States.

The American wing of the ALF was formed in 1981. Since spokespersons remain anonymous, the names of individuals associated with this group are largely unknown. The number of its members is unknown, and pictures show only ALF members with masked faces. In the United States only one ALF member has served a prison term, several have in England. Only three convic-tions have resulted from illegal laboratory raids.

In 1986, the California attorney general declared the ALF a terrorist organiza-tion. Three ALF raids are listed in the FBI's 1990 publication *Terrorism in the United States*. These university raids are arson at Davis, California, 1987; arson in Tucson, Arizona, 1989; and "malicious destruction of property" at Lubbock, Texas, also in 1989 (the Orem case, see below).

PETA, while claiming that it does not participate in ALF operations, is pre-pared to publicize any documentation of improper use of animals that the ALF or any whistleblower uncovers. There is a very close association between the two organizations; they appear to work hand-in-glove. ALF does the raid, and PETA publicizes the results. PETA has therefore become the focus of antagonism voiced by the pro-animal research community.

Subsequent raids

Several raids followed. In 1984, the City of Hope Medical Center in Duarte, California, was raided and more than 100 animals stolen; the raiders alleged violations of the AWA, and following a subsequent investigation and surprise site visit by NIH staff, NIH suspended funding of approximately $5 million for animal research at this facility (problems were with veterinary care, physical environment, and administrative oversight). USDA also fined the City of Hope $11,000 for violations of the AWA.

In 1985, there was a raid at the University of California, Riverside in which the ALF stole at least 260 animals, including one infant monkey with sutured eyelids being used in a sensory deprivation experiment and test of the efficacy of an auditory aid. NIH investigated and found no problems with the facility except for the eye suturing procedure, which had been too deep and had caused potential corneal damage.

In 1986, NIH received photographs of alleged violations at Columbia University from the New York City ALF. NIH staff then made a surprise site visit and subsequently suspended funding for animal research at the facility (problems were insufficient veterinary care and other infractions). In each case of suspended funding, when deficiencies had been corrected, NIH restored funding.

The spate of suspended NIH funding ended, but not the raids. A sampling of other institutions raided includes the following: the University of Oregon, Eugene (1986, $38,000 worth of damage done and 125 animals stolen); SEMA Inc., of Rockville, Maryland, a facility under contract with NIH (1986, four baby chimps stolen, possibly harboring non-A non-B hepatitis); the University of California, Davis (1987, arson at the Veterinary Diagnostic Laboratory believed to be the work of the ALF with damage estimated at close to $5 million); the University of California, Irvine (1988, ALF stole thirteen beagles from the Air Pollution Health Effects Laboratory); the University of Arizona (1988, arson that took over fifty firefighters more than an hour to quell, vandalism, and over 1200 animals stolen by the ALF, some infected with a pathogenic organism that could cause a dangerous form of dysentery); the University of Pennsylvania, offices of Adrian R. Morrison, a sleep researcher (1990, files stolen, and later some rats stolen from another researcher's lab). In many of these raids, walls of the research facilities were defaced with spray-painted slogans. Typical are "We Shall Return," "Nowhere is Safe," "Vivisection Will End," "Stop the Torture," and "Scum." Another common feature has been destruction or theft of research results so that researchers were faced with the devastation of losing years of research data.

Damage to labs has been costly. According to data reported to the Association of American Medical Colleges in 1990, the cost of lost data, break-in damage, property defacement, and demonstrations has mounted to $3.5 million and 15,000 staff hours over the past five years (Holden, 1990). This information was based on a survey of 124 of the 126 American medical schools.

One immediate effect of the early raids, probably related to the suspension of government funding, was that institutional financial resources that were traditionally hard to obtain for improvement of animal facilities became more readily available.

Among some researchers, there has been widespread fear about which facility will be targeted next by the raiders. Shakespeare wrote, "In time we hate that which we often fear."

For the researchers, the raids have had a demoralizing effect. According to a study by Michele Trankina (1992), a feeling of frustration appears widespread in the scientific community. Trankina found that 50 percent of the scientists she surveyed were dissatisfied for a number of reasons with their work, but among the life scientists, respondents cited the animal rights movement as a major reason for their dissatisfaction. Commenting on this report, the Foundation for Biomedical Research says "animal rights activists have been able to wield tremendous influence" within the scientific community.

The National Association for Biomedical Research and other pro-research organizations have rallied support for their cause by emphasizing the fear of raids and deploring the property destruction and personal threats. Along with the American Physiological Society and other affiliates of the Federation of American Societies for Experimental Biology, NABR has launched public awareness campaigns about the benefits of animal research and has sponsored media training for researchers so that they can effectively explain their work. For instance, regional affiliates of NABR have produced films and other materials explaining why animal experiments are done and the resulting benefits to human health.

The Society for Neuroscience has also been active. It has coordinated a letter-writing campaign in support of animal research under siege and in 1989, their then-president, Nobel Laureate David Hubel, urged physician-members of the society to let their patients know about the benefits of animal research. Hubel wrote to members of the Society suggesting that a note to this effect should be added at the bottom of the doctor's bill or prescription form.

Before the raids, it was fairly easy for anyone to walk into animal holding facilities and laboratories, but this is no longer the case in many institutions. Entry can be highly restricted; it is common practice that special passes are needed to gain entry to key doorways. Commercial companies that specialize in security of facilities have discovered a new market. A typical ad for such a firm promises "to bring the full capacity of its worldwide security, consulting and investigative services to bear on animal rights terrorism." In some, but not all, labs, a sense of openness is gone.

Large amounts of money have been devoted to installing security systems. According to 1990 American Association of Medical Schools data, installation and maintenance of security systems intended to protect research facilities had cost the institutions $5.5 million over the past five years (Holden, 1990).

This high security awareness is not present at all facilities. Some labs, even after being raided, are not plagued with "fortress mentality." "We researchers have no desire to turn our public institution into a fortress," says one researcher. "We do what we do in the public interest. We are not reluctant to explain it."

NABR and NIH have been active in organizing conferences to discuss how security of animal labs should best be handled. Typical of the topics covered are risk assessment, perimeter security, internal controls, and education and training of personnel. At one of the early NABR conferences on security, it was an embarrassment that the conference itself was infiltrated by an animal rights person. Since then, security about who can attend has been tightened.

Personnel screening and security checks on applicants for jobs have become important. PETA openly encourages its constituency to get a job in a lab (Brebner and Baer, undated). Also the Progressive Animal Welfare Society has issued a notice stating, "Do you work with research animals and deplore the cruelty? Are you an office worker with access to information?" Insiders are then encouraged to forward the facts to PAWS.

At an NIH conference on lab security, one administrator at an animal facility described the failure to check on a new employee who later turned out to be an animal rights person gathering intelligence with professional surveillance equipment. He said that the institution had ignored something that should have tipped them off: the new hire was a vegetarian. "Do your background checks and do 'em good," he urged (Powledge, 1989). Presumably, the message was that vegetarians may need close observation, not that all vegetarians make unreliable lab workers.

In a constructive approach, several research facilities have now established in-house policies designed to curb whistleblowing and to provide formal channels for reporting allegations of animal abuse.

NABR has been in the forefront of pressing for enactment of special criminal laws against laboratory break-ins. As of June, 1992, twenty-four states now have specifically outlawed such activities as entering a laboratory without permission, releasing animals, disrupting experiments, and removing documents and photographs related to research. Legislation is pending in nine other states. The penalties vary from state to state; for instance, Washington state provides for fines up to $100,000 in a civil lawsuit in addition to any actual damages awarded.

At the federal level, a Farm Animal and Research Facilities Protection Act of 1992 has been sponsored by Representative Charles Stenholm (D-TX) in the House and Senator Howell Heflin (D-AL) in the Senate. This proposed legislation would make it a federal crime (and thus trigger investigation by the FBI) to steal, to cause unauthorized release or intentional loss of any laboratory animal, to break and enter a research facility, or to receive, conceal, or retain any material from a raid. These bills have received wide support from the research community including the AVMA, FASEB, and many others.

Animal welfare and animal rights groups have generally opposed the legislation as unnecessary, unfair to laboratory employees, and believe it would stop individuals from calling public attention to improper animal treatment. They hold that the law should protect whistleblowers who report improprieties in laboratory animal use. The American Civil Liberties Union (ACLU) has agreed with this assessment, asserting that the individual worker's right to report sub-standard laboratory employees needs to be protected. The ACLU was also concerned that this legislation would prohibit the news media from publishing leaked information. Certain significant amendments were made in the wording of the bill to accommodate these objections. Under the new name Animal Enterprise Protection Act of 1992, President George Bush signed the measure into law on August 7.

The issue of violence

The use of violence (bombs, arson, and personal harassment) by extremists has brought criticism to the animal rights movement. In England there have been several episodes involving bombs both with intent to destroy property and to cause personal injury, in one case injuring a baby in a pram nearby. In the United States, bombs have been used to destroy laboratory property.

Arson has been used frequently against a number of U.S. animal facilities including Michigan State University (see Figure 11.1). On one occasion, six fires were set in one night in various parts of England during ALF actions against furriers. Although no one has been hurt as a result of the use of arson, it is obviously a dangerous tactic. It is highly questionable that much of the public would go along with setting fires as a justifiable means of protest.

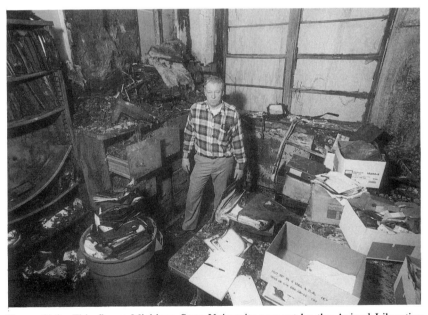

Figure 11.1 This fire at Michigan State University was set by the Animal Liberation Front on February 28, 1992, and caused $75,000 worth of damage according to a university spokesperson. Richard Aulerich, shown in his office, conducts toxicology and nutrition research using mink as experimental animals. This raid is the third of a series targeting mink research over the last year.

Even animal rights advocates themselves are questioning the use of violence in raids. For instance, critical comments appeared in the pages of the animal rights magazine *The Animals' Agenda* about the arson and vandalism at Michigan State University (Melville, 1992). The writer asked to open up a general discussion on the use of violence in raids and asked, "If the ALF care so much about life, why would they set a fire which might endanger others?"

Personal harassment of research investigators seems to have increased in recent years. Some investigators have, with good reason, feared not only for themselves but for the lives of their families. Death threats have been received. On occasion, animal rights groups have targeted investigators' homes—a form of personal harassment that brings with it great fear to the families concerned. Under this extreme duress, some investigators have changed their method or area of experimentation or have left research.

One case marked by egregious personal harassment involved John M. Orem, a professor of physiology at Texas Tech University. The case received considerable attention in *The Chronicle of Higher Education* (Mangan, 1990) and caused outrage in the scientific community. According to Orem, his NIH-funded cat research was relevant to sleep disorders such as apnea and Sudden Infant Death Syndrome (SIDS), although the relevance of Orem's work to SIDS has been disputed by animal rights groups. Approximately 5,000 children die of sleep breathing disorders each year, and methods to control these deaths are much needed.

On July 4, 1989, the ALF broke into Orem's laboratory and stole five cats and research data and destroyed equipment estimated to be worth between $50,000 and $70,000. The ALF said in a prepared statement (provided by PETA) that Orem's research techniques, such as bolting the cats' heads into steel clamps, were inhumane. Orem responded at a press conference, saying, "This is all sensational nonsense. The techniques we use are standard neurological procedures that are done under anesthesia. There is nothing gruesome, despicable, wasteful or barbaric about it. . . . The cats are given great care." According to *The Chronicle,* Orem received several death threats and thousands of pieces of hate mail. He told reporters, "Every move I make, I have to inform the police. The entire atmosphere is unpleasant."

Such tactics are as offensive to those who believe in the animal welfare cause as they are to scientists. Such intimidation and violence have undermined whatever effectiveness the raids initially had in winning public sympathy for the animal rights crusade.

Some allies of the Animal Liberation Front speak up in defense of violence, including the use of life-threatening tactics. According to one commentator, a leading ALF member in England, "I can support petrol bombing, bombs under cars, and probably shootings at a later stage. It's a war" (Henshaw, 1989). Vickie

Miller (1986), founder of an animal rights group in Canada, wrote, "This decade will see the first acts of true violence. Some may be accidental—like a bystander killed in a bomb blast. Some will be deliberate like a vivisector shot in the streets. The violence will confuse and divide us, but it will be a temporary adjustment and then we will learn to live with it as has every social movement before us." Sometimes veiled threats are apparent, as in the words of Steve Siegel (1989), director of Trans-Species Unlimited: "We must refuse to accept limits being placed on the lengths to which we will go to save [laboratory animals]."

In a series of articles on civil disobedience in the Hastings Center Report, Christine M. Jackson (1989), the senior correspondent for PETA, wrote, "ALF has expressed repeatedly, through anonymous representatives, its policy of non-violence." She quoted one spokesperson for the ALF as saying, "It is one of the rules of ALF that no one will be injured. Property yes, people, no. No one has ever been harmed in an ALF raid." It need hardly be pointed out that the use of arson would not qualify for many people as "nonviolent."

Five well-known leaders in the animal rights movement have condemned violence. Writing in *The Animals' Agenda* in May 1985, Singer, Spira, Michael W. Fox, Holly Jensen, and Patty Mark stated their position: "We do not place animals before people; all should be given fair consideration. Threatening the lives and health of any human or non-human is an act of unjustified violence and contrary to our basic beliefs."

The Animal Rights Direct Action Group of San Francisco has issued a "Nonviolence Agreement" (undated). Participants in their "actions" agree to comply with the following:

1. Our attitude will be one of openness and respect toward all whom we encounter.
2. We will use no violence, physical or verbal.
3. We will not damage property.
4. We will not run or use threatening motions.
5. We will carry no weapons.
6. We will not bring or use any drugs, including alcohol.

Some humane organizations also have condemned violence. For instance, a resolution drafted in 1990 by the ASPCA, Massachusetts SPCA, and the Humane Society of the United States proclaimed: "[W]e oppose threats and acts of violence against people and willful destruction and theft of property. . . . We shall energetically work to reduce [the use of animals as experimental subjects] through non-violent means" (Hoyt and Stephens, 1990). Also, the International Association Against Painful Experiments on Animals, an organization representing sixty groups worldwide, expressed the view that "the recent bomb outrages against researchers [in England] must surely be condemned by all responsible organisations working for the better treatment of animals. Certainly this Association . . . utterly repudiates this form of activity" (Anonymous, 1990).

In advice to the animal rights movement, Regan (1987) says

Many activists, understandably impatient with the pace of change, are ready to commit acts of violence. Whilst sympathizing with their frustration, we all need to recognize that there are *other* steps that can be taken. There are steps leading to nonviolent civil disobedience. The time has come for every person seriously committed to the struggle for animal rights to consider taking these steps. . . . I am a strong supporter of civil disobedience. I engage in it myself. As a strategy, Civil Disobedience is the last, not the first, choice. Other nonviolent methods for effecting social change—discussions and boycotts, for example—must first be tried. Only when these approaches have met with unresponsiveness should Civil Disobedience be used. . . .

I was one of the 101 people who occupied the eighth floor of Building 39 at the National Institutes of Health [in the Gennarelli case]. I don't think the media presented us poorly there at all. I think the media presented us as a real triumph. And that was because the CD was *very* well chosen, was *very* well organized, *very* well focused. . . . When we left NIH, we ran the sweepers, we washed the windows, we cleaned up, we polished. We made it as clean as it could be. All the signs were taken down, no spray paint, none of that stuff. It would just be detrimental.

There appears to have been an overall decline in public support for laboratory raids. At least two factors have contributed: the increased use of violence, and the decrease in public outrage about conditions uncovered in the raids. In recent years, raids have not uncovered evidence of such poor conditions as in previous raids. I believe there is now a general sense that whatever contribution raids made in the early 1980s to alerting NIH to be more vigilant and to persuading Congress to enact stronger legislation, the impact of raids has waned. Perhaps raids have now run their course. I and many others hope so.

12

The Use of Animals in Education

In the United States, the use of animals in education has been largely uncontrolled by legislation, and national policy on the subject is in its infancy. The Animal Welfare Act specifically exempts elementary and secondary schools from its provisions and, historically, has barely touched the use of animals at the college level. Although, strictly speaking, colleges that use any of the AWA protected species do fall within the province of the law, until recently enforcement mechanisms for control over student projects have been so weak that there has been no meaningful oversight. Since no educational use of animals in the elementary and secondary schools and virtually none at college levels receives Public Health Service funding, these schools fall outside the purview of PHS policy. A tiny fraction of PHS funds does go to support training in universities, and this is the only area in education where PHS policy applies.

A new rule was issued by the USDA in 1989 that has the effect of law. For the first time, it makes college-level instruction involving animal experimentation subject to review by Institutional Animal Care and Use Committees. The new rule requires that all activities, including "those elements of . . . teaching procedures that involve the care and use of animals," be reviewed by an institutional oversight committee for compliance with nationally accepted standards (Federal Register, 1989).

This regulation affects student use of animals in all facilities that fall under the AWA and therefore are registered with and inspected by the USDA. This includes all major universities. But many educational institutions are not affected because they do not use any of the regulated species—that is, they use only rats, mice, birds, and cold-blooded species, the species most commonly used for educational purposes. This is true of many smaller colleges and community colleges.

Despite these exclusions, this strengthening of the law is having an influence. The major universities have a dominant role in setting standards. The improvements they make in the use of animals tend eventually to raise standards in other educational establishments.

Review practices at the college level

Review practices for animal experiments vary according to whether or not the institution is subject to the provisions of the AWA. Those educational institutions that fall outside the AWA would rarely, if ever, have an IACUC, and the animal procedures would not be open to federal inspection. Decisions regarding what animal experiments are to be included in student training are made largely by individual faculty members, or by the faculty within a particular department. Generally, decisions are based on perceived educational value and budgetary considerations. It would be up to these institutions themselves to establish formal in-house policies regarding humane use of animals. Any failures to maintain proper standards in animal housing or experimental procedures would be corrected as a result of individual conscience, peer pressure from other teachers, from students, or from the public.

On the other hand, educational institutions that fall under the AWA have to have an IACUC. These committees now require both researchers and teachers to submit written protocols of proposed animal experiments for approval prior to proceeding. This extension to include teachers affects both undergraduate and graduate student use of animals. It also extends the range of issues open to question and review. Since 1989, these issues include such controversial questions as: Should a medical student whose career objective does not include animal surgery receive such training? Should a veterinary student induce pathological conditions and/or surgically manipulate a normal, healthy animal, or should naturally occurring clinical cases be substituted? Does a student have a right to conscientious objection from lab exercises that involve harming or destroying animals? In what situations can alternative exercises be substituted that do not inflict pain or death on sentient animals but that achieve the same or similar educational objectives? Teachers of the biological sciences continue to maintain strongly the need to experiment on, and sometimes to kill animals for the purposes of education. But the expansion of the review process has already resulted in more careful examination of what is done in the name of biology education.

Animals are used in a wide variety of ways in undergraduate courses in biology, zoology, psychology, physiology, pharmacology, and nursing. Live animal studies can range from observation of opened-up turtles to giving electric shocks to rats to study their behavior. Many animals also are used in dissection after death.

Not much information is available on the numbers of animals used in education at the undergraduate and graduate levels of education. Perhaps the most informative survey in the United States was conducted by the Association of American Medical Colleges during the school year 1983 to 1984 in 16 accredited medical schools (out of a total of 127 such schools). The 16 were selected to achieve balance in ownership, geographic region, and research expenditure. The AAMC found that all 16 used animals in some disciplines, the most common being physiology (10 of 16 schools), surgery (10 of 16), and pharmacology (8 of 16). So even in medical schools there are wide differences in opinion on when animal experimentation is essential and when it is not. In all, 7,274 animals were used that year, comprising 14 primates, 1,771 dogs, 279 cats, 64 pigs, 378 rabbits, and 5,172 rats, mice, guinea pigs, hamsters, and other species.

Universities are not always willing to cooperate in such surveys. In England, the prestigious Institute of Medical Ethics failed in their recent attempt to survey universities about the use of animals in education; an inquiry circulated to all U.K. universities yielded only one reply (Smith and Boyd, 1991).

Professional training: veterinary and medical schools

Traditionally in medical and veterinary schools animals have been used for physiology and pharmacology demonstrations (so-called "dog labs"). Often these are acute studies (no recovery of consciousness). Also, many species of animals have been commonly used for practice surgery, and these can involve recovery from the anesthetic. The surgery can range from practice in sewing up incisions to removal of vital organs and practice repair procedures. Another type of study that is quite common in emergency medical training is allowing different students to intubate a live cat repeatedly. The rationale is that since it is harder to intubate a cat than a baby, then to do it on a cat is good practice. The insertion of a large tube down the windpipe can be painful for the cat and damage can result. Sometimes the same animals are used over and over again. Alternatives exist for all these exercises (see, for instance, USDA/AWIC, 1989, Dunayer 1990, and PCRM undated).

A few medical, veterinary, and nursing students have been vocal in protesting these practices. Some have refused to participate and have objected that these labs can desensitize students to non-human suffering, and that harming healthy animals is not consistent with the goals of being a caring physician, veterinarian, or nurse. Some veterinary students are now saying that they will conduct surgery only when it benefits the animal, such as using client animals for spaying and neutering and correcting naturally occurring pathological states. It is thus that many human surgeons are trained. At North Carolina State University and the University of Illinois, plastic bones are now used by veterinary students to learn to drill, pin, and wire instead of using actual dog bones. Combining this method with operating on thawed frozen chickens in junior surgery, the University of Illinois saves about 100 dogs a year while cutting costs.

A number of medical schools have also adopted alternatives to live animal studies. According to the Physicians Committee for Responsible Medicine (1992), twelve medical schools have no animal laboratory exercises in their regular curriculum for medical students. The list includes Ohio State, Tufts, Michigan State, SUNY-Stony Brook, and the University of Washington. This same source indicates that "at nearly all the remaining medical schools, participation in animal laboratory exercises is optional."

John S. Najarian, M.D., in his 1989 presidential address to the American Surgical Association said, "In the past, many have felt that the craft of surgery can be best learned in the animal laboratory. But with decreasing surgical research with large animals, the so-called 'dog surgery' experience is becoming more and more a thing of the past. The actual craft is now learned in the operating room through assistance, followed by progressive, guided, direct experience, and eventually more independence."

In recent years there has been a considerable shift in interest among scientists to the cell and molecular rather than organ levels. This makes it easier to find suitable student projects that do not require whole animal experimentation.

Formal policies to permit conscientious objection have been adopted by educational institutions at all levels. They are probably most frequently encountered in veterinary schools. Nine out of the 27 veterinary schools in the United States have announced formal policies that permit students to use alternatives to harmful use of animals in their training. They are Colorado State, Tufts, Pennsylvania, Cornell, Minnesota, Washington State, Michigan State, Florida, and the University of California at Davis. One of the leading schools in this movement was Tufts whose dean, Franklin M. Loew, has written, "Our students were like conscientious objectors in time of war—they felt they couldn't work on animals whose only purpose was to be killed for teaching students. I don't view this as an assault on standard practice; I think it's a reflection of the times and the mind-set of the students now in veterinary school" (quoted in Boddy, 1989).

Very occasionally, universities have resisted when an individual student has requested an alternative study. When a court challenge has ensued, the student's right to object has invariably been upheld. A hard line has been taken by a military medical school, the Uniformed Services University of the Health Sciences, in Bethesda, Maryland, where students are required to sign away their rights of conscientious objection to pedagogic animal experiments on admittance. This has raised objections among some members of Congress.

Increasingly it has become standard practice for universities and colleges to announce ahead of time if animal use is involved in any particular course. Most universities include information in the course announcement. If a student objects to the animal project, then he must negotiate with the teacher for alternative studies.

High school dissection and alternatives

At the high school level, it was the issue of conscientious objection that first focused attention on dissection. In the mid-1980s, some teenagers began to refuse to dissect frogs, fetal pigs, cats, and other species in their high school biology classes because they had a moral objection. The issue of whether or not dissections of vertebrate animals should be retained, cut back, or omitted from pre-college education has now grown into a major controversy.

Steps to reduce and even to phase out dissection of frogs, fetal pigs, cats, dogs, and other species have been taken by some junior and senior high schools. This change in curriculum is being hailed by some as a much-needed reform that will make room for more pertinent labs better suited to today's educational needs. Voicing such a view, Juliana Texley (1987), a high school teacher and editor of *The Science Teacher* wrote, "Teachers have to ask themselves what laboratory experiences will be most valuable to the majority of tomorrow's adults." She concluded "Perhaps it's time to cut dissection down to size."

But to others, dissection represents far more than just a worthwhile student exercise: the retention of dissection is a cause that must be supported because it is part of a fight for the defense of animal experimentation as a whole—a fight of science versus antiscience. From this point of view, to give up any dissections is to cave in to the antivivisectionist and animal welfare causes. One biology teacher has damned a booklet that includes suggestions for alternatives to dissection as an "antiscience tract" and "evil" (Bentley, 1991). Groups that have previously not been noted for their interest in high school biology education have taken up the cause. As reported on the front page of *USA Today,* the American Medical Association announced at a press conference on April 2, 1991 that they will step up efforts to keep dissection in the classroom. Several animal rights groups and antivivisection groups have established programs to stop dissection in the high schools. Underlying these initiatives may be a belief that questioning animal dissection may lead to questioning of other human uses of animals. So a modest change in curriculum has been escalated into a major ideological battle. The issue is being redefined; it is no longer the pros and cons of conscientious objection, but rather animal experimentation versus antivivisection.

Frog dissection seems to have started in the 1920s (Orlans, 1988). It has been part of the curriculum for over fifty years and has become a rite of passage in high school biology. In 1969, approximately nine million wild-caught frogs were shipped by U.S. suppliers to educational institutions; just under half of them were preserved preparations, the remainder being alive (Gibbs et al., 1971). In the late 1980s, according to several leading educators, approximately 75 to 80 percent of the total of four million high school students participate in frog dissection (Orlans, 1988). If each student has one frog, then approximately three million frogs are destroyed each year for high school use alone (not counting use at other educational levels). Recently, fetal pigs, obtained as a side product from abatoirs, have also become popular for dissection; and in some high schools, cats and dogs are used also. Sometimes more than one vertebrate animal is dissected in addition to some invertebrate animals like worms.

The recent controversy dates back to April 1987, when Jenifer Graham, a 15-year-old student in Victorville, California, refused to dissect a frog because she had moral objections. She was told by her school that she would fail the course if she refused the dissection. She asked to be given an alternative study but this was refused because dissection was part of the curriculum. She persisted in her views and was initially given a "D" grade—later upgraded to a "C"—for this class. Jenifer was an "A" student, so this low grade was not acceptable and she took the matter to court, helped by the Humane Society of the United States. She contended that her ethical beliefs are equivalent to a religion and that the school district had violated her right to freedom of religion under the First Amendment.

Several court hearings occurred. In June 1988 the court ruled that the state education system does not require dissection for preparation for admission to California colleges or universities. This undermined one of the high school's major arguments in its refusal to allow Jenifer to receive credit for alternative study. In August 1988, a federal judge dismissed the case and offered a compromise; Jenifer's knowledge of frog anatomy should be tested by using a frog that had died of natural causes. The judge apparently did not know how extraordinarily difficult it is to find a whole dead frog in the wild. This unfeasible "solution" upholds Jenifer's right to refuse to dissect a frog, while it also upholds the school's view that it can insist on testing knowledge of frog anatomy on a real frog, not on a model as had been proposed. The school never did come up with a frog that had died a natural death, and Jenifer left high school with the matter unresolved.

Jenifer's case marked the beginning of several campaigns by student groups, humane societies, and animal rights groups. They used slogans such as "Say No to Dissection" and "Don't Cut the Frog, Cut the Class."

Among the several ensuing court cases was one in 1989 in Frankville, New Jersey, where 15-year-old Maggie McCool refused to participate in biology labs that involved dissection of frogs, fetal pigs, and other animals. As a result, she received an "F" grade for this class. Protesting this grade, she went to court. The American Civil Liberties Union joined the case on the side of the student. An out-of-court settlement required the school to recalculate Maggie's grade excluding the lab section of the course, and the school board to issue a statement in the student handbook that any students with sincere religious beliefs about dissection must be offered alternative course work.

Jenifer Graham's case also led to the enactment of the 1988 California Students' Rights Law, which upholds the right of a student under the age of 18 to conscientious objection to dissection—specifically to educational projects "involving the harmful or destructive use of animals." If the teacher believes that an adequate alternative is possible, then the student and teacher must work together to develop an alternative. The passage of this law attracted national attention.

Three other states, Florida, Maine, and Pennsylvania, have also taken action to permit students in elementary and secondary schools to refuse participation in dissection. Florida was the first state to pass such a law in 1985. It allows such students to be excused from dissection of a dead animal upon written request of a parent or guardian. This law also prohibits surgery or dissection on living mammals in elementary and secondary schools and specifically prohibits experiments that would cause "physiological harm" on live vertebrate animals. In Maine, the state's commissioner of education sent out a policy advisory in 1989 to the superintendents of public schools suggesting that teachers inform students they can choose not to dissect and can do an alternative project. The Pennsylvania Student Rights Option Law of 1992 grants kindergarten through 12th grade students the right to refuse to participate in dissection.

Jenifer later made a television commercial for Apple Computers. Apple markets a dissection program called "Operation Frog" which is often cited and used as an alternative to actual dissection. The ad, which lasts 30 seconds, was spoken by Jenifer. The full text was: "Last year in my biology class, I refused to dissect a frog. I didn't want to hurt a living thing. I said I would be happy to do it on an Apple computer. That way, I can learn and the frog lives. But that got me into a lot of trouble, and I got a lower grade. So this year, I'm using my Apple II to study something entirely new—constitutional law." (This last was said with a twinkle in her eye, and was an obvious reference to her then ongoing court battle).

This message was greeted with alarm by the California Biomedical Research Association, an affiliate of NABR, which circulated an "action alert" urging people to protest to Apple President John Sculley. This alert said that the ad was "in very poor taste and offensive" to science educators, that it "advances the cause of fanatics," and that Apple was contributing to "dangerous and simpleminded thinking." A spokesperson for the Association of American Universities said that the ad "was a cute marketable commercial for anti-vivisection." A spokesperson for iiFAR (incurably ill For Animal Research) called the ad "harmful" and wrote, "Campaigns by various animal rights and anti-vivisectionist organizations to eliminate the dissection of animals in high school class rooms have only one purpose—to produce future generations of animal activists, and to discourage young people from making animal research a vocational choice."

The ad was withdrawn after it had been running for several weeks.

CBS made a movie for national television recounting Jenifer's story. It was presented as a case study on the theme of the price paid for standing up for your beliefs and challenging the establishment. The movie was first aired in October, 1989, and was also distributed along with a teacher's handbook to be used for classroom debates on the issue of conscientious objection. It showed the harassment by the school administration and the ridicule of her classmates. This was balanced against the success of getting the California Students' Rights law passed, in which hearings Jenifer played an important role.

Meanwhile, the Animal Legal Defense Fund established a program to help students to exert their rights to conscientious objection, to learn about alternatives to dissection, and to provide legal counsel where needed. This included a hotline toll-free number (1-800-922-FROG) and brochures for both teachers and students advising them how to proceed if faced with these issues. The hotline received an average of 800 to 1000 calls per month in 1991.

The harvesting of wild native frogs is not without problems. Conservationists first became concerned about the depletion of native frogs in the late 1960s and cited the over-collection of *Rana pipiens* for use in biology classes as one of he causes (Gibbs et al., 1971). More recent evidence shows continued depletion of these valuable species (Barinaga, 1990).

There is also concern about the capture and transportation methods, which can cause disease and death. After capture, the frogs are stored in sackloads, often for protracted periods, before arriving at the biological supply house. During this period, they may develop red leg disease from overcrowding or may die from dehydration. No economic incentive works in the animals' favor since they can be sold alive and healthy, diseased, or dead.

The methods of capturing and killing cats destined for dissection have also been a matter of concern. In 1990, media attention was given to an exposé of a major supplier, Carolina Biological Supply Company of Burlington, North Carolina. In a national TV news report, live cats were seen being delivered to the supply house by a dealer who had previously been convicted of stealing pet animals. The cats were brutally beaten on the head with sticks and forced into a gas chamber. Several high school teachers have told me that some of the cats they have received for dissection show signs of bruising and that the students inquire where these bruises have come from.

Educators who want to keep dissection in the high school classroom offer a number of arguments in favor of this position. They contend that dissection enables students to learn about internal structures, the interrelationships among tissues, and the physical placement of organs, and helps them to develop manipulative skills.

Supporters of dissection often stress the benefits of hands-on experience. The hands-on argument holds that the knowledge gained thereby has more impact, is retained longer, or is understood better than if models, charts, or learning from textbooks are substituted. A literature search yielded little evidence that this widely held view is substantiated by rigorous educational testing. Indeed, considering the widespread use and long history of dissection, it is surprising how little educational evaluation of the practice has been done.

It is believed by some that dissection has a hardening effect on attitudes toward animals. An experienced biology teacher reports that he has observed a wide variety of student behavior ranging from "excitement to revulsion and fear" (Lieb, 1985). He has seen some students physically shaking while handling dead animals and has noticed that others cut dissection classes entirely.

There has been widespread media attention to the sense of moral offense that some students feel. Even cartoons depict this (see for instance Figure 12.1). For those who saw the movie *E.T.*, some will remember the scene where children, under E.T.'s influence, release frogs intended for the dissection knife.

It is inevitable that some student dissections will be done poorly. The additional disfigurement that comes from poorly performed dissection only adds to the sense of desecration felt by objectors. Disrespectful attitudes and larking around—a frequent human behavioral response to stressful situations—can amplify the unease of some students.

It has been claimed by both sides that teenagers' career choices can be affected by dissection—for some it attracts them to a career in science, for others it turns them off. It would seem though that there are many ways to present science as a worthwhile career to teenagers without involving animal death.

At one time, one dissection in the upper grade levels at high school was the norm. But now, multiple dissections of vertebrate animals are not uncommon in some school systems despite the availability of alternatives. In recent years, dissections have become more common in junior high and middle schools, and even in elementary schools. A number of parents whose young children have

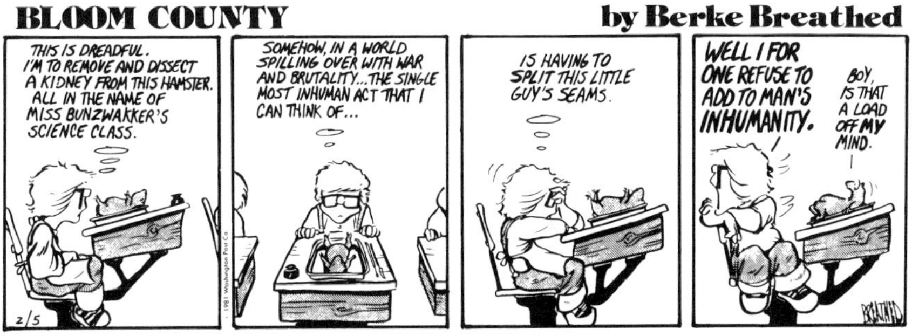

Figure 12.1 This Bloom County cartoon by Berke Breathed was first published in 1981 and carries an animal rights message of sympathy toward animals. This is an early example of what has later become widespread in popular culture. Examples of animal rights messages can now be found in movies (such as *E.T.*), television shows, fiction, rock music, etc.

been given dissections to do in class have voiced their objections. According to Pat Graham, the director of the dissection hotline, approximately 300 phone calls per month (a third of the total) are received from parents of elementary school students who hold such views.

An informal survey of teachers in Ohio showed that for many middle and high school teachers, dissection of dead animals is the *only* way they use animals (Mayer and Hinton, 1990). How can biology be taught properly if the students never study anything living? William V. Mayer (1973), the late director of the Biological Science Curriculum Study, said, "It is unfortunate to find in many schools that laboratory exercises in biology, which is defined as the study of life, are confined to the dissection of pickled specimens." It would seem that teachers are not adequately encouraged to maintain and study live creatures in the classroom.

The current over-reliance of some teachers on dissection comes at the expense of other laboratory studies. While instruction in mathematics and other sciences seems to have kept reasonable pace with advances in knowledge and broadening of perspectives, one wonders whether, in some respects, instruction in biology is not overly preoccupied with anatomical structure and memorization of details that will soon be forgotten. The new attention being given to high school biology instruction by professional scientific associations may well have a beneficial effect in keeping teachers abreast of the volume of new scientific information that has accumulated over recent years.

On a practical note, since only a very small percentage of students will need dissection skills in future careers, teachers and parents may ask why bother to do something that causes problems and is against the conscience of some when viable alternatives exist.

A significant event occurred in 1989 when the NABT announced an official policy that "recommends, where appropriate, alternatives to dissection and viv-isection in life science classrooms in schools and colleges" (NABT 1989 and a clarification 1990). NABT has organized a number of workshops to help teachers introduce alternatives and has also issued a monograph of suggested lesson plans for alternatives to dissection and other projects that do not harm or destroy animal life (Hairston, 1990). Included are lessons on teaching ethics as related to animal experimentation.

Among the most useful alternatives to dissection suggested by NABT and others are studies of human anatomy from X rays, movies of the gastrointestinal tract after barium meals, pyelograms of the kidney, CAT scans and magnetic resonance images of the heart and brain; various observational anatomical pro-jects of live animals; frog dissection videos; take-apart frog models; student-made models of stomach, livers, and other internal organs; student-made skele-tons of fish and other creatures; and dissection of chicken wings and slaughterhouse material. The new interactive videodisks that provide high quality video and computer graphics with interactive capabilities provide a valuable tool for teaching anatomy. According to Strauss and Kinzie (1991), "Research suggests that IVD-based [interactive video disk] simulations can be just as effective as the performance of actual activities . . . and perhaps more efficient."

Not all members of NABT have been happy with this encouragement of alternatives to dissection—some have protested as perhaps was inevitable.

In July, 1991, the board of Directors of the National Science Teachers Association adopted guidelines setting limits on the use of dissection at the precollege level. They state that the objectives of the study "must be appropriate to the maturity level of the student" and that a student's "views or beliefs must be considered." The context of these guidelines is generally one of approval of some high school dissection.

This policy was not satisfactory to some teachers. A science education specialist David A. Harbster (1992) wrote: "I find the NSTA's Guidelines for Responsible Use of Animals in the Classroom contrary to the standards, practices, and possibilities of quality education for students entering the 21st century. As a former advocate for animal dissection, I came to believe that my dissection units contrasted, paradoxically, with our labs in biochemistry, genetics, and ecology. . . . Dissection was certainly the easiest unit to teach and seemed to further indict me as a teacher who taught as he was taught." A consensus has yet to be reached among teachers on this issue.

One of the most interesting results of this conflict over dissection is that a number of high school and college teachers are spending the time normally spent on dissection on a class discussion of the boundaries of use of animals for educational and research purposes. What should and should not students or professional scientists be permitted to do? What are the relevant differences between professional use of animals and student use of animals that affect the justification of infliction of harm? Should precollege students be permitted to induce painful pathological conditions or demonstrate well-known deleterious effects of poisons on vertebrate animals for science fair projects? How can you tell if something hurts an animal? What is the relationship of humans to other animals? What is your value judgment on what justifies killing or harming animals? On what criteria are these judgments made? These challenging questions produce lively and worthwhile discussions.

The overall trend is to reduce or to phase out dissections, especially at the precollege and to some extent at the college level. The age and career commitment of a student are important considerations in any assessment of the justification for dissection. The emotional maturity and educational level of the student determine to a large extent the positive or negative effects. The older the student, the more meaningful the exercise is likely to be.

The use of live animals in high schools: science fairs

When animals are used for dissection, nowadays they usually are dead on arrival in the classroom—they have been killed by someone other than the teacher or student and have been shipped to the classroom. Another set of issues emerges when live animals are used, especially if they are vertebrates about which there is the greatest public concern. Since no federal policies apply to the use of live vertebrate animals in secondary schools, and few states have laws, voluntary codes generally prevail nowadays.

But historically, there was a time when even voluntary codes did not exist—youngsters with even minimal skills could virtually do what they liked. In the United States teenage students experimented on sentient animals in their homes—basements, bedrooms, and garages were common sites. Surgery on rabbits, mice, and even cats was not uncommon. Documented accounts date back to the 1930s of animals being subjected to crude experimentation by untrained youths. This type of activity ran unchecked for many decades.

In these unethical experiments, conditions were below acceptable standards and animal suffering was high. The experimenters were novices with poorly developed skills; their knowledge about anesthetics was faulty or entirely absent; their equipment could be defective and unsterilized; and supervision was cursory or nonexistent—youngsters with chutzpah worked unaided. Teachers and professional scientists were involved to the extent that they knew about these goings-on, they did not protest against them, and indeed sometimes encouraged them as a way to a career in the sciences.

By the 1940s, this type of activity received a considerable boost with the establishment of science fairs that encouraged home experiments. Now these home experiments received official sanction in that these projects were publicly exhibited and some were rewarded with prizes. Science fairs are high school science competitions in which teenagers conduct extracurricular projects for monetary awards and prestige. Some of these projects have been exceptionally well conceived, especially in the physical sciences, but in the medical sciences they have been largely responsible for the animal abuse encountered at this level of education. Estimates suggest that over one million youngsters, aged about 10 to 18 years, participate annually in science fairs. The fairs have been endorsed by several professional teachers' associations because some teachers believe that these competitions encourage interest in science. Competitors conduct their projects after school hours either at their homes or schools, or very occasionally in research institutions. Exhibition of the results of highly invasive animal experiments has been a regular feature of many of these fairs. With the addition of a competitive aspect, youngsters' projects became bolder and even more inhumane.

As Andrew Rowan (1984) of Tufts University tells the story, "The Mississippi 1968 award winner used 25 squirrel monkeys to demonstrate 'neuroelectrotele-

stimulation and electric form reactions' [sic]. Four relics of the student's attempts, including one animal dying with suppurating holes in its head, were
photographed and displayed at that year's International Science and Engineering
Fair (ISEF) in Detroit. The monkey displayed at the fair died of a variety of ills.
The necropsy disclosed large areas of sloughed and necrotic skin and demonstrated that the electrodes had not passed through the holes in the skull into the
brain. The only change instituted by the ISEF organizers after this particular
horror was a prohibition of the display of live, warm-blooded animals at the
competition."

Unlike some other countries, the United States has no law that requires a level
of competency before a person is allowed to conduct animal experiments. In
Germany, England, Sweden, Denmark, the Netherlands, and Switzerland, animal experimentation by high school students is prohibited by law. For instance,
the 1986 German law states, "Only persons with the requisite expertise may
conduct experiments on animals. Only persons who have completed university
studies in veterinary medicine, medicine or natural sciences may conduct experiments on vertebrates" (German Law, 1986, page 38).

In the United States, a watershed event occurred in 1969 when a seventeen-
year-old student from Richmond, Virginia, entered in the Westinghouse Science
Talent Search a project that involved blinding sparrows and then starving them to
death. The student blinded the birds by removing their eyeballs. This was done
because she wanted to test the light perception of non-seeing birds; she starved
them because she used food as a reward for the birds making the "correct" choice
of moving toward light in a dark/light choice situation. But because she could
not get the birds to respond—they just stood still—she withheld food for increasingly long periods until some starved to death.

I saw this exhibit and was appalled. Apparently none of the teachers or judges
had questioned the treatment of the birds. Indeed, they had awarded the project a
top prize of $250.

A number of journalists voiced their protests. Bob Cromie of the *Chicago
Tribune* wrote a series of articles protesting this and similar activities; the *New
York Times* ran an editorial, "Prizes for Torture," which started, "There is a
growing fad among high school students to perform heart transplants, brain
surgery and other radical experiments on animals"; an article in the *Christian
Science Monitor* was headlined " 'Research' by the Unskilled." A spokesperson
for Westinghouse Electric, the sponsors of the competition, wrote that the
sparrow-blinding project was "an isolated incident which slipped past the safe-
guards" of the rules. In fact, there was nothing in the rules that prohibited such
projects.

As a result of the sparrow-blinding project, the Westinghouse rules were
drastically changed in 1969 to permit only observational studies of vertebrate
animals; pain-inflicting projects were forthwith prohibited. Since these rules

were established, no public protests have occurred. The Canada-Wide Science Fair has rules virtually identical to those of the Westinghouse Science Talent Search since 1975. Organizers of the Canadian fair have repeatedly expressed satisfaction with their rules.

But another fair exists that has not followed these reforms—the International Science and Engineering Fair (ISEF). At first this fair had no rules on animal experimentation, but public protests in the 1960s made Science Service, the organizers, seek advice. They asked the National Society for Medical Research to prepare rules. The rules that emerged, however, permitted the infliction of animal pain and suffering—even severe pain is allowed (procedures that would fall into categories D and E on the pain scale presented in Table 6.1). Indeed, some traumatic procedures, such as induction of cancer and irradiation, were specifically mentioned, thus tending to encourage them.

For decades some science fair projects have endlessly documented the harmful effects of tobacco smoke, psychedelic drugs, and other well-known deleterious substances on sentient vertebrate animals such as hamsters, gerbils, rats, and mice. A home-rigged apparatus used to give electric shocks to animals was relatively common. Other projects involved feeding nutritionally deprived diets to small mammals such as guinea pigs. Sometimes these diets were maintained until the animals became seriously ill or died. Another project has been to force small mammals to consume alcohol—forced inasmuch as the animals are given no choice. These projects, intended to teach youngsters to eat balanced diets and not to drink alcohol, have been popular for several decades. A more recent vogue has been to administer already well-documented harms (such as radiation or poisons like carbon tetrachloride) to pregnant small mammals to see how many dead and deformed babies emerge. Often these projects are crudely performed, and all involve significant animal suffering. Protests about such projects have repeatedly been made by a number of animal welfare organizations.

The factors that contributed to this bad situation were several: inadequate rules that permit invasive animal experiments by beginning students, a lack of ethical education about animal issues, a lack of technical skill, inadequate supervision, unsuitable facilities, and the historical fact that highly invasive animal experiments receive a disproportionate share of prizes.

A certain amount of progress has been made since the 1960s in tightening up the rules. Animal surgery in students' homes is no longer allowed; adult supervision is required; some limits have been placed on the severity level of animal harm resulting from nutritional deprivation and of induction of pathological lesions; use of the LD50 test has been banned; and the killing of small mammals has to be humanely done. Recently, better efforts have been made to enforce these rules, but rules allowing beginning students to inflict pain and suffering on vertebrate animals remain to this day. The basic argument used by ISEF to justify these rules is that bright students must be motivated via encouragement to pursue extracurricular studies to pursue careers in the life sciences, and excessive restrictions will undermine their motivation, a disputed contention.

The standards at the International Science and Engineering Fair are still inadequate. A 1985 survey of this fair showed that when vertebrate animals were chosen for study, four out of five projects did some harm to the animals (Orlans, 1985). This predominance of harm-inflicting projects has been repeatedly documented. A recent example is a 1989 prize-winning project that involved burning hamsters with an electric soldering iron. Twenty-eight animals were used; the purpose was to observe burn healing. Is it essential to burn animals for a teenager's competition?

What is lacking is an understanding of the range of useful studies that involve neither harming nor destroying sentient life. In teacher training little or no attention is given to educating the teachers about how to maintain suitable classroom organisms that will help students understand life processes. There are many suitable classroom animal studies, including those of protozoa, worms, insects, and fish, and non-harmful studies of small mammals and of human beings. Thousands of sound educational exercises can be conducted that do not involve infliction of pain or death on highly sentient creatures (see, for instance, Orlans, 1977, and Kramer, 1989). Biology teaching would surely be enhanced if it involved more observation of living organisms.

Among the many non-harmful projects suitable for high school students, professional associations of biology teachers have recommended observations of normal living functions such as feeding, growth, reproduction, activity cycles, communication, behavior, and interrelationships of organisms, and the study of normal living patterns of wild animals in their natural habitats or in zoological parks or aquariums. None of these studies need involve harming or destroying sentient animal life. By studying a wide range of creatures from protozoa to human beings, a sense of biodiversity would be conveyed. Some have urged that studies of human behavior, circulation, special senses, growth, and so on could use the students themselves as the experimental subjects. Biology education could thereby by made more relevant to a student's life and future adult needs.

Leading educators are alert to these needs, and major overhauls are now under way in the high school biology curriculum.

Current policies and policy reforms

In response to public protests about practices in science fairs, several states enacted laws during the period 1973 to 1985. Typical is that of Massachusetts (1979), which states in part, "No school principal, administrator or teacher shall allow any live vertebrate to be used in any elementary or high school . . . [to be] experimentally drugged in a manner to cause painful reactions or to induce painful or lethal pathological conditions, or in which said vertebrates are injured through any other type of treatment, experiment or procedure including but not limited to anesthetization or electric shock, or where the normal health of said animal is interfered with or where pain or distress is caused."

Similar wording is found in four other state laws and in voluntary policies issued by various groups. The rationale is that:

1. Morally, it is indefensible to hurt or kill animals unless original contributions that will advance human health and welfare can be expected. Elementary and secondary school studies do not meet this test.
2. Psychologically, it can be emotionally upsetting for youngsters to participate in harming or killing animals; even worse, it may be emotionally desensitizing or hardening to immature minds.
3. Socially, in these days of widespread violence, fostering personal acquaintance with inflicting pain on lesser creatures should be avoided.
4. Educationally, teaching about abnormal states before the student has a sound grasp of normal physiology is against common sense and does not advance scientific education.
5. Scientifically, promoting teenage animal surgery or induction of painful pathological conditions fosters an improper regard for animal life and an unbalanced view of biology that will rebound adversely when the next generation of scientists comes of age.

In the United States, some professional teachers' associations have promulgated rules on live animal studies. A consensus has not yet emerged. There are two major professional associations of science teachers, and there have been differences in the course each has taken. Since 1980, one organization has espoused different basic concepts about the permissibility of infliction of pain at different times; the other organization has consistently been against the infliction of pain on vertebrate animals by elementary and high school students.

With the National Science Teachers Association (NSTA), which comprises teachers of all the sciences, the pendulum has swung. Most of the time, their guidelines have permitted infliction of pain. The first NSTA policy to break away from this stance was announced in 1980 (NSTA, 1980). It encouraged study of living organisms, suggested many avenues for humane biological studies, and specifically prohibited any infliction of pain on a vertebrate animal or interference with its health. In 1986, this policy was changed to permit once again infliction of pain on vertebrates, specifically sanctioning "use of pathogens, ionizing radiation, toxic chemicals, and chemicals producing birth defects" as long as the junior or senior high school students' projects are done under supervision by a qualified person. The question arises whether supervision of any caliber brings with it justification for a highly invasive procedure conducted as a pre-college exercise.

The other key organization, the National Association of Biology Teachers (NABT), comprising only biology teachers, issued a policy in 1980 that was compatible with that of the 1980 policy of the NSTA—it did not allow vertebrate animals to be subjected to "pain or distinct discomfort" and promoted observational studies. The NABT has consistently held this position since. In 1989, they went a step further by issuing an official policy that included the following words: "NABT supports alternatives to dissection and vivisection wherever possible in the biology curricula. These alternatives must satisfy the objectives of teaching scientific methodology and fundamental biological concepts."

In another statement issued in 1990, NABT stated firmly that lab activities "should not cause the loss of an animal's life." Furthermore, this policy echoed the Canadian position in stating that vertebrate animals can only be used in the following situations: (1) for observations of normal living patterns of wild animals in their natural habitat or in zoological parks; (2) observations of normal living functions such as feeding, growth, reproduction, activity cycles, etc.; and (3) observations of biological phenomenon among and between species such as communication and reproduction. All invasive studies are in violation of this code.

For five years, NABT had been awarding prizes at the International Science and Engineering Fair, as do several professional organizations. After adoption of the new code on animals, NABT sought to use this as the basis for judging these awards. No NABT awards would go to any project in which an animal was harmed or killed. The International Science and Engineering Fair responded by banning NABT from giving any awards.

A recent development is that the International Science and Engineering Fair is requiring that teenagers who experiment on animals establish a sort of informal, three-person mini-IACUC to review their work. However, the success of this scheme is uncertain. Instructions are provided in an article of how to put together a rubber-stamp committee; it is advised that persons who are likely to object be excluded from committee service and that disapprovals of the proposed project "should be used sparingly" (Snyder et al., 1992). It seems to me that this is inappropriate acculturation for a young person embarking on a career in which public accountability is important. Given the history of poor humane standards in science fairs and the persistence of rules that permit students to inflict pain on sentient animals, it is arguable that this new system will solve many problems.

Perhaps the slow pace of policy reform in the use of animals in education is partly attributable to the way mandated national policies have, in the past, been worded. In contrast to the many voluntary guidelines that have been promulgated that specifically state that they apply to the use of animals in education, the mandated policies have not given such a clear picture—they mix together the use of animals in research and in education with no distinction being made between the two. Indeed, both the PHS and AWA policies leave the impression that the same rules apply in both situations, and this could have caused confusion. In the PHS policy, for instance, it is specifically stated that certain basic principles apply "in testing, research, and education" (PHS Guide 1985, pages 81–83).

Similar phrases can be found in the AWA. No mention is made of the need to assess the experimenter's competency level and to match this against the degree of permissible infliction of animal harm. The idea that different and more stringent limits should be set on the infliction of vertebrate animal pain and suffering in education is missing. A false impression exists among some people that untrained youths should follow the same rules as highly trained researchers—no additional constraints are necessary. In fact, at one point, a committee of NSTA charged with establishing rules for high school students proposed that the PHS policy be adopted, as if that were all that was needed!

The development of national policies has now matured to the point where some refinements are needed to separate the use of animals in education from that of research. It would be helpful if the standards of both PHS and AWA addressed as a separate issue the use of animals in education.

A new general policy is needed on the use of animals in education that relates the educational level of the student to the justification for inflicting pain and death on a sentient animal. Novices should start with studies of non-vertebrate creatures and vertebrate studies that do not involve pain or lingering death. Thus, at the secondary school level, projects involving vertebrate animal pain would not be permitted. Only as their educational level advances should students be permitted to progress to vertebrate studies involving minimal animal pain. At a later point in the students' training, the goal of the experiment shifts from being solely educational to involving the search for new knowledge. Most commonly this occurs at the graduate school level. In any particular instance, judgment of what is appropriate must be left to the students' supervisors and the federally required IACUC. Before any student is allowed to conduct intrusive animal experiments, training in humane techniques should be a requirement. Procedures involving moderate or significant vertebrate animal pain should be reserved for the acquisition of new knowledge, that is, for research. Injurious procedures are not justified in education because alternatives that teach the same things without harming or killing are available.

Adoption of a policy that relates educational level and competency of the student with the justification for inflicting harms on animals, as proposed here, is already a reality in the secondary schools of New South Wales, Australia (NSW, 1991). Guidelines of the NSW Department of School Education divide animal projects into categories 1 to 4, each category involving increasingly harmful animal procedures. Increasingly stringent restraints are placed on each category, with category 4 covering prohibited procedures. Examples of category 4 include induction of infectious diseases, administration of ionizing radiation or other stimuli causing distress, among others. (The International Science and Engineering Fair specifically permits these). This innovative Australian policy is the first example that I know of where educational policy has been framed around use of a pain-and-harm scale.

13

The Source of Laboratory Dogs and Cats: Pound versus Purpose-Bred Animals

A major question in the debate over the use of animals in research is where laboratory dogs and cats should come from—from city pounds and animal shelters, or solely from animal breeders? For the last seventy years, the American biomedical community has fought hard for the continued use of pound and shelter animals with no restrictions, while the animal welfarists and antivivisectionists generally oppose such use. The laboratory use of specially-bred dogs and cats obtained from animal dealers (so-called purpose-bred animals) is much less controversial except among those who are opposed to all animal experimentation.

The reliance of the biomedical community on pound dogs (so-called "random-source" animals) was at an all-time high in the 1950s but has been diminishing. At the NIH research facility during 1964, 100 percent of all animals used were random source, but by 1973 this had fallen to 85 percent of all dogs used (Potkay and Bacher, 1973). By 1989, it was estimated that nationally about 60 percent of all animals used were pound animals (roughly 94,000 dogs); the rest, 40 percent, come from commercial breeders (Wolfle, 1989).

As discussed in chapter 5, the total number of dogs and cats from all sources used in biomedical research has decreased somewhat in recent years, the most notable decline being in dogs (see Figure 5.3 and Appendix A). In 1991, 108,000 dogs were used and 35,000 cats. Dogs and cats together comprise only a small proportion of the total number for all species, estimated to be over twenty million animals.

Random-source animals are used for a wide variety of experimental purposes in all three categories of research, testing, and education. They are used for research on cardiovascular disease, bone injuries, hearing loss, blindness, lung disorders, and infectious diseases; for testing involving drug reactions and birth defects; and for educational purposes to demonstrate basic physiological and pharmacological principles and for practice surgery.

Rowan (1991) estimated that in 1990, nationwide, pounds and shelters handle about six million animals each year and of these, probably some three million animals are killed. Other animals are returned to their owners or adopted, and others go live to laboratories for experimentation.

Nowadays, there is no hard-and-fast distinction between "pound" and "shelter"—the terms are used interchangeably. Traditionally, pounds are facilities established and financed by local or municipal ordinance for animal control purposes and shelters are operated by humane societies. But these distinctions have become blurred over time.

According to The Humane Society of the United States (HSUS) in 1989, of the 2500 animal control facilities (called either pounds or shelters) in the United States, some 2000 are run by towns and municipalities, and 500 are privately operated. As far as the law is concerned, publicly financed pounds must of course obey public laws, whether these are to provide or not to provide animals for research. Where no local ordinance or law pertains, publicly financed pounds are the most likely to voluntarily provide animals for experimentation.

The influential HSUS urges animal control facilities to stop providing animals for research. Indeed, in the early 1980s, HSUS made abolition of the release of animals to research institutions a major priority of their organization. Shelters that are financed exclusively by private funds (operated by humane societies) can usually set their own policies regarding handing over animals to research facilities, and overwhelmingly they opt to refuse. Only a small handful of shelters funded entirely by private funds provide animals for research, and they are atypical.

Trading in dogs and cats

Dogs and cats currently come from several sources and arrive at the laboratories by several routes. Figure 13.1 depicts both major and minor routes. Random-source animals are largely strays and abandoned or unclaimed pets. These animals are first handled through pounds and then commonly through animal dealers, though a few go directly from the pound to the laboratory. In contrast, purpose-bred animals typically go directly from the commercial breeders to the laboratory in a single step. The figure clearly illustrates that random-source animals are subject to far more trading by multiple handlers and live in numerous holding facilities before arriving at a laboratory. As a result, the potential for

SOURCE AND TRADING ROUTES OF
LABORATORY DOGS AND CATS

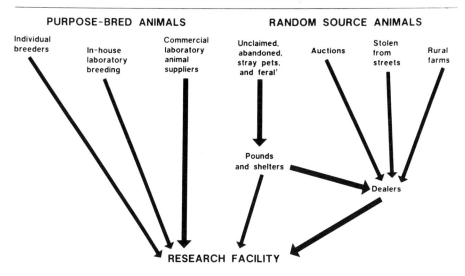

PURPOSE-BRED ANIMALS   **RANDOM SOURCE ANIMALS**

Individual breeders | In-house laboratory breeding | Commercial laboratory animal suppliers | Unclaimed, abandoned, stray pets, and feral[1] | Auctions | Stolen from streets | Rural farms

Pounds and shelters

Dealers

RESEARCH FACILITY

Figure 13.1   In this schematic representation, two major and several minor routes by which dogs and cats arrive at the laboratory door are shown. The actual width of the bars does not indicate the relative importance of the routes in terms of numbers of animals involved. An additional source, not shown here, is retired greyhounds from the race track.

1. In the absence of identifying tags on the animals, it may be difficult to differentiate between these groups unless other sources of information are available. For instance, the animals' behavior, such as obeying human commands, can help identify a one-time pet.

neglect and mistreatment is much greater for random-source than for purpose-bred animals.

Animal dealers act as middle men, purchasing dogs and cats from many sources including some pounds and shelters, farms, breeders, animal traders, and persons who advertise animals for sale, for instance, in local newspapers. Some unscrupulous dealers resort to theft of pet animals from home properties and the streets, and some have been convicted for this. Dealers also obtain animals from so-called "puppy mills," where animals are bred repeatedly; the inhumane conditions encountered in some "puppy mills" have been a matter of concern for several national humane societies, including HSUS. "Bunchers" (not shown in the figure) arc people who obtain animals for sale to animal dealers.

Dealers who sell animals to research institutions have to be licensed under the AWA as Class B dealers. This means that their facilities are subject to USDA inspection and that the transportation of animals must comply with federal standards. Also, dealers are technically required to document the source of the animal, but enforcement is woefully inadequate. Judging from the number of convictions for violation of humane standards, bunchers, puppy mills, and some dealers are far more likely to treat animals poorly than do commercial breeders of purpose-bred animals.

The expected time sequence in the life of a typical pound animal is as follows. A dog or cat that arrives in a pound can expect to spend from three to seven days at the pound before its fate is decided (the holding period is sometimes mandated by state or local policy). Those animals destined for laboratories through a dealer will then typically spend from 5 to 30 days in the dealer's facility. Transportation time to the laboratory can take from one to several additional days. During the time at the dealer's facility and during transportation, the animals are subjected to several environmental and food changes, and possible contact with sick animals and exposure to pathogenic agents.

Once having arrived at the laboratory, dogs and cats commonly enter a pre-paratory period before experimentation. They are quarantined (or conditioned) for various periods of time, usually from several weeks to two months. Eckstein (1987) determined that for dogs used in research, the length of laboratory experiments ranged from less than 24 hours to 5.5 years, with an average of 9 to 11 days. One third of experiments lasted one month or longer. These figures are based on an analysis of fifty-two journal articles published during 1985 to 1987 in which mongrel dogs were used. To summarize, the range of time for a pound animal from the point of arrival at a pound to death in a laboratory can be as short as 7 days or as long as 5 years.

The beginnings of pound animal use

During the 1920s, the research community increasingly relied on dogs and cats obtained from city pounds as a convenient source of cheap animals. In 1921, when the Humane Society of Missouri gained control of the local animal shelter, they refused to provide stray animals to the local medical schools (Lederer, 1992). The Dean of the Washington University School of Medicine led the campaign to continue their use. Public hearings ended in victory for the medical schools and passage of a law providing that dogs from the pound be delivered to the medical schools for the unit price of 75 cents. This success encouraged research advocacy groups in other cities to attempt similar tactics. Later the biomedical community established national lobbying groups to pursue these ends: in 1945 the National Society for Medical Research, and in 1979 the National Association for Biomedical Research. These organizations coordinated, expanded, and intensified the efforts to retain the use of pound animals for research.

After World War II, the United States embarked on an accelerated program of biomedical research. Federal funding disbursed through the agency of NIH rose rapidly: $0.7 million in 1945, $98 million in 1956, and $2,000 million in 1988. Along with this acceleration came an increased demand for laboratory animals.

In the early days of expanding federal funding for biomedical research, rats and mice became firmly established as the most frequently used species, and the commercial animal-breeding industry was built around these species. Initially, because of the easy access to pound animals, only a relatively small market for purpose-bred dogs and cats existed. For commercial suppliers, it is a lengthy, demanding, and expensive undertaking to develop a colony of breeding dogs or cats; not many have made this investment.

The rising affluence in post-war years resulted in an increase in the number of household pets in the United States—estimated in 1987 at about 52 million dogs and 56 million cats. During this period, there was a growth in irresponsible pet ownership and consequent uncontrolled pet breeding. The humane societies tried to control the vast overpopulation of dogs and cats that started to develop in the 1950s. They launched public education programs and low-cost spay-and-neuter clinics to help control this tide, but soon the problem was out of hand and great numbers of puppies, kittens, and adult animals had to be killed because no one wanted them. So it came about that one of the major tasks for city pounds and shelters was to destroy animals—a total of approximately three million unwanted dogs and cats in 1990. Approximately fifty percent of these are stray animals and another fifty percent are relinquished pets, according to a 1985 survey by the American Humane Association (Anonymous, 1985). When an animal arrives at a pound, it may be returned to its owner, adopted by a new owner, or killed. Estimates of the American Humane Association suggest that with dogs, roughly some 25 percent are returned to their original owner, another 20 percent are adopted, and the remaining 55 percent killed. There are no reliable figures to my knowledge on the number of pound animals that end up in research.

Along with more refined research methods and increased federal funding came the need for higher quality animals. Researchers began to prefer purpose-bred animals for certain investigations, so research establishments started developing their own breeding colonies. For instance, in the late 1960s and early 1970s, NIH began its own breeding colonies of beagles and foxhounds. Also, in the 1980s, a number of commercial breeders stepped up their dog-breeding programs, presumably in response to demand. In 1984, for instance, Hazelton Laboratories started a purpose-bred dog colony in Cumberland, Virginia. By 1989, this facility alone was producing approximately 13,000 animals per year.

Both individual investigator preference and various mandates against use of pound animals have encouraged the switch from pound animals to purpose-bred animals. In an article in the *New Scientist* entitled "Bad animals mean bad science," a switch from pound to purpose-bred animals from an accredited source was urged by geneticist Michael Festing (1977) because to do otherwise can compromise the reliability of research results. According to Festing, upgrading the quality of biomedical research involves also upgrading the quality of the animals used, and it is a mistaken belief that buying cheap animals is an economy. Other scientists apparently agree. In Canada, the use of pound animals has decreased considerably in recent years and reliance on purpose-bred animals increased. In England, Sweden, Holland, and Denmark, there has been a long-term tradition of relying exclusively on purpose-bred animals. In the United States, Hoffmann-La Roche, the pharmaceutical company, gave up using pound animals in 1989. In Japan, Kobe University gave it up in 1992.

In the United States, for seventy years legislative battles have been fought between the biomedical community and humane organizations over whether pound animals should or should not be allowed to be used for research (see Chapter 4). By 1991, fourteen states had enacted laws that forbid the use of pound animals; six states specifically affirm use of pound animals; six states have laws that permit it. In the other states without specific laws, the use of pound animals can occur.

To lobby on these issues at both the state and federal level, an unprecedented cooperation developed between long-established humane and antivivisection societies. In 1985, eleven leading societies formed a coalition called ProPets (The National Coalition to Protect Our Pets) (Giannelli, 1985). Among these were the American Anti-Vivisection Society, The American Humane Association, American SPCA, Animal Protection Institute, Fund for Animals, The Humane Society of the United States, International Society for Animal Rights, Massachusetts SPCA, The Michigan Humane Society, The National Anti-Vivisection Society, and the New England Anti-Vivisection Society—a coalition representing substantial legislative expertise and financial resources.

The ProPets coalition lobbied for a federal bill that would prohibit the use of pound animals in NIH-funded research. The Pet Protection Act (H.R. 778) was first introduced in Congress in 1987 and attracted considerable support in the House and Senate before finally dying. ProPets noted accurately that NIH does not prohibit grantee institutions from using pound animals, and claimed that NIH "has not used pound animals in their own research for over a decade." At issue was whether NIH should prescribe what animals should be used in the institutions receiving NIH funds.

The bill became a target for opposition by the biomedical community and their lobbying group, NABR. Congressman Robert J. Mrazek (D-NY, who introduced the bill) and Michael E. DeBakey, M.D. (the internationally famous heart surgeon, and president of the Foundation for Biomedical Research, the sister organization of NABR) argued this issue in the pages of the *New York Times, Washington Post,* and other leading newspapers, (Mrazek, 1987, and DeBakey, 1987a and b). The opposing arguments are presented below.

Arguments for and against the use of pound animals

The major arguments in favor of continuing the use of pound animals are that pound animals are suitable for many kinds of research; without pound animals biomedical research would be impeded and costs would rise; most of these animals are not really pets but are abandoned animals; in any case, people do not mind if their unwanted pets are used in research; two animals would die instead of one (a purpose-bred animal and the pound animal); and the animals will be killed anyway (because they are part of an excess population) and if used in research at least they will have a socially useful end.

Lobbyists for the biomedical community have predicted dire consequences if researchers do not have access to pound animals. Michael DeBakey asserted that stopping the use of pound animals will "prevent or slow" medical research, and that the "future of biomedical research—and ultimately human health" will be compromised. According to AMA officials, stopping the use of pound animals for research "would dismantle medical research . . . medical advances would be compromised" (Smith and Hendee, 1988). A representative of the Society for Neuroscience wrote that not using pound animals would be "a major loss for the future of health and society" (Burke, 1985). Since substitutes for pound animals are available, these predictions are extreme.

The major arguments against the use of pound and shelter animals are that this practice undermines the central concept that shelters shall be sanctuaries for lost and abandoned animals; it impedes the acceptance of alternatives that have lesser ethical costs, such as substitution of purpose-bred animals; pet owners should not have to face the double calamity, for some, of pet loss followed by an uncertain fate of the animal in a laboratory; it is ethically improper to treat the pet overpopulation problem as a resource to be exploited; and spurious scientific results could occur because pound animals can be stressed animals, lacking physiological normality, and they may even exhibit long-term pathological damage (e.g., heart-worm that would make them less than ideal for cardiac research).

On behalf of ProPets, former director Michael Giannelli wrote that use of pound animals for research "is a direct invasion of the heart of the animal protection movement, a breach in the wall of what were intended to be places of last refuge and protective sanctuary for animals." Taking pound animals for research "interferes with everything humane societies represent and attempt to accomplish" said John McArdle (1985) of The Humane Society of the United States. Humane societies argue that they have a hard enough job in persuading the public to bring in unwanted pets to local shelters rather than abandoning them to the streets. Even more difficult is their task if the animals coming in through the front door are known to be shipped out the back door for sale to laboratories.

Humane associations conducted surveys that came up with the answer they sought—that public confidence in their local shelters would be undermined by taking pound animals for research (McArdle, 1985, and AHA, 1988). In an AHA survey, shelter clients were asked if they would bring a lost animal to a shelter that released animals to research. Of the 2,438 responses, 2,273 (or 93 percent) said they would not. Public attitudes in support of biomedical research do not appear to mesh with these results.

Who has the right to direct what happens to unwanted pets? The humane societies who have physical possession of the animals and devote a large share of their resources to deal with pet animal issues? Research labs that want the animals for experimentation? Or is it for the public to decide? Inasmuch as humane societies are built on the concept of providing sanctuary for animals, should these societies control the fate of all animals that pass through their doors, even those whom they have to kill? Since the pet overpopulation is a social problem brought about by irresponsible members of the public, could not these animals be viewed as part of public property to be used for the socially useful purpose of medical research?

An argument used by the biomedical community is that costs would rise if pound animals were not available because it would be necessary to breed additional animals at greater expense. In 1987, pound dogs typically cost around $35 per animal, and purpose-bred dogs of specific breeds ranged from around $300 to $500, less for a mongrel. According to DeBakey's 1987 figures, a total ban on pound animals would add $90 million per year to research costs, thus reducing the amount of money available for research each year. Neurosurgeon Robert J. White wrote in a 1988 *Reader's Digest* article, "If medical centers are prohibited from purchasing pound animals, many researchers will not be able to afford to continue their work."

Experience at the NIH facility some twenty years ago showed that the cost differential between pound and random-source animals is minimal; the most important cost factor was the stamina and vitality of the animal (Zinn, 1968; Potkay and Bacher, 1973; and Palmer, 1973). This conclusion was backed up with detailed data. Although the high proportion of deaths and disease among random-source animals reported by these authors, all NIH personnel, may not hold for today's conditions because of better conditioning procedures at the receiving lab, the general point that random-source animals may be a poor economy may hold some truth. As Festing (1977) pointed out, buying cheap animals may not be an economy. Not only may the validity of the research results be compromised, but also the uncertain and often inferior health status of random-source animals means that more of them are likely to die than with purpose-bred animals. These sicknesses and deaths add to the cost of using pound animals because greater numbers have to be used.

The true cost of using research animals is the acquisition cost plus the utilization cost. The longer the animal lives, the higher the utilization cost and the less significant proportionally becomes the purchase price. Dogs are maintained for weeks or sometimes even years in research institutions. Utilization costs comprise, in part, routine maintenance which, according to NIH figures, amounts to approximately $1000 to $1500 per year, depending upon the size of the dog (Potkay, 1989). In addition, the costs of surgery or other experimental procedures, special veterinary care, and facility overhead for the experiment add substantially to utilization costs. So, for any animals kept for any length of time, the initial purchase price becomes less important in relation to the over-whelmingly larger utilization costs.

Substituting purpose-bred animals

Would the overall situation be worse or better if purpose-bred animals were substituted for pound animals? Opinions are divided.

Purpose-breeding, according to its proponents, offers higher-quality animals whose health status, age, and genetic background are known, thus helping to make the experimental sample more uniform. Selecting a uniform subject sample is often (albeit not invariably) very desirable or essential to an experimental design. Random-source animals, on the other hand, are usually of unknown age and genetics. Also from a purely practical standpoint, using purpose-bred animals avoids controversy with the humane movement—a desirable end that should not be overlooked.

From an ethical standpoint, the Foundation for Biomedical Research (FBR) implies that a worse situation would prevail. If a pound animal is not used, then two animals die instead of one—a purpose-bred animal and a pound animal. This is the first listed consequence of a ban on pound animal use appearing in a 1990 document from the FBR establishing the case for continued use of pound animals. The intended implication is that the use of a pound animal (which will die anyhow) saves another animal from being born and killed for human use, and thus it is ethically more justified.

To accept this "two deaths are worse than one death" argument suggests that one dog death equals another dog death and that one dog life equals another dog life, and the ethical responsibility of society in all cases is the same. Not every-one holds this view. Some believe that there are different qualities of life among individual animals, and different levels of human responsibilities toward animals in different circumstances. These factors influence human choice in making life-and-death decisions about the animal. Our responsibilities toward one dog are not necessarily the same as our responsibilities toward another. There are many different subsets of dogs in general—wild, specially bred and captive but not a pet, pet, etc.—and human beings do not have the same degree of responsibility to all these subsets.

Similar ethical dilemmas of using wild-caught rather than purpose-bred animals are posed with other species and in other contexts. Is the ethical cost of using a monkey specially bred for experimental use equal to taking a wild-caught monkey? There is no simple answer, but I believe a number of people prefer the purpose-bred alternative just as they prefer purpose-bred dogs. In a number of countries a recent trend has been to stop the use of both wild-caught monkeys (France, for instance) and random-source dogs (several European countries and

Canada). In their place, purpose-bred animals are being used. Another example is the use of wild-caught birds for the pet trade rather than using purpose-bred birds. There is strong pressure to stop the importation of wild-caught birds (who die in their thousands at every stage of their journey) and in their place rely on the commercially bred popular species that are available from breeders. The Wild Bird Conservation Act of 1992 seeks to ban the importation of wild birds, and two of the largest pet chains in America will not sell wild birds in their stores.

The view that using purpose-bred animals imposes lesser ethical costs rests in part on the ground that pound animals have a life that preceeds their laboratory life, and this preceding life should be a factor in determining the animal's fate.

But some would argue that pound animals used for research are not prior pets at all. For instance, literature from the National Association for Biomedical Research (1987) states categorically that "shelter animals used for research and education are not people's pets." But unless the animals are second- or third-generation feral individuals, pound animals have indeed been one-time pets. Pound animals frequently show unmistakable signs of close association with humans in their friendliness and obedience to human commands. Inasmuch as there are many more pound animals available than are ever needed for research, there is a selection process to identify the preferred animals. Based on common sense and evidence, the animals that are the friendliest and most easy to handle are more likely to be chosen. Whatever mix of animals exist in pounds, from highly socialized to somewhat wild, the former pet animals typically end up in the laboratories.

In general, pet animals are used to considerable freedom of movement; they have probably never lived in a cage alone. Their life has been rich in stimulus; they have known affection from humans and have had social relations with other animals; they are used to variety in their environment and food. When they enter a laboratory, most of this is lost. They suffer deprivation because there is little or no opportunity to express their previously learned behavioral repertoire.

Dogs, as pets, have established behavior patterns. For instance, it is their natural behavior to mark their territory by frequent urination to leave scents, but when held in a laboratory cage, this behavior has to be suppressed because of space confinement—indeed, some cages have not allowed room for a dog to lift its leg to urinate.

Adapting to an environment that permits lesser freedoms can be traumatic. Humans subjected to incarceration suffer anxiety, depression, hopelessness, and anger. Although this is somewhat speculative, it is reasonable to believe that animals can suffer these same responses. Certainly there are variations in people's ability to adjust to being held captive, and individual animals also respond differently to becoming a laboratory subject. To the degree that loss of freedom is traumatic to the pound animal on becoming an experimental subject, there is an ethical cost.

On the other hand, the fact that purpose-bred animals have been born and raised for laboratory purposes has determined every part of their lives and their status in relation to humans. Purpose-bred animals have never known certain freedoms or any life other than being captive. They have always been subject to considerable restrictions in living space, social contact, diet, reproduction, and so on. Thus they have less to be deprived of when they are used for research.

It was over the issue of substitution of purpose-bred animals that the ProPets coalition became divided and fell. In 1985, pressed by the antivivisection members, ProPets declared that it "will not advocate or condone, as an alternative [to shelter animals] the use of any other source, type, or species of animal" (Giannelli, 1985). This was pressing the point for some coalition members who held that substitution of pound animals with purpose-bred animals more truly represented their viewpoint. Approximately four years after the coalition had first been formed, ProPets quietly disbanded largely because of disagreement over this issue.

After the disbandment of ProPets, the majority of the individual associations represented in this coalition have remained silent on the issue of purpose-bred animals. Indeed, it is rare for any organization to publicly advocate substituting purpose-bred for pound animals. It is more politic for humane societies to publicly ignore the issue lest the advocacy of purpose-bred animals give the appearance of promoting animal experimentation, which would risk losing members and financial support.

An exception is the American Humane Association (AHA), an original member of ProPets. Their representative, Richard Meyer, testified in 1989 hearings before the Virginia state legislature that AHA supported the use of purpose-bred animals as a preferred alternative to pound animals.

The lobbying groups for the biomedical community are not drawn into promoting purpose-bred animals. Their stance has been to retain the status quo and even to expand the availability of pound animals. Commercial breeders (who would stand to benefit financially from increased use of purpose-bred animals) may have recently increased their advertising for purpose-bred dogs and cats, but their political cohesion with the rest of the biomedical community prevents open declarations of any advocacy of purpose-bred animals at the expense of any other source.

A compromise recommendation

The polarization of viewpoints on pound animal use and the political nature of the battles have hampered exploration of practical solutions. A compromise solution not substantially tried in the United States is to retain the use of pound animals for certain purposes—for short-term, non-survival experiments in which the animal is dead, for instance, within 24 hours of leaving the pound. The rationale is that, from the animal's perspective, there is little difference in terms of pain or suffering. The animal is going to die soon anyhow, and providing that high standards of humaneness are maintained after leaving the pound for transportation and overnight housing, then death in the laboratory is really only a slightly delayed euthanasia.

For the policy to work as a compromise certain restrictions would have to apply: (1) the animal should be used, say, within 24 hours of leaving the pound and only used for non-survival experiments in which the animal is either killed immediately or fully anesthetized and never allowed to recover consciousness until death; (2) the animals should be obtained directly by the USDA-registered research facility from the pound, not through a dealer; and (3) this policy should not apply to shelters that fund animal-control programs with private funds, but only to facilities such as pounds that receive public funds to operate animal-control programs (this condition is included for the purely practical reason of acceptability by the private sector). Such a proposal has been made by Stevens (1988) in an individual statement that was part of National Academy of Sciences' report on animal experimentation.

A system similar to that described here was in operation in Ottawa, Canada, for several years, where such use of pound animals was, at the time, authorized. Typically, the animals scheduled for euthanasia were picked up around 5 P.M. from the pound, taken to the University of Ottawa, and used for experimentation under full anesthesia the next day. They were dead at the latest by that evening. This supply of animals to the University of Ottawa was terminated by the local humane society in 1989).

The advantages of this "acute-study" recommendation are that (1) the animals' measure of suffering is not appreciably increased; (2) an inexpensive source of dogs and cats is provided that is suitable for some purposes; and (3) because of this availability, some investigators might be encouraged to turn to acute experiments in preference to chronic studies. As a way to minimize animal pain—a mandate of the AWA—acute studies are more desirable than chronic studies. In general, the earlier the endpoint of death, the better it is for the animals. Various types of studies can be done under short-term conditions, including research studies of intervention in myocardial infarction, drug and certain neurological studies, and acute toxicity testing, among others.

It seems to me that this is a compromise that calls for serious consideration.

14

Editorial Responsibilities and Issues

When a piece of work is complete, the researcher writes up the findings. Publications are an indispensable part of the scientific endeavor. They document scientific thinking and discovery. Publications are the way scientists communicate with each other and with the public. They are the way investigators inform colleagues of the results of their research, command attention, and build a reputation. The number and quality of publications are a key factor in career advancement. Publications document the state of science, and implicitly they also reveal its ethical standards.

Historically, scientific journals have given little attention to reviewing the humaneness of animal experiments. Although peer review is well-developed for such matters as scientific merit, compliance with the journal's style, completeness of citations, clarity of expression, and accuracy of identifying animal stock source, sex, and numbers used, it usually does not take into account ethical aspects of animal experimentation. In general, editors have been passive, and editorial boards and professional societies have failed to develop policies and formal mechanisms on these matters.

But attitudes are gradually changing. Over the last decade, a number of journals have adopted policies stating that the results of any research based on animal experiments will not be published unless the experiments are in compliance with certain specified standard of humaneness. This chapter will describe these changes, explore the reasons why some editors have assumed and others have resisted these editorial responsibilities, and make some recommendations for change.

Publication of the controversial English *Handbook for the Physiologists* in 1873 revealed the embarrassing lack of ethical standards in animal research and publication at that time (see Chapter 1). The book's failure to mention the need to use anesthetics for painful procedures caused a public uproar and contributed substantially to the passage of the 1876 legislation controlling animal experimentation.

The first indication of American concern over editorial responsibilities about animal experiments occurred in 1914 when Walter Bradford Cannon, head of physiology at Harvard and a leader in fighting the antivivisectionists, circulated a letter among editors of medical journals (1914a). He urged that considerable care be exercised in the publication of research involving animals and human beings because "the omission or vague statement of the facts that an anesthetic was used in experimentation upon animals . . . is seized upon and only too often serves as a text or basis of a diatribe against scientific research" (1914b). He wanted investigators to demonstrate in whatever they published that they had followed ethical principles such as the 1909 code that Cannon himself had drawn up.

Several decades later, Cannon's code formed the basis for the "Guiding Principles in the Care and Use of Animals," a five-paragraph statement prepared by the American Physiological Society (APS) in 1953 as their official policy (Brobeck et al., 1987). These principles required that animals be lawfully acquired, receive every consideration for their bodily comfort, and be properly fed, that operative procedures must be done under anesthetic, that post-operative care shall minimize discomfort during convalescence, and that humane killing methods must be used. Students were required to be supervised.

A few years later, the APS took the further step of adopting the policy that "articles based on experiments violating the Guiding Principles shall not be acceptable for publication in the journals of the Society" (Anonymous, 1959). Furthermore, APS has also proclaimed that adherence to the guiding principles is an obligation of membership in the society.

The APS appears to be the first professional association in the United States to establish either general or editorial policies and is deservedly praised for its leadership. It has become established policy of the *American Journal of Physiology* (*AJP*), the APS's journal, to charge peer reviewers of manuscripts with this responsibility. Like other refereed journals, the *AJP* uses a peer-review process in which senior people are called upon to provide review comments. Their advice is critical to the editor. In current *AJP* instructions, reviewers are asked to answer in their written report, "Is any question raised of violation of the American Physiological Society's guiding principles for experimental procedures?" The reviewer has to answer yes or a no. If the answer is no, then the editor-in-chief is obliged to find out what the concern is and either to reject the paper on that basis or to have the investigators revise or explain why they had to use that procedure. The APS maintains a standing committee to deal with animal experimentation concerns, and editors-in-chief of their journals can refer manuscripts that raise ethical questions on animal issues to this committee for review. M. Virginia Miller, the 1992 chair on this Animal Care and Experimentation Committee, says that in these cases (of which there have been about five in the last two years) all members of the committee receive copies of the manuscript for comment. Manuscripts have occasionally been rejected for noncompliance with APS animal policies. This formal procedure also serves an educational purpose in constantly bringing the matter of humaneness of animal experimentation to the fore in the planning and conduct of research projects.

Despite the great burgeoning of scientific publications that occurred during the 1960s and 1970s, many years elapsed before any other journal followed the lead of APS. The silence was broken by Patrick D. Wall, professor of anatomy at University College London, the editor of the new journal *Pain,* who established an editorial policy on animal experimentation in the very first issue in 1975: "We shall refuse to publish any reports where the animal was unable to indicate or arrest the onset of suffering." Wall was criticized by one pain researcher for using such "emotion-laden terms as 'suffering,'" which carried with it "connotations of evil-doing" on the part of the investigator; Wall's words smacked of a "stern and moralistic view which rings with the uncompromising judgment of an Old Testament prophet" (Sternbach, 1976). Despite this adverse comment, the issuance of this editorial policy helped set in motion the establishment of first-ever official guidelines for the pain research constituency. These guidelines, issued in 1980, were published in *Pain* (Zimmerman, 1980). On several occasions over succeeding years, this constituency has publicly addressed the issue of professional guidelines on animal use, and the policies appear to be meaningful to the researchers.

Editorial policy changes since 1980

The next constituency to take action was veterinarians. In the early 1980s, three veterinary journals established editorial policies: the *American Journal of Veterinary Research* (published by the American Veterinary Medical Association), the *Canadian Veterinary Journal* (published by the Canadian Veterinary Medical Association), and the *Veterinary Quarterly* (published in the Netherlands). The policy of the American journal, one sentence long, was that "harsh conditions or treatment" of animals have to be justified (Anonymous, 1980). The Canadian journal required authors to adhere to national guidelines established by the Canadian Council on Animal Care.

In 1985, the editors-in-chief of the Dutch *Quarterly* issued thoughtful guidelines for authors and editorial boards, stipulating that research that involves harm to animals should be published only if the experiment cannot be replaced by scientifically responsible research that does not use animals (Report of Editors-in-Chief, 1985). In the case of contentious cases, it recommended that advice be sought from a consultant editorial board and authorities on ethics and be transmitted to the author. The report says, "In general, acceptance of a contentious article, published together with editorial comment, is to be preferred to rejection: the latter does little to change attitudes. This general rule has one exception, namely that an article which clearly transgresses the borders of ethical responsibility may be rejected on the grounds that acceptance might imply recognition of totally unacceptable research methods, in the same way as publications which are of no merit on scientific or technical grounds are rejected."

The issue was given a little boost in 1983 when the influential style manual of the Council of Biology Editors addressed animal experimentation for the first time. The Council is an umbrella organization for over four hundred professional journals in the life sciences. The statement is brief—it mentions anesthesia, review by institutional committees, and the need for the author to verify that "the care of animals followed accepted standards" (Council of Biology Editors, 1983). Regrettably, the manual's instructions to reviewers call no attention to these matters.

The vast majority of journals still had not adopted any editorial policy on animal experimentation. In 1986, an informal study of journal practices was made by M. Ian Phillips, professor and chair of Physiology at the University of Florida, who reported the results at a conference sponsored by the University of Texas at Houston. Of the manuscripts from thirteen different journals he had recently reviewed he was "surprised" to find that "only two [journals] asked any question about compliance with ethical standards of animal experimentation." There were the *American Journal of Physiology* and *Hypertension* (published by the American Heart Association). Phillips recommended a more widespread adoption of editorial policies on animal welfare issues.

Spurred perhaps by the strengthening amendments to the AWA and increasing public concern about laboratory standards, several prestigious journals that publish the results of animal experiments began to establish policies on animal welfare. Table 14.1 provides a listing compiled in 1991 of some major journals that currently have editorial policies on animal experimentation. The journals were selected in an attempt to be somewhat broad-ranging in discipline and to include those fields likely to be involved with invasive animal experimentation.

It is one thing to have a policy, and another to take measures to enforce it. Some journals, including those published by the American Psychological Association and APS, require both the authors submitting manuscripts and the reviewers to provide written assurance of compliance with the journal's ethical standards of animal experimentation. Others do not. The Society for Neuroscience has quite a detailed policy on animal experimentation that runs to almost a page of fine print, but the impact is somewhat dissipated by the statement in their instructions to authors that "in submitting a paper to the Journal [of Neuro-

TABLE 14.1   A sample listing of journals with editorial policies
on animal experimentation

Journal	Publisher	Editorial Policy
Am J Physiol, J Neurophysiol, and other APS journals	Am Physiological Society '59	Detailed
Pain	Internat Assoc Study Pain '75	Detailed
Am J Veterinary Research	Am Veterinary Medical Assoc '80	Brief
Canadian Veterinary J	Canadian Veterinary Med Assoc '80	National
Veterinary Quarterly	Royal Netherlands Vet Assoc '85	Brief
J Neuroscience	Soc Neuroscience U.S. '82 rev '86	Detailed
Animal Behavior	Animal Behav Soc U.K./U.S. '84 rev '86	Detailed
Laboratory Animal Science	Am Assoc Lab Animal Science '84	National
Hypertension, Arteriosclerosis, and all other AHA journals	Am Heart Association '85	Detailed
Clinical Diabetes	Am Diabetes Association '85	Detailed
J Mammalogy	Am Society Mammalogists '85	Detailed
J Comparative Psychology and all other APA journals	Am Psychological Association '86	Detailed
J Pharmacol and Exp Therap	Am Soc Pharmacol Exp Therap '86	National
Science	Am Assoc Advancement Science '87	Brief
Neuroscience Letters	Elsevier Scientific Publ '87	IASP policy
British J Cancer	Cancer Research Campaign '87 rev '91*	Brief
British J Radiology	British Inst Radiology uses British Biological Council policy '88*	Detailed
J National Cancer Institute	Superintendent of Documents, U.S. Government '88	Brief
Laboratory Animals	Laboratory Animals, Ltd, U.K. '88	National
Cancer Research	Am Assoc Cancer Research '88 uses N.Y. Acad Sc policy	Detailed
J Neurosurgery	Am Assoc Neurological Surgeons '90	National

The journals are listed in approximate chronological order based on the year when an editorial policy on animal experimentation was first established. There was a considerable time lag between the first policy in 1959 and the second in 1975. The 1980s have seen an increasing number of journals adopting policies.

The editorial policies are grouped into three types according to content and effectiveness. These policies are: (a) Detailed, which amplifies prevailing nationally mandated standards, commonly prepared by the professional association that publishes the journal. In one case (*Cancer Research*), a policy prepared by an association other than the publishing association is used.

(b) National, which requires compliance with the national standards of the country of publication.

(c) Brief, which are the journal's own brief remarks (usually one or two sentences).

*The *British Journal of Cancer* and the *British Journal of Radiology* endorse the United Kingdom Coordinating Committee on Cancer Research 1988 Guidelines. These guidelines require, among other things, that animals should be killed before predictable death occurs, before they get into poor condition, or before the tumor mass becomes overly large—"tumor burden should not usually exceed 10% of the host animal's normal body weight." They are obtainable from UKCCCR, 20 Park Crescent, London WIN 4AL, UK.

science], each author will be assumed to have conscientiously abided by these principles" (Anonymous, 1990). It is highly unusual to obtain 100 percent compliance with any policy unless there is some sort of check, and there is no indication that such a check is made. In mid-1992, the society was working toward a much more specific policy which was due to be announced in the September/October 1992 *Neuroscience Newsletter* (personal communication, Nancy Beang, Executive Director, Society for Neuroscience, June 11, 1992).

Not surprisingly, some associations have not established their own policies but instead rely on compliance with established national policy. All journals that have elected this route merely include a note saying that the law must be followed; key parts of the federal law are not restated. Animal experiments in the United States cannot legally be started unless they are in compliance with federal standards on using anesthetics and minimizing pain, so such a journal policy is feeble, but better than nothing. It is a step up for a journal to use an association policy because such policies usually amplify the national policies in helpful ways that are specific to their constituencies.

Differences in attitudes among journal editors are reflected in responses to my queries, which ranged from expressions of thanks for bringing the matters to their attention (some leading to subsequent clarifications and revisions) to an angry retort from an editor who enclosed a copy of the First Amendment guarantee of free speech in his defense of having no policy. This journal later enunciated a strong policy that requires a statement of compliance.

As of June 1991, a number of journals still do not carry a stated policy on ethical standards. This does not necessarily mean that these issues are ignored, but merely that no formal mechanism for checking humane standards is in place other than those outside the purview of the journal itself. Among these journals are some that carry reports of highly invasive animal experiments. Some examples are:

1. The *Journal of the American Medical Association*, published by the American Medical Association, an organization that has been very active in fighting both the animal welfare and animal rights organizations. (See for instance the American Medical Association "Animal Research Action Plan," 1989, which describes aggressive campaign tactics to be used in this fight). The AMA is not deficient in dealing with all ethical issues—quite the contrary. The AMA is in the forefront in dealing with ethical issues such as responsible authorship, financial disclosure of commercial interests, and informed consent of human subjects of experiments, but they have not extended their concerns to matters of animal experimentation.

2. The *American Journal of Psychiatry*, published by the American Psychiatric Association and notable because it publishes results of attempts to induce aversive and psychotic mental states in monkeys and other animal species. This journal has policies on many other ethical issues, including disclosure of

commercial interest, patient anonymity, and informed consent, and four
pages of fine print of instructions to authors.
3. *Cancer,* published by the American Cancer Society, which carries two pages
   of small-print instructions to authors but makes no mention of ethical issues.
4. *The Journal of Trauma,* sponsored by the American Association for Surgery
   and Trauma, which publishes research on trauma. Journal staff report that
   reviewers are not specifically charged with the task of ethical review, but in
   practice authors may include statements in their articles that their animal work
   is in compliance with PHS standards and has been approved by their Institutional Animal Care and Use Committee. This can occur either voluntarily or
   on request from the editors.

Challenges to ethics of published research

Over the years, critics of animal experimentation have turned to published accounts of animal experiments as an important source of information. Published
accounts of traumatic animal experiments have often been cited in congressional
testimony on legislation aimed at strengthening the standards of laboratory animal use.

Until recently, scientists were not among those who voiced ethical objections
to practices in experimentation—at least not in print; critical comments invariably came only from antivivisectionists, humane societies, philosophers and other
outsiders. Gradually, this situation is changing. For instance, in "Letter to the
Editor" in 1986 and 1987, W. Jean Dodds, a hematologist and veterinarian,
challenged the humaneness of two studies published in the *American Journal of
Veterinary Research* and questioned the journal's editorial policy. One involved
induction of the rare disease of pancreatitis in six healthy cats, and the other used
death as an endpoint in an induced pathological state in six ponies. In 1990, Neal
Barnard, a psychiatrist and president of the Physicians Committee for Responsible Research, criticized a study published in the *American Journal of Psychiatry*
of drug-induced panic reaction in monkeys on the grounds that using human
subjects in which these events were occurring spontaneously would have made
more sense. In all three cases, the authors of the original articles responded in
their own defense and no further discussion took place. However, it was significant that the objections were published at all.

Some journals are reluctant to publish comment challenging political stances
of the biomedical community, or discussion challenging methods used in housing
or experimenting on animals on ethical grounds. A recent instance involved a
proposed response to an original article that had been published in *Science* that
commented on recent laboratory animal legislation and also described the benefits that have resulted from research using primates. It was written by five staff
members of the Yerkes Regional Primate Center (King et al., 1988). The point of
contention was these authors' negative attitudes toward new legislation that

required that the care of primates should address their psychological well-being. The critic, whose comments were submitted to *Science,* was Mary Midgley, chair of the Animal Experimentation Advisory Committee of the Royal Society for the Prevention of Cruelty to Animals and a leading professor of philosophy in the U.K. Midgley's argument was that zoos had been transformed in the last few decades by attention to the psychological well-being of captive animals. Zoo-keepers, she said, have noted that "close confinement, monotonous surround-ings, solitude, or forced contiguity with unchosen companions, depressed and damaged their animals in specific observable ways—producing such symptoms as aggression, inactivity, stereotypic behaviours, sometimes death. Their change in policy has not flowed from what [King et al] so oddly call 'well-intentioned legislation based on emotional rather than empirical arguments,' but from empir-ical study of the facts." *Science* parleyed several letters between the RSPCA and the original authors, but none of these exchanges were published by *Science.* They were however subsequently published by the RSPCA in 1988.

A cause célèbre in the pages of *Nature*

In 1989, *Nature* published some monkey research that touched off a storm of controversy, with letters to the editor coming in for almost a year (see all refer-ences listed under *Nature, 1989*). To complicate this debate, a few months after it began, the laboratory where this work had been conducted was raided by animal rights activists, although the connection, if any, with the *Nature* debate was unclear since other explanations were available.

The experiments were conducted in France and the article's authors included two researchers in France, one in England, and one in the United States. The experiments were intended to assess the influence of retinal input on cortical development. Fetuses were surgically removed from two anesthetized pregnant macaque monkeys and then both the eyes were removed from the fetuses. The fetuses were returned to the uterus and the pregnancies later terminated by caesarean section. The baby monkeys were allowed to survive for some weeks and then killed for tests.

The debate was started by Clive Hollands (1989) of the Committee for the Reform of Animal Experimentation (an activist group in Scotland), who strongly criticized the humaneness of these experiments: "Such gross interference with a highly intelligent species requires overwhelming justification—if it can ever be justified. . . . To my knowledge, no other reputable scientific journal published in this country [England] will accept any reports of work which clearly would not have been authorized under British law."

In subsequent correspondence, just about every viewpoint on animal experi-mentation was aired, from extremists at both ends to moderate middle ground. One correspondent charged that in even publishing Hollands's complaint, *"Na-*

ture has done a great disservice to biomedical research." An ardent pro-researcher, whose own work has been under attack by animal rightists in England, was outraged that Hollands should "pontificate" about the legality of French experiments as if they were to be conducted in England. (Hollands serves as a member of the national oversight committee for experiments conducted in Great Britain—the Scientific Procedures Committee—although it was not in this capacity that he was speaking on this occasion.) This researcher suggested that letters of condemnation be sent to the Home Office about Hollands. An American questioned whether persons from "reform" groups should "serve on [oversight] committees that regulate animal research." But of course this respected oversight committee is constituted so that a broad spectrum of views is represented and members include some leading scientists, members of the upper chamber of parliament, lawyers, public members, etc. Several correspondents wrote in support of Hollands. The fires were rekindled when a leading article in *Nature* suggested that "given anesthesia, there is hardly ever any pain" in animal experimentation, a view that was roundly challenged.

More temperate discussion also took place, particularly about the role of editors in publishing reports on research conducted under ethically questionable conditions. The editors of *Nature* stated, "The complaint [made by Hollands] is fairly, even temperately, made. It deserves an answer" (*Nature*, 1989:339:324, 1 June). They defended publication of the questioned research on the grounds of freedom of the press. "The most obvious weakness of the complaint is that it conflates two disparate issues—animal experimentation, which in most places requires regulation, and publication, which everywhere should be free from it." What is illegal in one country may be legal in another, they argue, but the press should be free to report what has happened.

Nature's editors continued, "That there should be variations of practice from one country to another, in relation both to the press and to animal experiments, is inevitable and unavoidable; legal systems differ. But even where, as in Britain, Japan and the United States (the three countries in which this journal is equivalently published), the press is free from formal regulation, it is wise that it should conduct itself in a seemly fashion. The editors' rule of thumb for at least a quarter of a century has been that the results of animal experiments that would not easily win general regulatory consent had better be of *exceptional interest* if they are to be published" (emphasis added). They concluded, "The obvious counter-argument, that a refusal to publish will ensure that contentious experiments arc not undertaken in the first place, might have more force if there were not, for other good reasons, such a variety of journals." *Nature* not only lacks a formal policy on animal experimentation to which they could refer, but its editors do not ask their reviewers to comment on ethical concerns even in a general way.

During this debate, David G. Porter, chair of the department of biomedical sciences at the University of Guelph argued that a journal can no more escape the moral responsibility when it publishes research involving animals than can the investigator (Porter, 1989). Noting that an author is rewarded by publication, he contended that *Nature* "has at least the duty not to undermine the morality of the society in which it publishes. Indeed it can be argued that it has a duty to promote it."

On two grounds, the argument of "exceptional interest" is an inadequate response. First, *Nature* offered no evidence that this criterion is explicitly taken into account. Regarding the article under debate, neither the authors nor *Nature*'s editors directly addressed this point, nor was there any direct acknowledgement of the highly traumatic procedures used. Yet both the significance of the results and the trauma to the animals have to be identified in order to weigh the justification for conducting the experiments. The exceptional interest of retinal input and cortical development should not be assumed to be apparent to all readers without an explicit statement accompanying the article. Second, *Nature*'s "rule of thumb" does not incorporate the idea that some procedures are unacceptable irrespective of possible scientific merit.

It is true that an editor cannot stop the publication of unethical work. An editor can only control what is published in her own journal. Bad papers are often published sooner or later. They may be turned down by the better journals, but if their authors persist, they are likely to find an outlet elsewhere. The considerable number of biomedical science journals in existence—over 3,600 according to the 1992 indexing system of the National Library of Medicine—makes that result likely.

Once an article is published, editors are limited in what they can do. John Maddox, editor of *Nature,* says editors cannot be expected to investigate ethical concerns raised such as plagiarism, fraudulent research, and challenges to the humaneness of animal research. They have neither the resources nor authority to conduct such investigations. "Even now, there are many journals that do not entertain the idea that they should publish letters from correspondents complaining that material already published should not have seen the light of day. Others publish comments on material already published but only after the original authors have responded" (Maddox, 1989). As a result, he says, you usually cannot tell which is correct! This is all too true. But certainly the case of the year-long *Nature* correspondence illustrates how provocative, and in the end, how educationally useful discussion of a particular piece of research can be. Better surely to have these letters to the editor than to cover up the issues.

Problems of journals with diffuse constituencies

In general, the more narrowly defined the constituency, the easier it is to set standards; the more diffuse the constituency, the more constrains there are. *Nature,* for instance, is a highly respected international journal, with an extremely broad scope, and it is commercially published. Commercial journals do not have a defined "membership" nor an association structure (of committees charged with specific tasks) that can be called upon to help resolve issues. The paucity of policies in such journals should be understood in the context of these constraints.

The International Committee of Medical Journal Editors, which represents a group of over 300 journals, has a weak policy that states in its entirety: "When reporting experiments on animals indicate whether the institution's or the National Research Council's guide for, or any national law on, the care and use of laboratory animals was followed" (International Committee, 1988).

A look at international journals shows that the degree of effort to address animal issues varies widely. International journals with no stated policy include *Nature*, as mentioned, and *Neuroscience*, published by the International Brain Research Organization. Some international journals have modest policies. *Toxicology*, an international commercial publication with managing editors in Germany and the United States, has a policy that states in its entirety: "It is expected from the authors that they submit only data that have arisen from animal experimentation carried out in an ethically proper way. The Editors will not accept manuscripts which violate these principles." Just what these principles are is hard to fathom.

The policy of the British journal *Medical Science Research* about accepting articles from abroad for publication states: "Only those papers reporting work which conforms to high ethical standards will be considered for publication. In general, these standards are those which are governed by statute in the United Kingdom, but the Editor reserves the right to apply more stringent criteria where these are felt to be appropriate. The fact that the country of origin of a particular study does not have legislation governing animal or human experimentation which is as stringent as that operating in the UK, will not be relevant to the editorial decision" (Dixon, undated). Bernard Dixon, editor of *Medical Science Research*, says that "wherever in doubt about an author's protocols, I always consult a member of our Editorial Board who is a former member of the Home Office Advisory Committee on animal experimentation and who in turn remains closely and actively interested in these matters" (personal communication, December 24, 1991). Several British journals, including *Animal Behaviour, British Journal of Pharmacology, Journal of Physiology, Journal of Small Animal Practice,* and *Veterinary Record* have adopted the same policy.

Scientific journal editors have been quickly responsive to many ethical issues—they do what they can. This is true of ethical concerns about human experimentation and about disclosure of financial interests in the products being discussed. Some researchers have financial holdings, for instance, in drug companies that produce the drugs about which they are reporting. Nowadays, a number of journals require an author to declare that financial interest.

After some highly publicized incidents involving publication of fraudulent results, the attention of editors to the issue of fraud in science has been remarkably fast and thorough. In the last few years, the American Association for the Advancement of Science has organized several workshops and special sessions addressing this issue at their annual meetings. In 1988, journal editors from around the world convened for a conference, "Ethics and Policy in Scientific Publication," sponsored by the Council of Biology Editors in Washington, D.C. Although they recognized that editors are limited in what they can do, they agreed that they should not be content with a passive role. A consensus of the conference was that journal editors should require authors and co-authors to take public responsibility for their authorship and the validity of the manuscript and that authors should be required to provide access to raw data during the peer review process. If fraud is uncovered after publication, they agreed that editors have the responsibility to publish retractions, and that this information should be linked with the original computerized and other citation indexes thereafter. Many journal editors have established policies that follow these recommendations.

The response of journal editors to issues involving violations of animal welfare standards has been far less concerted.

Formal policies and editors' notes

Since life science journals—especially the prestigious journals—do affect the general standards of conduct, a strong case can be made that more editors should take an active role in animal experimentation issues. This is especially true for editors of journals published by professional associations because of the immediate beneficial influence that is possible with a narrowly defined constituency.

The rationale for establishing formal editorial policies is that publication of an article implies scientific approval and tends to legitimize the work. If authors are told what standards to comply with, then this provides a formal framework for reference. Furthermore, if the reviewers are specifically charged with watching out for unethical treatment of animals, then it is more likely that it will be identified. Scrutiny for ethical concerns does not just happen automatically in the review of manuscripts.

The *American Journal of Physiology, Pain,* and *Animal Behaviour* are among the journals most advanced in developing policies on animal experimentation. In these cases, the relevant professional associations have drawn up meaningful guidelines specific for that discipline; the guidelines are included or fully cited in instructions to authors; reviewers are charged with ensuring their compliance; and manuscripts identified as involving questionable animal procedures are referred to special committees for determination.

In the event that the committee receives a manuscript for determination, they have three options, depending on the seriousness of the concern:

1. Reject the manuscript on humane grounds with a clear statement to the author describing the areas of concern.
2. Require modification of the manuscript by the investigator to include any or all of the following: justification of the importance of the work; a description of the severity and duration of animal pain; a description of the procedures taken to alleviate the animal's pain or suffering.
3. Publish the article with an editor's note drawing attention to the concerns.

The case for journals publishing ethically borderline work is that, once published, the work is open for scientific and public scrutiny. An editor's note is essential for helping to stimulate further discussion of the issues by other contributors. Indeed, publication provokes discussion in a way that is probably unmatched by any other means. In the areas of fraud and in human experimentation, the publication of unethical or borderline ethical results has had a powerful effect in bringing about needed reforms.

An editor's note accompanying a published article and drawing attention to ethical concerns about animal welfare issues is a rare event. It did happen in 1984 in the journal *Animal Behaviour*. The editor's note stated, in toto: "The Ethical Committee of [the Association for the Study of Animal Behaviour] considered this paper and was satisfied that the killing of the pups was instantaneous and that no suffering was involved." The article in question, "Does copulation inhibit infanticide in male rodents?" described how the investigators offered newborn mice pups to forty-two individually tested adult mice to see if they would kill the babies. The incidence of infanticide was recorded and a comparison made of adults that had recently copulated and those that had not. At that time, there was a vogue among animal behaviorists for conducting infanticide studies and a number of papers were published on this topic.

In 1986, a detailed official policy was adopted by *Animal Behaviour* that addressed, among other things, staged infanticide. The policy requires that "wherever possible" field studies of natural encounters should be used in preference to staged encounters, and that where staged encounters are necessary, the use of models or alternative experimental designs should be considered (*Anonymous*, 1986). Furthermore, a formal review mechanism involving a special ethics committee was established to advise the editor about any submitted papers that appear to violate the spirit of the guidelines.

Patrick Bateson, professor of ethology at the University of Cambridge and secretary of this special ethics committee, has written: "If suffering was likely to be intense, we would not regard work as acceptable and would recommend rejection [for publication] even if the work was of high standard" (personal communication, 28 October, 1985).

In a subsequent 1988 article reporting results of staged infanticide published in that journal, the authors themselves included a section headed "Ethical Considerations." They discussed the issues in some detail and demonstrated that they had designed their experiments with ethical concerns about animal experimentation in mind.

Control of article content by editors

From the viewpoint of animal welfarists, the stylized presentation of scientific articles tends to downplay the level of animal pain and other harms involved, and fails to address the justification for inflicting these harms. Omissions in content and the choice of language also contribute to the downplaying of animal harms. Although it is common practice to include methodological details such as the dosage of anesthetic and analgesics, many aspects of the condition of the animal remain unstated. The animal's deviations from normal behavior, adverse responses, and descriptions of any severely deleterious condition are often omitted. Indeed, on reading some reports of research that involved slow and painful deaths for animals, one who is unfamiliar with the particular procedure would find it hard to detect the level of animal suffering. It is either omitted or glossed over.

This difficulty is illustrated by a paper describing the effects of ampicillin toxicity in guinea pigs (Young et al., 1987). I happened to read this shortly after emerging from a month-long stay in a hospital due to suffering the toxic effects of this drug. What happens is that administration of the antibiotic ampicillin can disturb the balance of the normal intestinal flora, thus permitting an overgrowth of enterotoxin-producing *Clostridium difficile*. As the authors of the study state, "The resulting enterocolitis often is fatal." The animals suffer diarrhea and are moribund, say the authors, but they do not indicate how much pain is involved. For me, the pain associated with ampicillin toxicity was the greatest I have ever suffered in my life, more than gall stones or childbirth. Human patients are treated around the clock with Demerol (meperidine hydrochloride) to control the pain. The guinea pigs received no pain-relieving treatment. For at least five of them, the endpoint of the study was a painful death.

Editors should assure that for all articles published (not only those of questionable ethics) sufficient information is provided so that the amount of harm done to the animals can be assessed. If a researcher specifically justifies the use of certain traumatic procedures instead of taking it for granted that such use is justified, then reviewers and other readers have a means of making up their own minds on the matter. The more traumatic the procedure, the more important it is that authors provide justification. If death is used as an endpoint, then the rationale for this, rather than an earlier and therefore more humane death, should be part of the paper. If the instructions to authors require that the infliction of moderate to severe animal harm must be justified, then it is likely that this would be complied with. As Maddox says, "Authors will go to endless trouble to meet conditions laid down by journals."

Another common omission is a description of the methods of housing and handling, yet these can have profound effects on the physiological and psychological state of the animal, which can translate into profound effects on the research results. Good discussions of these aspects are found in Bustad (1987) and Barnard and Hou (1988). The notion that methods of housing and handling animals do not belong in scientific papers may be justified by some in the interests of brevity—competition for space in journals is intense, so scientific papers have to be economical. But what is indispensable in a scientific paper is detail adequate for replication of the crucial experiment. Since differences in housing and handling can profoundly affect research results (as is being increasingly documented), then the rationale for this omission is brought into question.

Professor David Morton (1992) has commented on this issue in an article "A Fair Press for Animals" in the *New Scientist*. He describes a survey made by the RSPCA and FRAME of some 300 papers published in the late 1980s including experiments on monkeys in Britain. He writes: "More than one paper failed to reveal which species of monkey had been experimented upon . . . [and other] scientific omissions. Information about animal handling and care was often incomplete, or obscure, or so bland as to be meaningless; certainly it would be impossible for any researchers reading the paper to repeat the work accurately in their own laboratory. By not giving adequate information about the species, strain, and sex of animals, as well as husbandry and caging conditions, the animal "model" cannot be effectively reproduced elsewhere. And because scientific papers also neglect to give details of successes and failures encountered in early stages, other scientists using the model may well be unaware of what is likely to go wrong, leading to needless animal suffering." Morton recommends that authors "should pass on to readers any scoring systems [of animal harms] or special signs" by which animals were judged to be suffering. Authors should discuss the effectiveness of any scoring system to assess suffering, painkillers used, whether the experiment was correctly assigned a "severity banding." I fully endorse Professor Morton's recommendations.

Choice of language and format

There is a tradition that scientists downplay animal suffering and depersonalize their language. In the acculturation that takes place during a scientist's education, one learns that only "objective" facts are to be mentioned, not "emotional" aspects of the study. This impersonal style is part of the language of science, but to some extent it has been imposed by editors.

Jane Goodall was incensed when, at the beginning of her career, the editor of a scientific journal to which she had submitted a paper for publication demanded that every *he* or *she* (of her observed chimpanzees) be replaced with *it*, and every *who* be replaced with *which* (Goodall, 1990). Apparently the editor was so wedded to the impersonal language tradition that this was to take precedence over the readers' understanding of Goodall's scientific results. This editorial practice of using the word *it* when referring to an animal has still not died out, as was seen in the April 1992 issue of *Lab Animal*. The exchange was as follows. A letter to the editor quoted from a previously published article, "Evidently, the administered anesthetic did not successfully depress the animal's respiratory function enough so that it (*sic*) needed breathing assistance [*Editors' Note:* The decision to refer to the animal as "it" is a function of the editorial style of this journal, and was not the authors' original wording]."

The tradition of an impersonal style of scientific writing goes back many decades. It can be attributed in part to efforts of the biomedical community to avoid conflict with antivivisectionists. Susan E. Lederer (1992), a historian at Penn State medical school, describes some early editorial practices of textual revisions in her article "Political Animals: The Shaping of Biomedical Research Literature in Twentieth-Century America" published in *ISIS*, a leading journal of the history of medicine. In an effort to address problems with misrepresentation by antivivisectionists, Walter Bradford Cannon, in his capacity as chair on the Council on the Defense of Medical Research, circulated a letter among editors of medical journals in 1914 noting instances "in which it is claimed that, as there is no mention of anaesthetics, animals have been experimented on without anaesthesia." Cannon asked that "expressions which are likely to be misunderstood" be eliminated from publications of original papers. According to Lederer, Cannon received replies from more than twenty editors who agreed to comply with his suggestions.

Following Cannon's lead, Francis Peyton Rous went many steps further when he was editor of the *Journal of Experimental Medicine* from 1921 to 1946. Rous developed in-house guidelines for his editorial staff regarding textual revisions prior to publication. Always deleted was information that dogs had been obtained from a municipal pound (a common practice at that time); the use of personal names for animals such as Whitie or Mother was not allowed. Word substitutions were made: *animal* for *dog, fasting* for *starving, hemorrhaging* for *bleeding, intoxicant* for *poison,* and *pronounced* instead of *severe.* Rous's guidelines, writes Lederer, "dictated the avoidance of such qualifying descriptions as 'acute,' 'intense,' and 'severe,' or 'anything describing suffering or weakness too graphically.' Instead, 'impersonal medical terms' were preferable." The substitution of objective medical descriptions was intended to convey the idea of minimal animal suffering in the course of laboratory experimentation. Furthermore, details of animal activity or distress before or during an experimental procedure were proscribed as were details of an animal's struggle during the procedure. "Expressive features of an animal's vocalizations during an experiment were also omitted, as in the case of a 1934 article in which a reference to the 'almost continuous moaning' of ferrets, 'whining as though the animal was in pain' were eliminated from the text." The range and detail of the textual revisions in the *Journal* were

so great that, in the words of Lederer, the effect was to "scramble" the communication of laboratory data, "skewing expectations, replications, and results."
(What is extracted here is but a part of the editorial practices of the *Journal;* the
reader should go to Lederer's article for a fuller account).

Before these in-house policies had been established, both Rous personally and
the *Journal* had been subject to criticisms from the antivivisectionists. *Journal*
editorial staff had been sensitized by several episodes involving abuses of human
subjects, writes Lederer, in which antivivisectionist complaints about research
appearing in the *Journal* had generated considerable public discussion. Also,
Rous himself had been sensitized to issues of lay perceptions of animal experiments because extracts of a 1908 article in which he had reported his studies of
production of lymphocytosis in adult dogs had been criticized in antivivisection
literature.

Rous' editorial practices were doubtless successful in diverting antivivisection
comment from articles published in the *Journal of Experimental Medicine,* but
they also had other effects. A style of obfuscation of animal pain became established for scientific journals and remains to this day. Scientific language entails a
distancing of the researcher from the subject. Scientists may write about "collecting" animals from the wild when they really mean capturing and killing. This is
akin to military language where euphemisms (such as "body count") make it
easier for one side to inflict harm on the other. It is open to question just what
effect this imposed writing style has had on investigators and their attitudes
toward their experimental subjects.

According to Broad and Wade (1982) in *Betrayers of the Truth,* "The conven-
tions of scientific reporting require the writer to be totally impersonal, so as to
give the appearance of objectivity." A style that would make the material accessi-
ble to a wider audience is frowned upon because it "leads the reader to feel
uncertain concerning the rigor with which the experiments were performed"
(Wolff and Hunt, 1990).

Broad and Wade have also commented on the rigid rules of composition in
scientific publications: in the introduction, only in the most formalized way may
a scientist allude to his reasons for undertaking an investigation; then comes the
"materials and methods" section where the ingredients are described in tele-
graphic form; the "results" section is a dry tabulation of the data produced by the
given techniques; last comes the "conclusions" in which the researcher indicates
how his data confirm, refute, or extend current theory. Who did what, why, and
when have to be jettisoned from the start. In the name of logic, the historical path
to understanding must pass unmentioned, they say. The literary framework of a
scientific paper is a "fiction designed to perpetuate a myth."

This rigid format may have much to commend it in terms of ensuring completeness of scientific data for the purposes of possible replication of results.
Nevertheless, it is a format that can limit what can be said: it tends to bypass

discussion of ethical issues and the broader social implications of the work. How bereft we would be if Charles Darwin or Claude Bernard had had to conform to this format. We would have less appreciation of their literary talent and scientific genius, and also of the social controversies their work evoked. A broader perspective of current editors about inclusion of discussion of socially relevant ethical issues would be enlightened.

The need for ethical discussion in mainstream scientific literature

Currently, there is virtually a complete separation between journals that report the results of animal experiments and those that discuss ethical issues. As a result, the majority of bench scientists never read any discussions of the ethical issues in their professional publications. I have known of articles that address ethical concerns of animal experimentation that have been rejected despite highly favorable comments by several reviewers because the editor believed he should only publish animal research results.

Criticisms about unethical practices do not receive much welcome from editors and therefore do not often get published in the scientific literature. It should be noted that Beecher's influential article (1966) describing twenty-two publications in which he held that ethical norms had been breached in human experimentation was first rejected by the *Journal of the American Medical Association* before being published in the *New England Journal of Medicine*. It is still rare for an author to get comments on the ethical issues of animal experimentation published in mainstream literature.

Given the vast amount of research to be reported, specialization for journal content is inevitable. But given the inseparability of scientific results and the methods that are used to obtain them, inclusion of occasional articles on ethical issues in the journals that are primarily devoted to reporting research results would be welcome.

A few scientific publications are exceptional in their readiness to give space to animal welfare positions. Outstanding is the *New Scientist,* a commercially published science news magazine based in the U.K. that views itself as a bridge between scientists and non-scientists. In 1992, the *New Scientist* ran an unusual series of eighteen articles on the ethical issues of animal experimentation in which frequently a moderate stance of an animal welfare perspective was presented (see listing under the heading *New Scientist,* 1992). The stated editorial purpose was "to air many points of view in the hope of breaking down . . . polarities and promoting a climate of reasoned debate. We argue that animal experimentation is a legitimate topic of public debate, and that the public has a right to know what is done in its name. We call for greater openness on the part of scientists and civil servants as the only effective way to allay public concern." These articles stand as a model for journals and magazines in other countries.

In one of the contributions Mary Ann Elston, a sociologist at the University of London, reports on an inquiry into the relatively extensive attention given by the *New Scientist* to animal experimentation issues. By analyzing the articles published during the period 1970 to 1991, the magazine ran a total of 398 items on the animal experimentation debate, a mean of one item for every 2.8 issues (Elston, 1992). All items that referred to, or that generated comment of the scientific value or ethics of animal experimentation or laboratory animal welfare were included. By comparison, this was more than twice as many as *Nature* carried and over four times as many as the *British Medical Journal*.

Elston found that in 65 percent of the 398 items published in the *New Scientist* authors explicitly took a stance for or against some aspect of animal experimentation (the others were neutral). In 81 percent of those that took a stance (54 percent of the total) "the stance was more or less critical of some aspect of the practice, at least as currently organised." Elston writes that the *New Scientist* accepts "the value (and, implicitly, the necessity) of animal experimentation in the pursuit of scientific knowledge—a goal to which the magazine is clearly committed— while also accepting the right of critics to be heard and the legitimacy of at least some of the criticisms." Such a forum is missing in the United States, where the scientific literature tends to run an occasional strongly pro-animal experimentation article and very little involving any criticism.

In summary, high among the policy challenges facing journal editors today are establishing an explicit journal policy on animal use standards and a review mechanism to see that the policy is enforced; assuring completeness of information about both the harms and the justifications of performing traumatic animal procedures; and relaxing the current rigid journal format to permit wider discussion of ethical issues.

15

Looking Ahead

There are several broad fields of influence that impact on shaping public attitudes and public policy. They stem from academia, the legislature, the courts, and from the individual agendas of the protagonist parties. Some highlights from these influences can give a glimpse of what lies ahead.

New academic courses and appointments

Recent innovative developments in academia can serve as useful prototypes for broadening the discussion of animal issues in a less partisan environment. They range from the introduction of animal issues into the undergraduate curriculum, the establishment of academic chairs in the field of animal welfare, and courses on ethical concerns in veterinary schools, to the establishment of academic centers on alternatives.

At East Tennessee State University a scientist engaged in animal experimentation and a philosopher who is an antivivisectionist and an animal rights activist have established a course on ethical issues arising from use of animals for human purposes. The course, first offered in 1990, was repeated in 1991. To assure that the students are exposed to different perspectives, Anthony J. DeLucia, professor of surgery, and Hugh LaFollette, professor of philosophy, take turns in giving the lectures and also bring in guest lecturers. The topics covered include animal experimentation practices, alternatives, factory farming, hunting, wildlife issues, and so on. The leading philosophic and religious views about animals are

240

presented in an effort to help students clarify their own set of values. Along the way, the students learn by professorial example about mutual respect and about the problems of establishing public policy in areas involving moral issues. Premed students who have taken this course have voiced their appreciation to the faculty and have said they are pleased to be challenged on these issues now rather than in mid-career, as is most common.

Purdue University introduced an undergraduate course in 1991 leading to an animal welfare minor or subspecialty; a future graduate degree program is planned. Two faculty members, Lawrence Glickman, head of the department of veterinary pathology, and Alan Beck, director of the Center for Applied Ethology and Human-Animal Interaction, started the program. Participating faculty represent a broad spectrum of disciplines—veterinary medicine, agriculture, consumer and family sciences, liberal arts, and science. There will be courses on ethics, the biological basis of animal behavior, animal issues and the media, and human-animal interaction. Representatives of all parts of the animal welfare political spectrum, including the biomedical community, livestock producers, zoo staff members, and animal rights proponents, will give guest lectures. Students will also do field work at zoos, farms, and other animal sites. Since the courses are available only to upper-class students, the first graduates will enter the work force in about 1993 when it is expected that they will take jobs educating consumers, scientists, legislators, and animal owners about animal welfare issues.

A third new initiative is the intensive course on the ethics of animal experimentation that was given in the spring of 1991 at the Kennedy Institute of Ethics at Georgetown University. Philosophers with varying perspectives presented their views on such topics as who or what has moral standing, the rights of humans and other animals, and reassessing Darwin. Useful discussion took place among animal experimenters, veterinarians, philosophers, and animal rights activists. The courses at these three universities could serve as useful examples of what could take place in many academic settings.

Progress has also been made in the attainment of academic recognition of the field. By mid-1992, four academic chairs had been established on animal issues, three in Europe and one in Canada. The first, in the early 1980s, was the Chair of Ethics and Animals at the University of Leiden, The Netherlands, held by Tjard de Cock Buning, whose interest is in philosophical issues of animal experimentation. Shortly thereafter, the Colleen Macleod Chair in Animal Welfare was established at Cambridge University, England, and is occupied by Donald M. Broom, an animal behaviorist whose work focuses on agricultural animal welfare. In 1989, David B. Morton, a veterinarian and researcher, was appointed the head of department in a newly created Department of Biomedical Science and Biomedical Ethics at the University of Birmingham, England. This appointment combines the practical base of direction of laboratory animal resources with study of ethical issues—a unique linkage with value in enacting ethical decisions. Also, the Ontario Veterinary College (OVC) has established the Col. K. L. Campbell Chair in Animal Welfare, and its first holder is Professor Ronald S. Downey, a veterinarian and assistant dean at OVC, who assumed the position on July 1, 1992. He will explore ways to encourage and support alternatives and will investigate methods that reduce, refine, and replace the use of animals in research, including research that is aimed at improving the quality of life of animals in general. Part of Professor Downey's job will be to promote the interests of the Center for the Study of Animal Welfare, which was established at the University of Guelph in 1990.

In the United States three academic centers dealing with the use of animals in toxicity testing (as distinct from research and education) have been established. In the order in which they were founded they are: the In Vitro Toxicology Laboratory at Rockefeller University, first headed by Dennis Stark, and since June 1991 by Michael D. Hayre, both veterinarians; the Center for Alternatives to Animal Testing at Johns Hopkins University, headed by Alan M. Goldberg, a toxicologist; and the Center for Animals and Public Policy at Tufts University School of Veterinary Medicine under the direction of biochemist Andrew N. Rowan. In addition, on the initiative of Dean Borje Gustavsson, the Center for Animal Well-being has recently been established at the College of Veterinary Medicine at Washington State University at Pullman.

The courses at East Tennessee State, Purdue, and Georgetown are unusual, but there is additional instruction going on in American colleges about animal issues. Tom Regan estimates that well over 100,000 philosophy students each year are challenged with ethical dilemmas involving animals in their course work. Typically, in a fifteen-week course on contemporary moral issues, one or two weeks will be devoted to animal topics, and a range of contrasting viewpoints presented. Moral concern about animals is now a classroom topic as never before.

Textbooks have been developed for these courses. Most notable for comprehensiveness, balance, and usefulness is *Animal Rights and Human Obligations* edited by Regan and Singer, which is an anthology of writings about moral views on animals ranging from the Bible, Aristotle, Saint Thomas Aquinas, Descartes, Voltaire, Hume, Darwin, Kant, Schweitzer, Salt, and so on through contemporary times (Regan and Singer, 1976, 1989). Other texts which also present opposing sides are available (for instance, Levine, 1989, and Baird and Rosenbaum, 1991).

Moral concerns about animals have also become a topic for doctoral dissertations. Georgetown University, Princeton, and the University of Rochester are among the universities where philosophy students have graduated with doctorates on animal issues. This is a worldwide trend; examples could also be cited from Australia, Poland, South Africa, and throughout Europe.

Overall, the increase in academic instruction and research on animal issues is a hopeful sign because it helps promote fair discussion with all points of view being debated. As a result, a more informed and thoughtful process of developing public policy could emerge than is currently the case.

In departments of biological science, instruction on ethical aspects of human-animal interaction is becoming fairly well established in veterinary schools. The pioneering efforts of Bernard Rollin, professor of philosophy at Colorado State University, and Jerrold Tannenbaum, J.D., of the veterinary school at Tufts to promote instruction in veterinary ethics are having some effect. Typically, veterinary students are now presented with the problems of making value judgments on such topics as animal experimentation and the use of animals in veterinary and other education, mutilation procedures (such as debeaking of hens), cosmetic alteration of pet animals (such as ear cropping), detrimental inbreeding of show dogs, and other situations where the welfare and interests of the animal are in conflict with the wishes of the animal's owner.

It appears that medical schools have been generally less receptive than veterinary schools to discussions of animal experimentation. Instruction is less frequently offered and it tends to be narrow, covering primarily the case for animal experimentation; a fair presentation of contrary moral positions is unusual. Yet informing these students about various perspectives on these ethical issues is highly relevant to their future careers. It would be a mark of progress if instruction on the ethical aspects of animal experimentation became an established part of the curriculum in the biomedical sciences generally, not just for veterinary students.

The political and legal arenas

Major social influences flow not only from academia but also, of course from the political arena. An important law, the Animal Enterprise Protection Act, was passed in 1992. This law amends Title 18 of the United States Code by creating a new section 43, Animal Enterprise Terrorism. The law stipulates that any activity against an animal enterprise that results in economic loss greater than $10,000 would become a federal offense punishable by fines and/or imprisonment. The law also imposes stiffer penalties if people are seriously injured or killed. Because of the change in wording in the bill before passage it was considered unnecessary to address whistle-blower protection. The intent of this law is to reduce the violence and frequency of raids, and the intimidation of scientific investigators. By bringing in the FBI when a lab raid has occurred, it is hoped that more offenders would be brought to justice—something that happened rarely under previous laws.

The federal and state legislatures have before them a number of issues that are controversial. These include fostering alternatives to the LD50 and Draize tests, controlling toxicity testing of cosmetic and household products on animals, and controlling the military use of animals for weapons testing. In addition, still waiting for resolution is the question of using pound animals for research.

In recent years, animal rights groups have been paying greater attention to the political platform of candidates on animal and environmental issues. Recommendations for voting on presidential and other candidates is now within their compass. This development is still in its infancy, however. Few candidates for political office have established much of a record on animal experimentation issues. On the other hand, lobbying activities are well established and well financed by groups representing different positions.

A third major social influence flows from the courts. So far, several legal disputes regarding the use of animals in education have been decided. A student's right to choose an alternative study not involving harming an animal has been repeatedly upheld. Many institutions are voluntarily developing their own policies to deal with conscientious objection.

Awaiting USDA action are several issues involving the Animal Welfare Act—inclusion of rats, mice, and birds under provisions of the Act, and the adequacy of the USDA regulations on environmental enrichment of primates and exercise for dogs. Also unresolved in several jurisdictions is the issue of public attendance at, and access to records of Institutional Animal Care and Use Committee meetings. Court battles are likely to continue.

It seems to me that these three influences (trends in academia, in the Congress and legislatures, and in the courts) are working together in the same direction—to increase the awareness of animal welfare issues. As a result, much is being accomplished through voluntary efforts. An increasing concern for the limits of responsible animal experimentation in research, in testing, and in education is emerging.

But currently emotions remain so high that on some issues no quick resolution is in sight. Improvements in the environment for discussion of animal welfare issues do not, unfortunately, signify a softening in the positions taken at both ends of the spectrum of opinion. The search for solutions is not a welcome addition to the agenda of diehard polemicists at either extreme who are more preoccupied with defending established positions—either total approval or total disapproval of animal experiments. They fear that any concession will encourage further pressure and further retreats. There is little recognition that serious and objective examination of major issues and an effort to arrive at an accommodation will redound to society's benefit and their own.

For an improved environment, there needs to be a softening of the counterproductive strategies used by both extremes. There is too much emphasis on strategies intended to obscure the issue and to pose false alternatives. For example, the first line of defense against any reform has been to portray it as an attack on biomedical research, if not on science in general. This tactic serves to obscure the specific issues that are under examination. Similarly, any evidence of animal suffering is generalized to support a charge that all animal experimentation is needlessly cruel and that all investigators lack sensitivity to ethical concerns for laboratory animals.

Equally visible is the resort to "stonewalling"—so evident throughout all segments of society and most prominently in politics. It includes the automatic denial of all charges, the insistence that everything is perfect, and the attempt to block all access to information unless it is compelled. A scientist who happens to take a view that wavers from the establishment position can count on being misrepresented and given the kind of treatment usually reserved for whistle-blowers. At the other extreme, the conspiratorial approach of some activists serves the same purpose of evading responsibility for antisocial acts and the destruction of legitimate scientific endeavor.

Thus optimism that the future will bring further definition of the reasonable limits on animal experimentation needs to be tempered. I am cheered that in the field of cosmetic safety testing, for example, scientific investigators for consumer products have cut substantially their reliance on painful animal tests and they did so with no apparent detriment to their own work or to product development. Some states recognize the right of students to escape compulsory dissection as conscientious objectors, and the sky has not fallen. Some veterinary schools now allow students to qualify professionally without resort to harming healthy animals for pedagogic exercises. Thanks to the influence of Institutional Animal Care and Use Committees, the use of proper anesthetics, improved post-surgical care, and use of approved euthanasia procedures is now becoming routine. Also, as these committees gain experience, review for animal welfare concerns is becoming better defined and investigators are more carefully justifying the animal procedures they use. Although the general direction seems clear, progress depends on a growing willingness of partisans to seek solutions.

An agenda for some future progress has been proposed throughout this book. A few of the recommendations merit reiteration.

Summary of major recommendations

1. Adopt a meaningful pain scale

A classification system to denote severity of animal harms would be a welcome addition to public policy in the United States. Such a classification system could be used by Institutional Animal Care and Use Committees in their review process and as a basis for reporting annual statistics for animal experimentation.

2. Improve national data collection

Three major revisions are needed in the way national statistics on the use of laboratory animals are compiled. In addition to the one mentioned above, these are to report the purpose of the experiment according to principal categories, and to provide details about primate use by major species.

3. Strengthen policies on animals in education

National policies on the use of animals in education require strengthening. At the secondary school level there should be no killing or harming of vertebrate animals for classroom or home projects. For grade school extracurricular projects (as in science competitions), as a general rule, only observational studies of pets, wild animals, and zoo animals should be permitted.

National policies in the United States should be refined to address more effectively the use of animals in higher education. Instead of treating all types of animal use as if they were equally justified, as the current policies do, the Animal Welfare Act and the Public Health Service policies should separate the use of animals in education from their use in research or in testing. New policies are needed that encourage avoidance of harming or killing vertebrate animals for educational purposes wherever possible and that allow student conscientious objection to animal experiments.

4. Heighten awareness of animal issues among editors

Where editorial policies are lacking, scientific journal editors should establish guidelines on the ethical conduct of animal experimentation that provide (a) a stated policy of standards of animal experimentation for their journal and (b) a review mechanism to see that these standards are complied with. In addition, the guidelines should require full information within the text of a research article about the degree of animal harms inflicted and the justification for performing traumatic procedures. Editors should be encouraged to be more open to publishing occasional discussions of ethical issues.

5. Foster an "acute study" policy for pound animals

A compromise should be sought to end current polarized battles over the use of pound animals. An "acute study" policy that releases pound animals for painless experimental studies offers a reasonable alternative to the "free access" and "no access" extremes. Controlled conditions could be established that would ensure that the animal (a) travels directly from the pound to the USDA-registered laboratory facility with no involvement of animal dealers, (b) is used for acute, nonsurvival experiments that permit no recovery of consciousness after anesthesia, and (c) is dead within 24 hours of leaving the pound. This policy would not be forced on shelters unwilling to cooperate. This would not lessen the opposition of antivivisectionists, but it would address the concerns of those who support animal experimentation but object strongly to the possible use of pets in research.

6. Establish a national commission

A national commission, fairly representing the spectrum of viewpoints, like the highly influential one on ethical issues of human experimentation issues, could tackle some of the thorny problems now besetting the conduct of animal research. Its charge could include provision of additional protection of non-human primates used in research, training needs of those who conduct animal experiments, research needs to foster better pain relief in laboratory animals, improved methods of collecting national data on animal experiments, development of special policies on student use of animals, mechanisms to enhance the public's involvement in decision-making regarding animal experiments, and gaining public confidence in animal experiments that are being conducted.

Inasmuch as Institutional Animal Care and Use Committees represent a key mechanism of control of animal experiments in the United States, research on their functioning is needed. Depending on available resources, the proposed commission could either contract out such studies, or could achieve this objective by some other means. The purpose of the research would be to provide a national picture of the range of current practices and to explore ways to strengthen their influence and public accountability. Findings about the practices of the most effective committees should be publicized. Results of such studies might be instructive for developing more informed public policy on such issues as the role of the community member, increased representation of the animal protection constituency in decision-making, problems of inconsistencies in approving certain experimental procedures between committees of different institutions, and clarifying the scope of authority of the committees.

The timing of when to establish a commission is critical to its success. The 1978 National Commission for the Protection of Human Subjects carried with it widespread public support for resolving what appeared at that time to be intractable problems. Similarly, an animal experimentation commission would need a high level of public support for finding solutions in order to make it worthwhile. Without such support, its recommendations could be ignored. The idea of having an animal experimentation commission has been around for several years, and is mentioned here again, not because the time is yet ripe, but because the idea should be kept alive as a mechanism worth using at the right time.

Conclusion

One of the stated purposes of this book was to make recommendations for policy changes that are achievable within the foreseeable future that would improve the lot of animals used for experimentation without stultifying scientific progress. When recommendations for change are made about highly controversial subjects, they are likely to be misunderstood and misrepresented—they may even arouse antagonism between groups whose views are polarized. Any proposed compromise between the extremes is subject to challenge from both extremes. Despite the hazards of addressing these issues, I believe that open debate is a constructive route. This book reflects a modest effort in that direction.

Appendix A
Animals Used in Experimentation, (in thousands)
FY 1973–1990

FY	Primates	Dogs	Cats	Guinea pigs	Hamsters	Rabbits	Other	Total
1973	42	195	66	NA	NA	NA	1350	1653
1974	51	199	74	NA	NA	NA	1368	1693
1975	36	154	51	NA	NA	NA	1136	1378
1976	50	210	70	NA	NA	NA	1458	1780
1977	53	176	62	349	394	439	47	1520
1978	57	197	66	419	414	475	58	1687
1979	59	211	69	457	420	540	76	1832
1980	56	189	68	422	406	471	49	1662
1981	58	189	58	433	398	474	50	1658
1982	46	161	50	459	338	454	69	1577
1983	55	175	53	485	337	467	109	1680
1984	55	202	57	561	437	529	233	2074
1985	57	195	59	599	414	545	284	2154
1986	49	176	54	463	371	522	144	1778
1987	61	180	50	539	416	554	168	1969
1988	52	140	42	431	332	459	178	1635
1989	52	156	51	482	389	471	154	1754
1990	47	110	33	353	311	399	324	1578
1991	43	108	35	379	304	396	578	1842

The years represent all years for which USDA data are available. Figures are rounded to the nearest thousand. The total represents all "AWA-Protected Animals." During all years, primates, dogs, cats, guinea pigs, rabbits, and hamsters, and certain other species are included, but the "other" has varied over time.

For all years, rats, mice, and birds are excluded. For years 1973 through 1989, agricultural animals (pigs, sheep, and calves) are excluded. In 1990, agricultural animals (comprising 66,702) were counted for the first time and are included here in "other."

NA = not available; for these years, guinea pigs, hamsters, and rabbits are included in "other."

Source: APHIS, USDA.

Appendix B
Funding Sources for Targeted Programs
to Promote Alternatives

Note: This chronological listing by year of inception represents two types of entry: (a) grant-giving organizations for which persons or organizations in the United States qualify for funding (no asterisk) and (b) organizations for whose funding U.S. applicants do not qualify (asterisk).

* 1961. The Lawson Tait Trust in the U.K. in association with three leading antivivisection societies was established to promote research into the development and dissemination of human techniques, such as tissue and organ cultures, or the use of films and models in teaching.

* 1970. The Dr. Hadwen Trust for Humane Research, 22 Bancroft, Hitchin, Herts SG5 1JW, England, established by the British Union for the Abolition of Vivisection, gives small-scale funds for scientists to develop techniques and procedures that will "replace or reduce current usage of animals." In 1992–1993, the Trust awarded in excess of £60,000 sterling, and its research budget is due to expand.

* 1973. The Air Chief Marshall Lord Dowding Fund in England was established by the National Anti-Vivisection Society along similar lines to that of the Hadwen Trust, see above.

* 1972. The Felix-Wankel-Tierschutz-Forschungspreis award, West Germany.

* 1979. The Swedish government awarded approximately $90,000 for alternatives research.

* 1981. The BMJFFG (German Ministry for Youth, Family, Women, and Health) research award, West Germany.

1981. The Johns Hopkins University Center for Alternatives to Animal Testing, School of Hygiene and Public Health, 615 N. Wolfe St., Baltimore, MD 21205-2179. Director, Alan Goldberg, Ph.D. This Center was established with a one million dollar donation from the Cosmetic, Toiletry and Fragrance Association Inc., Avon Products Inc., Bristol Myers Company, and other companies. The Center provides grant support for *in vitro* research in testing and has proved to be an important source of funds in the United States.

1981. American Fund for Alternatives to Animal Research (AFAAR), 175

West 12th St., Suite 16G, New York, NY 10011. Director, Dr. Ethel Thurston. The first grant went to Joseph Leighton, M.D., at the Medical College of Pennsylvania, Philadelphia to develop *in vitro* alternatives to the Draize test. This grant program has proliferated over the years. In 1990, AFAAR, responding to industry claims that alternative tests although available are still at the prevalidation stage and therefore not usable, starting funding a validation project at the Multicenter Evaluation of In Vitro Cytoxicity, which operates in twenty laboratories in nine countries.

1982. Geraldine R. Dodge Foundation, 95 Madison Avenue, P.O. Box 1239, Morristown, NJ 07960. Executive Director, Scott McVay. One of the program areas is "Welfare of Animals." As an indication of size, in 1991, a total of forty-eight grants were awarded, amounting to over $750,000.

1983. New England Anti-Vivisection Society, 333 Washington Street, Suite 850, Boston, MA 02108-5100. Executive Director, Frank Cullen. They have supported tissue culture alternatives to the Draize test, and other projects.

* 1984. The British government Home Office started awarding grants to support research into the use of alternatives. Recipients have included the Fund for the Replacement of Animals in Medical Experiments (FRAME), Nottingham, England (£185,000) and the Universities Federation for Animal Welfare (£30,000). Lesser amounts were awarded in subsequent years so that in 1989, for instance, the entire government funding was four grants (out of 124 applicants) for a total of £70,000. The RSPCA considered this to be a "paltry sum when compared to the vast amounts spent on research using animals and in comparison to the £1,000,000 from the West German government to validate alternatives to the Draize test."

* 1985. Platform for Alternatives, Dr. P. de Greéve, Veterinary Public Health Inspectorate, Department of Animal Experimentation, P.O. Box 5406, 2280 HK Rijswijk, The Netherlands. Seven government ministries, a number of pharmaceutical companies, and four animal protection organizations participate in this endeavor to "coordinate and stimulate the national efforts in the area of alternatives." In 1989, awards totalled 1.5 million guilders (approximately $780,000).

* 1985. The European Federation of Pharmaceutical Industries Associations (EFPIA), Avenue Louise 250, Bte 91, B-1050 Brussels, Belgium, makes an annual award of 25,000 Swiss francs for recognition of research contributing to the development of non-animal methods of experimentation. EFPIA represents the pharmaceutical industry in sixteen European countries.

1986. Hildegard Doerenkamp and Gerhard Zbinden Foundation Awards, c/o Gerhard Zbinden, M.D., F.R.C. Pathology, Professor of Toxicology, Institute of Toxicology, University of Zurich, CH-8603 Schwerzenbach, Switzerland. Awards a number of annual prizes for scientific contributions to reduction of animal experimentation. The focus for each year's prize is announced.

1986. The William and Charlotte Parks Foundation for Animal Welfare, c/o Fleet Investment, One City Center, P.O. Box 9791-MEPM005, Portland, Maine 04104. In 1990, a total of twenty-five awards were made, totaling $186,000.

1986. Marchig Animal Welfare Award, c/o World Society for the Protection of Animals Headquarters, Park Place, Lawn Lane, London SW8 IUD, England, and also WSPCA, Western Hemisphere Office, 29 Perkins Street, Boston, MA 02130. Provides an internationally competitive annual award of S. Frs. 40,000 for any one of the following program areas: (1) the development of new alternative methods to the use of animals in experimental situations; (2) practical implementation of an alternative method in a scientific or manufacturing procedure; or (3) for practical work in the field of animal welfare by a society or individual deserving of support anywhere in the world.

1987. National Institutes of Health, Department of Health and Human Services, Bethesda, MD 20892. This agency of the federal government first announced in January 1987 that NIH would award grants for "research into methods of research that do not use vertebrate animals, use fewer vertebrate animals, or produce less pain and distress in vertebrate animals used in research." By 1989, seventeen awards had been made. See discussion of this program in chapter 5.

* 1987. Fund for Experimental Animal-Free Research, Switzerland.

* 1988. Home Office, Room 971, Division E, 50 Queen Anne's Gate, London, SW1H 9AT, UK, provides grants for research to reduce, refine, or replace the use of living animals in scientific testing. This grant program was established in 1986 when the Animals (Scientific Procedures) Act was passed, and the first awards were made in 1988. In 1991, the Home Office announced preference will be given to proposals that have a good prospect of leading to the refinement or replacement of procedures that use large numbers of animals or that involve substantial suffering.

* 1988. Land-Government of Nordrhein-Westfalen Research Award, West Germany.

1988. International Foundation for Ethical Research, 53 West Jackson Boulevard, Suite 1542, Chicago, IL 60604. Executive Director, Michael J. Bello, Ph.D. Supports projects involving all three R's of refinement, replacement, and reduction. In 1989, three grants were awarded, totaling $55,000. This funding source was founded and is financed by the National Anti-Vivisection Society.

1988. Physicians Committee for Responsible Medicine, P.O. Box 6322, Washington, D.C., 20015. President, Neal D. Barnard, M.D. Summer fellowships for veterinary and medical students to conduct supervised independent projects critically evaluating animal research and non-animal methodologies. The stated purpose is to help build a bridge between organized medicine and the animal protection movement to help rectify the polarization on animal experimentation.

1988. Bristol-Myers Award for Distinguished Achievement in Pain Research,

345 Park Avenue, 43–38, New York, NY 10154. Annual award of $50,000.

1988. Medical Research Modernization Committee, P.O. Box 6036, Grand Central Station, New York, NY, 10163-6018. Vice Chairman, Stephen R. Kaufman, M.D. Awards research fellowships to evaluate the relevance of animal models for the diagnosis and treatment of human disease.

1989. Colgate Palmolive Postdoctoral Award, c/o Education Committee, Society of Toxicology, 1101 Fourteenth St., N.W., Suite 1100, Washington, D.C. 20005. One award of a fellowship in *in vitro* toxicology is made each year, and each recipient receives $33,500 for each of two years. The program has "particular interest in alternatives to animal studies for assessment of dermal and ocular toxicity and in technology that could be applicable to this goal."

1989. Animal Alternatives Program, Proctor and Gamble Company, Miami Valley Laboratories, P.O. Box 398707, Cincinnati, OH 45239-8707. In June 1989, the University Animal Alternatives Research Program (UAARP), a competitive awards program, was established. Its purpose is to encourage university investigators in the biological sciences to develop alternative methods (all three R's) for efficacy and safety testing. It provides up to three scientists with up to $50,000 annually for a maximum of three years' support. The first awards were announced in 1990.

1989. The American Anti-Vivisection Society, Alternatives Research Department, Suite 204 Noble Plaza, 801 Old York Road, Jenkintown, PA 19046-1685. Funding of grants up to a maximum of $50,000 each is available to U.S. universities and research institutions to "encourage the utilization of alternatives to traditional use of animals in biomedical research, product safety testing and educational demonstrations." In both 1990 and 1991, four grants were awarded each year.

1989. Johnson and Johnson, 401 George St., New Brunswick, NY 08901-2021. Vice President of Science and Technology, Dr. Robert Z. Gussin. Grants awarded to several university-based investigators for study of *in vitro* alternatives for evaluating ocular and dermal toxicity.

* 1989. Alternative Research Fund, Animal Defence League of Canada, P.O. Box 1880, Station C, Ottawa, Ontario, Canada KIY 4M5. Awards grants and bursaries to promote scientifically valid alternatives to the use of animals in research, testing, and teaching.

* 1990. Hugo van Poelgeest Prize (DFL. 15,000), administered by Professor Tjard de Cock Buning, Faculty of Medicine, P.O. Box 9606, 2300 RC, Leiden, The Netherlands. Awarded every four years to an investigator who succeeds in developing methods leading to outstanding scientific results without the use of animals, in a field where animal experimentation is the main option.

* 1990. Joseph F. Morgan Research Foundation, 205-151 Slater St., Ottawa, Ontario, Canada KIP 5N1. Established through an initiative of the Canadian Federation of Humane Societies, this program will in the future fund research

directed towards the refinement of controversial procedures such as those for acute toxicity and metabolism/function tests, and towards the reduction of animal use in chronic assays.

* 1990. Swiss Institute of Alternatives to Animal Testing (SIAT), Secretariat, Christoph A. Reinhardt, Dr. phil., Turnerstrasse 1, CH-8006 Zurich, Switzerland.

* 1990. Le A. L. Antivivisectionists in Italy funded six grants amounting to 6 million lire each.

1990. The Demeter Fund, The American Anti-Vivisection Society, Suite 204, Noble Plaza, 801 Old York Rd., Jenkintown, PA 19046-1685. Annual award of grants for research in the development and validation of non-animal methods. Three awards were made in 1992.

1991. Russell and Burch Award, The Humane Society of the United States, 2100 L St., N.W., Washington, D.C. 20037. A single award made annually of five thousand dollars to recognize a scientist who has made outstanding advances to promote the three R's of alternatives to the use of animals in research, testing, and education.

* 1992. NEAMS Trust (New Educational Aids in Medicine and Science), P.O. Box 516, Darlinghurst, New South Wales 2010, Australia. NEAMS is an autonomous charitable trust that aims to encourage the adoption of non-animal teaching methods in tertiary medical and science courses.

Appendix C
Sunshine Laws

"Sunshine laws" in the United States require that meetings of certain agencies be open to the public and that certain agency records be made available to the public. The laws are particularly pertinent to institutions that receive state funding. Broadly speaking, the intent is that policy-making decisions should not be made nor pertinent records held behind closed doors. Not all states have such laws and the terms of the laws vary.

The following listing is divided into two sections according to whether American state or Canadian provincial sunshine laws are upheld or not regarding activities of Institutional Animal Care and Use Committees. In each section, entries are listed in rough chronological order of when these committee meetings or records became open to the public, which could have happened either by a legal ruling or other event. In states not mentioned, it can be assumed that the IACUC meetings are closed. This could be because existing laws have not been tested.

Sunshine laws do apply

Florida

The IACUC of the University of Florida at Gainesville was probably the first to become open to the public, around 1985. This occurred with no legal challenge. To this day, all IACUC meetings are regularly attended by animal rights activists under provisions of the Florida sunshine law. (See Chapter 11, page 174, for additional comment.)

Washington

When a suit was brought to open the IACUC meetings of the state-supported University of Washington in Seattle, contentious litigation resulted. University officials maintained that the IACUC is an advisory body to the Vice President for Health Sciences and is not a governing body and therefore falls outside the Open

Public Meetings Act. In an April 29, 1987, ruling the Washington court however, found that the university's IACUC is, in fact, a governing body of the university with respect to issues of the use, care, and welfare of laboratory animals, and the IACUC meetings are within the scope of the state law. So now the meetings are open. The university was required to pay the animal welfare society that brought suit in excess of $5,000 in legal fees. Although the suit was concluded, the dispute continued and on November 2, 1987, King County Superior Court ruled that the University of Washington must release protocol review forms to the animal welfare society.

Texas

In 1990, Texas Attorney General Jim Mattox issued a decision that Texas Tech University Health Sciences Center must reveal the names of IACUC members and make public the IACUC minutes, records, and reports under the state Open Records Act. Texas Tech had argued that these records were protected under the Texas law because they contained protected opinion or scientific information that could be sold. The university also sought to prove that disclosure of the names of IACUC members would expose them to harassment or litigation, but both arguments were discounted.

North Carolina

A January 15, 1991, decision of the North Carolina Court of Appeals ruled that the University of North Carolina Chapel Hill had to disclose certain IACUC documents to the public under the state's public records law. Students for the Ethical Treatment of Animals had filed suit to force the disclosure of four animal research applications. The court ruled that the university could remove the names, addresses, phone numbers, departments, and experience levels of the researchers, and proposals not approved by the IACUC need not be revealed. The higher court ruled that information on animal research cannot be withheld from the public "merely because someone chooses to label it a 'trade secret.'" There was no evidence that trade secrets were involved, the court said, and furthermore, "academic freedom" was not a justification for keeping documents secret.

Vermont

An injunction issued in June 1991 requires the University of Vermont to open its IACUC meetings and make its records available to the public. This is unusual in that it allows members of the public to participate, not just to attend as observers. On August 28, 1992, the Vermont Supreme Court upheld the injunction.

Kentucky

In Kentucky, IACUC meetings are "open" with significant restrictions. In a ruling that became effective in January, 1989, a Kentucky state circuit court determined that the University of Kentucky's IACUC is subject to state open meetings and records laws. The court also determined that protocols submitted to the IACUC were exempt from disclosure to the public and were the individual property of the faculty member. The protocols are not final and may be modified by the IACUC, by the investigator, or by the funding agency, and are protected under the AWA, which precludes the release of confidential information. For similar reasons, IACUC minutes dealing with individual protocols were not to be disclosed. Finally, because the AWA makes it unlawful for the IACUC to disclose confidential information, those portions of the IACUC meetings where protocols are discussed are to be held in private.

Sunshine laws do not apply

California

On August 18, 1989, an Alameda County Superior Court judge dismissed a suit brought by Animal Allies against the University of California system. The judge ruled that the University of California's ten campuses are not subject to the state's open meeting law. An appeal brought by seven humane groups against this ruling failed in 1991. In a separate action brought under the Public Records Act by In Defense of Animals, the court ruled on November 4, 1992, that the University of California must copy and turn over to IDA uncensored autopsy reports on lab animals that had died in its care. Before this ruling, IDA had been able to obtain only censored reports.

Virginia

In 1989, the Virginia Supreme Court refused to overturn a Richmond circuit court decision denying Students for Animals access to meetings of the University of Virginia's Animal Research Committee. The court compared the Animal Research Committee to the Virginia National Guard planning committees and university basketball or football coaching staff meetings. The court wrote, "To require meetings of such groups to be treated as public meetings would be to carry the idea of government in the 'sunshine' to an absurd extreme."

New York

In 1991, the New York Supreme Court overturned a lower court's 1989 decision ordering the State University of New York Stony Brook's IACUC to open its meetings to the public. A four-judge panel of the Appellate Division, Second Department, unanimously decided that the committee is not a "public body" as defined by the law. The IACUC at Stony Brook acts only as an "advisory body" and it is "manifestly apparent" that the committee is not involved in "deliberations and decisions that go into the making of public policy" and therefore does not perform a "government function." Prior to this decision, the university said it had released 700 grant applications to animals welfare organizations, an action that is reportedly unprecedented for any college or university in the state.

Oregon

In 1991, Oregon circuit court judge George Woodrich ruled that PETA and Students for the Ethical Treatment of Animals lacked standing to seek judicial review of the University of Oregon's ban on public attendance at their IACUC.

Massachusetts

At first, a lower court and the Suffolk Superior Court of the Commonwealth of Massachusetts ruled that the open meeting law did apply to the University of Massachusetts' IACUC. But this decision was reversed on appeal. The Massachusetts state Appeals Court ruled on October 28, 1991, that since the committee meetings are held to ensure compliance with state and federal animal care and use regulations and not to discuss public policy, they are therefore exempt from the state open meeting laws.

Ontario, Canada

An appellant tried to obtain reports required by the Ontario Ministry of Agriculture and Food (OMAF) concerning IACUC members' "names and particulars" and number of species used by commercial research facilities in Ontario. Under Ontario provincial law, such information is contained in institutions' annual reports required by OMAF. A May 25, 1990, verdict denied access of this information because of possible vandalism by animal activists. According to the CCAC, Ontario is the only province to have such a Freedom of Information law.

References

Chapter 1 The beginnings

Anonymous, 1839. Experiments on Living animals. Editorial. *Lond. Med. Gaz.* 24:212–5, May 4.

———, 1840. Sketch of Magendie by an American. *The Medical Times,* 2(33):77, May 9.

———, 1863. The Discussion on Vivisections. *BMJ* ii:323–5, September 19.

Bell, C., 1824. Natural System. 29–30. Quoted by Olmsted J.M.D., 1944. *François Magendie,* Shuman's: New York, page 116.

Bentham, J., 1962. *The Works of Jeremy Bentham,* ed. J. Bowring. Russell and Russell: New York. Vol. 1, pages 142–3.

Bernard, C., 1865. *An Introduction to the Study of Experimental Medicine.* Originally published in France in 1865. Translated into English by Henry Copley Greene and republished in 1949 by Henry Schuman, Inc., in the United States (no city given). Pages 100–102.

Canadian Council on Animal Care, 1980. *Guide to the Care and Use of Experimental Animals,* volume 1, pages 65, 66, and 75.

Descartes, R. Selections from *Discourse on Method, Part 5.* In: *Philosophic Works of Descartes,* tr. E. S. Haldane and G.R.T. Ross, London: Cambridge University Press. Volume I, pages 115–8. Other selections reprinted in *Animal Rights and Human Obligations,* eds. T. Regan and P. Singer, second edition. Prentice Hall: Englewood Cliffs, New Jersey, 1989.

French, R. D., 1975. *Antivivisection and Medical Science in Victorian Society.* Princeton University Press: Princeton, NJ, and London. (a) page 107; (b) pages 20–1; (c) Appendix 11, pages 414–5; (d) page 48; (e) Appendix 1, page 413.

Fulton, J. F., 1966. *Selected Readings in the History of Physiology,* second edition. Thomas: Springfield, IL. Pages 280–5.

Gordon-Taylor, G., and Walls, E. W., 1958. *Sir Charles Bell: His Life and Times.* E. and S. Livingstone, Ltd.: Edinburgh and London. Page 129.

Holmes, F. L., 1974. *Claude Bernard and Animal Chemistry: The Emergence of a Scientist.* Harvard University Press: Cambridge, MA. Pages 126–7.

Jonas, H., 1969. Ethical Aspects of Experimentation with Human Subjects. *Daedalus, Journal of the American Academy of Arts and Sciences.* Spring issue, Volume 98, pages 219–47.

Olmsted, J.M.D., 1938. *Claude Bernard Physiologist.* Harper and Brothers: New York. Pages 34–35. Quoted from: Bernard, C., 1867. *Rapport sur les progrès et la* marche de la physiologie générale en France. Impr. impériale: Paris. Page 237 et seq.

————, 1939. Claude Bernard, Physiologist. Cassell: London. Pages 226, 233–9.

————, 1944. François Magendie. Schuman's: New York. (a) page 138; (b) page 222.

Perry, A., 1860. Vivisection Cruelties. The Lancet, Nov. 24, page 517.

Richards, S., 1987. Vicarious Suffering, Necessary Pain: Physiological Method in Late Nineteenth-century Britain. In: Rupke, N. A., ed. 1987, Vivisection in Historical Perspective. Croom Helm: London. Pages 125–48. (a) page 141; (b) page 125; (c) page 127; (d) page 140.

Sechzer, J. A., 1983. The Ethical Dilemma of Some Classical Animal Experiments. In: The Role of Animals in Biomedical Research. Annals of NY Acad. Sciences. ed. J. A. Sechzer, volume 406, pages 5–12.

Vyvyan, J., 1988. In Pity and in Anger: A Study of the Use of Animals in Science. Micah Publications: Marblehead, MA:. Page 43.

Chapter 2 Current attitudes and ethical arguments

Beauchamp, T. L., 1992. The Moral Standing of Animals in Medical Research. Journal of Law, Medicine and Ethics. 20(1–2):7–16.

Caplan, A. L., 1988. Just Like Us. A forum with other participants held in New York City. Harpers Magazine, August, pages 43–51.

Clarke, S.R.L., 1977. The Moral Status of Animals. Clarendon Press: Oxford, UK.

Cohen, C., 1986. The case for the use of animals in biomedical research. NEJM 315(14):865–70.

Darwin, C., 1871. The Descent of Man. The cited passages are found in T. Beauchamp, J. Feinberg, and J. M. Smith, eds., Philosophy and the Human Condition, 2d ed. Prentice Hall: Englewood Cliffs, NJ, 1989. Pages 107–110.

Donnelley, S., and Nolan, K., eds., 1990. Animals, science, and ethics. Special supplement to the Hastings Center Report, May/June, 32 pages.

Frey, R. G., 1980. Interests and rights: the case against animals. Clarendon Press, Oxford, UK.

————, 1989. The Case against Animal Rights. In: Animal Rights and Human Obligations, eds., T. Regan and P. Singer. Prentice Hall: Englewood Cliffs, NJ. Pages 115–8.

————, 1991. Rights, Responsibility, and Animal Experimentation. Transcript of lecture at a course at the Kennedy Institute of Ethics, Georgetown University, March 24–28.

Masserman, J. H., Wechkin, S., and Terris, W., 1964. Altruistic Behavior in Rhesus Monkeys. Amer J Psychiatry 121:584–85. Wechkin, S., Masserman, J. H., and Terris, W., 1964. Shock to a Conspecific as an Aversive Stimulus. Psychonomic Science 1:47–48.

Midgley, M., 1983. Animals and why they matter. University of Georgia Press: Athens, GA.

Miller, H. B., and Williams, W. H., 1983. Ethics and Animals. The Humana Press: Clifton, NJ.

Radner, D., and Radner, M., 1989. Animal Consciousness. Prometheus Books: Buffalo, NY. Page 8.

Regan, T., 1982. All That Dwell Therein: Essays on Animal Rights and Environmental Ethics. University of California Press: Berkeley, CA.

———, 1993. *The case for animal rights.* University of California Press: Berkeley, CA. 1983.

———, 1987. *The struggle for animal rights.* International Society for Animal Rights: Clarks Summit, PA.

Rollin, B. E., 1981. *Animal Rights and Human Morality.* Prometheus Books: New York.

Sagan, C., and Druyan, A., 1992. *Shadows of Forgotten Ancestors: A Search for Who We Are.* Random House: New York. Chapters 15–19, pages 267–383.

Sapontzis, S. F., 1987. *Morals, Reason, and Animals.* Temple University Press: Philadelphia.

Singer, P., 1975. *Animal Liberation,* 1st ed., 1975; 2d ed., 1990. Random House/New York Review of Books: New York, NY .

The Price of Knowledge, TV broadcast in New York, December 12, 1974, WNET/13, quoted by Peter Singer in *Animal Liberation,* 2d ed., from a transcript supplied courtesy of WNET/13, and reported in *Hastings Center Report* 1975: 5(1):6–8.

Thorpe, W. H., 1974. *Animal Nature and Human Nature.* Anchor Press/Doubleday: Garden City, NY. Chapters 3 and 8.

White, R. J., 1971. Antivivisection: The Reluctant Hydra. *The American Scholar* 40:503–7.

———, 1988. The Facts about Animal Research. *Readers Digest.* March, pages 127–32.

———, 1990. Animal Ethics? *Hastings Center Report* November/December, page 43.

Chapter 3 Major issues

Caplan, A. L., 1990. Innovation WNET/TV Channel 13. Animals in the Middle. Transcript. Washington, D.C.

Russell, W.M.S., and Burch, R.L., 1959. *The Principles of Humane Experimental Technique.* London: Methuen. Page 64. Reprinted 1992 by the Universities Federation for Animal Welfare, 8 Hamilton Close, South Mimms, Potters Bar, Herts, UK EN6 3QD.

Federal Republic of Germany Law on Animal Protection. Issued in Bonn on August 22, 1986, effective January 1, 1987. Reprinted in *Animals and Their Legal Rights,* 1990, 4th ed. Appendix, pages 336–52. Published by the Animal Welfare Institute, Washington, D.C.

Smith, J. A., and Boyd, K. M., 1991. *Lives in the Balance: The Ethics of Using Animals in Biomedical Research.* Oxford University Press: London. Page 37 et seq.

Sprigge, T.L.S., 1985. Philosophers and Antivivisectionism. *ATLA (Alternatives to Laboratory Animals)* 13:99–106. Published by FRAME, UK.

Chapter 4 Legislation and growth of protagonists

American Medical Association, 1989. *Animal Research Action Plan.* June, page 6.

Anderson, G. C., 1990. New Laws Divide Lawmakers. *Nature* 344:96. March 8.

Animal Welfare Legislation, 1990. Includes Animal Welfare Act as amended (7 U.S.C. §§2131–2157) P.L. 99-198. Title XVII, §1756(a), December 23, 1985, 99 Stat. 1650. Available from Animal Welfare Information Center, Series #4 (Annual Report), United States Department of Agriculture, Beltsville, MD 20705.

Anonymous, 1984. Double Talk on Animals; NIH seems more ready to risk its reputation than to meet serious critics on animal care. *Nature* 309:2.

————, 1989. Animal Welfare Regulations Reissued. *The Pharmacologist* Spring, page 58.

Bayne, K., Dexter, S., and Suomi, S., 1992. A Preliminary Survey of the Incidence of Abnormal Behavior in Rhesus Monkeys (*Macaca mulatta*) Relative to Housing Condition. *Lab Animal* May. Pages 38, 40, 42, 44–47.

Blumenstyk, G., 1989. With State Legislatures as the Battleground, Scientists and College Officials Fight Animal Welfare Groups. *The Chronicle of Higher Education* 35(30):25–26.

FASEB, 1989. Animal Welfare Regulations Reissued: Will Radically Affect Every Lab Using Animals; Major Costs Seen. *FASEB Newsletter* April, page 7. Federation of American Societies of Experimental Biology, Bethesda, MD.

Fox, G. J., Cohen, B. J., and Loew, F. M., eds., 1984. *Laboratory Animal Medicine.* Academic Press: Orlando, FL. Page 9.

Giannelli, M. A., 1986. The Decline and Fall of Pound Seizure. *The Animals' Agenda.* Monroe, CT. July/August. Pages 10–13, 36.

Jamieson, S. W., 1985. Animal Research in Development of Transplantation. In: *National Symposium on Imperatives in Research Animal Use: Scientific Needs and Animal Welfare.* Page 43. NIH Publication No. 85-2746.

Jaschik, S., 1990. Agriculture Department is Backing Away from Rules Governing the Care of Research Animals. *The Chronicle of Higher Education* June 20, page A29.

Jasny, B., 1988. Open Season on USDA. *Science* 241:1755, September 30.

King, F. A., Yarbrough, C. J., Anderson, D. C., Gordon, T. P., and Gould, K. G., 1988. Primates. *Science* 240:1475–1482.

Lindsey, J. R., 1980. NSMR: Its Image, Direction and Future. *Int. J. Study Animal Problems* 1:229–33. Originally dated November 10, 1979 and circulated privately.

Melcher, J., 1991. The Mental Health of Primates. *Washington Post,* September 8. Page C5.

Myers, 1990. U.S. Eases Proposed Regulations on Care of Laboratory Animals; Researchers are Relieved, but Welfare Groups are Critical. *The Chronicle of Higher Education* September 5, pages A20 and A26.

National Association for Biomedical Research, 1989, "Total Increased Costs for 9 C.F.R. All parts all regulated entities." June 22. Handouts distributed at conference "Canine Research Environment" organized by the Scientists Center for Animal Welfare by Barbara Rich staff person for NABR, June 23, 1989.

Public Health Service Guide for the Care and Use of Laboratory Animals. NIH Publication No. 86–23, revised 1985. Also, *Public Health Service Policy on Humane Care and Use of Laboratory Animals,* revised September 1986. Available from Office for Protection from Research Risks, National Institutes of Health, 900 Rockville Pike, Building 31, Room 4B09, Bethesda, MD 20892.

Richards, R. T., and Krannich, R. S., 1991. The Ideology of the Animal Rights Movement and Activists' Attitudes Toward Wildlife. *Trans. 56th N.A. Wildl. and Nat. Res. Conf.* Pages 363–371.

Singer, P., 1975. *Animal Liberation.* 1st ed., 1975; 2nd ed., 1990. Random House/New York Review of Books: New York, NY.

Stevens, C., 1990. Laboratory Animal Welfare. In: *Animals and Their Legal Rights.* Animal Welfare Institute: Washington, D.C. Pages 66–105.

Stone, C. D., 1972. *Should Trees have Standing: Toward Legal Rights for Natural Objects.* William Kaufmann: Los Altos, CA.

U.S. Department of Agriculture, 1989. Improved Standards for Laboratory Animals proposed regulations Parts 1, 2, and 3 in accordance with the 1985 amendments to the Animal Welfare Act (P.L. 99-198). *Federal Register,* Vol. 54, No. 49, March 15, pages 10822–10954.

United States District Court for the District of Columbia. Civil Action No. 90-1872 (CRR) Filed January 8, 1992. Animal Legal Defense Fund, *et al.,* Plaintiffs, v. Edward R. Madigan, *et al.,* Defendants. Opinion of Charles R. Richey, United States District Judge.

Wayman, S., 1966. Concentration Camps for Dogs. *Life* 60(5), February 4. Pages 22–29. A photo-article with photos by Wayman and author not stated.

Chapter 5 Animal subjects and alternatives

Abee, C. R., 1989. The squirrel monkey in biomedical research. *ILAR News* 31(1):11–20.

American Medical Association, 1989. Animals in research. Council report. *JAMA* 261(24):3602–06.

Anonymous, 1985. The ethics of animal research. *Health Sciences Report.* University of Utah. Spring.

———, 1990. Researchers Take Aim. *The AV.* Published by The American Anti-Vivisection Society, Jenkintown, PA. June, page 4.

Burke, R., 1989. Presentation by Robert Burke, M.D., In: *Animal Care and Use: Policy Issues in the 1990s.* Proceedings of an NIH OPRR/OACU conference held November 16–17, 1989. Pages 75–76.

CCAC, 1991/1992. Trends in Experimental Animal Use. *Resource,* 16(1), page 7. Canadian Council on Animal Care, 100–151 Slater St., Ottawa.

Colgate Palmolive Company 1989 Report of Laboratory Research with Animals. Colgate Palmolive Company, New York. February 1990.

Frame News, 1992. Animal experiment in the Netherlands: 1990. July, page 3.

Garattini, S., and van Bekkum, D. W., 1990. *The importance of animal experimentation for safety and biomedical research.* Kluwer Academic Publishers: Dordrecht, The Netherlands.

Goodwin, F. K., 1989. Interview by FASEB. *FASEB News* 3:2456.

Katterman, L., 1984. The controversy over animals in research. *The Research News,* The University of Michigan. October–December, 20 pages.

King, F. A., Yarbrough, C. J., Anderson, D. C., Gordon, T. P., and Gould, K. G., 1988. Primates. *Science* 240:1475–82.

McArdle, J., 1988. AV Fact Finding. *The AV.* Published by the American Anti-Vivisection Society. October, pages 14–15.

Miller, N. E., 1983. Understanding the use of animals in behavioral research: some central issues. *Ann. NY Acad. Sci.* 406:113–18.

Modeling in biomedical research: an assessment of current and potential approaches, 1989. Abstracts of meeting held May 1–3. Sponsored by the NIH, Bethesda, MD.

Morell, V., 1990. Gerontology research comes of age. *Science* 250:622–4.

NAS Report, 1988. *Use of laboratory animals in biomedical and behavioral research.* National Research Council, National Academy of Sciences, Washington, D.C. Pages 27–37.

NIH Guide for Grants and Contracts, 1987. Ongoing Program Announcements: Research into methods of research that do not use vertebrate animals, use fewer vertebrate animals, or produce less pain and distress in animal used in research. Vol. 16, No. 1, January 9, pages 6–7.

Roberts, L., 1990. The worm project. *Science* 248:1310–13.

Ryder, R. D., 1989. *Animal revolution.* Basil Blackwell: London. Page 251.

Sample, S., 1985. The ethics of animal research. *Health Sciences Report,* University of Utah. Spring, 40 pages.

Sharpe, R., 1988. *The Cruel Deception: the Use of Animals in Medical Research.* Thorsons Publishers Ltd.: Wellingborough, Northamptonshire, UK.

Spinelli, J. S., 1983. The use of laboratory animals. *California Veterinarian* 37(1):76–78, 102.

Statistics of Scientific Procedures on Living Animals: Great Britain, 1990. Home Office, London.

The Dr. Hadwen Trust for Humane Research, 1991. *Policy and conditions of support for research.* Leaflet distributed by the Trust, Hitchin, Herts, England.

U.S. Congress, Office of Technology Assessment, Alternatives to Animal Use in Research, Testing, and Education. Washington, DC: U.S. Government Printing Office, OTA-BA-273, February 1986.

Welsh, H. J., 1990. *Animal testing and consumer products.* Investigator Responsibility Research Center: Washington, D.C., 167 pages.

Zbinden, G., 1990a. Alternative methods, the present and future. *Therapie* 45(4):347–50. In French.

———, 1990b. In vitro methods, past successes and future challenges. *Acta Physiol. Scand.* 140: Supplement 592:9–12.

Zutphen, L.F.M., Rozemond, H., and Beynen, A. C., eds., 1989. *Animal Experimentation: Legislation and Education.* Pages 55, 69, and 70. Veterinary Health Inspectorate, P.O. Box 5406, 2280 HK Rijswijk, The Netherlands.

Chapter 6 Protocol review

American Psychological Association, 1985. *Guidelines for Ethical Conduct in the Care and Use of Animals.* Washington, D.C., page 6.

Australian code of practice for the care and use of animals for scientific purposes, 1990. Australian Government Publishing Service, GPO Box 84, Canberra ACT 2601. This code is not federal law, but compliance is a condition for receipt of all federal funds. This code is law only in New South Wales, where it has been incorporated under regulations as part of the Animal Research Act (1985). In Victoria, compliance with the code is mandated in their regulations but a person cannot be prosecuted for noncompliance. In South Australia, compliance with the code is a condition of licensing but it has no legal status. An authoritative source says that it is likely that in the future compliance with the code will become a legal requirement for all states and the commonwealth. Pages 30 and 27.

Canadian Council on Animal Care, 1980. *Guide to the Care and Use of Experimental Animals,* Volume I. Ottawa, Ontario, page 44.

Dresser, R., 1989. Developing Standards in Animal Research Review. *Am. J. Vet. Med. Assoc.* 194(9):1184–91.

———, 1990. Review standards for animal research: a closer look. *ILAR News* 32(4):2–7, Fall.

Institutional Animal Care and Use Committee Guidebook, 1992. Jointly produced by the Office for Protection from Research Risks, NIH, and Applied Research Ethics

National Association (ARENA). Pages B-B-1, 8. Copies available from National Institutes of Health, Office for Protection from Research Risks, Division of Animal Welfare, Building 31, Room 5B59, Bethesda, MD 20892.

Institutional Animal Care and Use Committee Guidebook, 1992. *op cit.* Section B-2-9, page 34.

Kallman, R. F., J. M. Brown, J. Denekamp, R. P. Hill, J. Kummermehr, K. R. Trott, 1985. The use of rodent tumors in experimental cancer therapy: conclusions and recommendations from an international workshop. *Cancer Research* 45:6541–45.

Krauss, R., 1984. Letter dated July 11 to Carol Young, NIH, reprinted in *FASEB Newsletter* 17(5):5: August. Federation of American Societies of Experimental Biology: Bethesda, MD.

National Institutes of Health Guide for Grants and Contracts, 1984. Special Edition Volume 13(5): pages 4, 10.

Orlans, F. B., 1987. Scientists' attitudes toward animal care and use committees. In: Effective Animal Care and Use Committees. Eds. F. B. Orlans, R. C. Simmonds, and W. J. Dodds. *Laboratory Animal Science,* January, pages 162–66.

PAWS, 1988. *News.* Issue 9, page 24. Progressive Animal Welfare Society: Lynnwood, WA.

Public Health Service Policy on Humane Care and Use of Laboratory Animals. Revised September 1986. Pages 6–7. National Institutes of Health, Bethesda, MD.

Report of the Animal Procedures Committee for 1990. Presented to Parliament by the Secretary of State for the Home Department by Command of Her Majesty. London: Her Majesty's Stationary Office CM1646, page 3.

Traystman, R. J., 1987. Who Needs It? Investigator's viewpoint. In: Orlans, F. B., Simmonds, R. C., Dodds, W. J., eds. Effective Animal Care and Use Committees. *Laboratory Animal Science.* Special Issue January 37:108–10.

University of California, San Francisco, 1984. UCSF policy on restraint of non-human primates. September 11.

Williams, J. F., 1987. Investigator Concerns. In: Orlans, F. B., Simmonds, R. C., and Dodds, W. J., eds. Effective Animal Care and Use Committees. *Laboratory Animal Science.* Special Issue January 37:113–14.

Chapter 7 Community members on animal review committees

Animal Welfare Institute, 1987. *A bibliography for the use of non-affiliated members of animal care and use committee.* Available from AWI, P.O. Box 3650, Washington, D.C. 20007.

Australian code of practice for the care and use of animals for scientific purposes, 1985 and revised 1990. Australian Government Publishing Service, GPO Box 84, Canberra ACT 2601. Page 11.

Blue Ribbon Committee Report on the Care and Use of Laboratory Animals in Cambridge, MA, 1989. Submitted to the Mayor and City Council by Steven M. Wise, J.D., John Moses, M.D., and Stuart E. Wiles, V.M.D. February 24.

Brobeck, J. R., Reynolds, O. E., and Appel, T. A., eds., 1987. *History of the American Physiological Society: The First Century,* 1857–1987. The American Physiological Society: Bethesda, MD. Page 402.

Canadian Federation of Humane Societies, 1985. *Guidelines for lay members of animal care committees.* Available from CFHS, 30 Concourse Gate, Suite 102, Nepean, Ontario K2E 7V7, Canada.

City of Cambridge, MA, 1989. Ordinance number 1085, final publication number 2453. Article IV, Ordinance for the care and use of laboratory animals in the city of Cambridge.

Hutchinson, J., 1985. Researchers and Animal Protectionists: Creating a New Partnership. *Lab Animal*. September, pages 37–9.

———, 1988. Thoughts on educating community members of animal care and use committees. In: *Science and Animals: Addressing contemporary issues*. H. N. Guttman, ed. SCAW conference proceedings, June 22–25.

Mench, J. A., and Stricklin, W. R., 1991. Institutional Animal Care and Use Committees: Who Should Serve? *ILAR News* 33(1–2):31–7. National Academy of Sciences: Washington, D.C.

Peck, J. D., 1987. Reflections of a public member. In: Orlans, F. B., Simmonds, R. C., Dodds, W. J., eds. Effective Animal Care and Use Committees. *Laboratory Animal Science*. Special Issue January 37:85–87.

Public Health Service Guide for the Care and Use of Laboratory Animals, NIH Publication No. 86-23, Revised 1985. Page 82, Principle II. National Institutes of Health, Bethesda, MD.

Roy, S., 1990. Army Drafts Stolen Dogs for Bone-Breaking Experiments. *PCRM Update*, pages 1–4. Physicians Committee for Responsible Medicine, Washington, D.C. July–August.

United Action for Animals, Inc., 1984. Mid-year 1984 report. Page 1. New York, NY.

United States Department of Agriculture, 1989. *Reference material for non-affiliated members of animal care and use committees*. Available from: Animal Welfare Information Center, National Agricultural Library, USDA, Beltsville, MD 20705.

University of Southern California, 1991. *Policies Governing the Use of Live Vertebrate Animals*. Revised July 1.

Wiemer, U., 1989. *Animal Experimentation: Legislation and Education*, edited by L.F.M. van Zutphen, H. Rozemond, and A. C. Beynen, Veterinary Public Health Inspectorate, Rijswik/Department of Laboratory Animal Science, Utrecht.

Wisconsin Regional Primate Research Center Policy Statement on Principles for the Ethical Use of Animals, 1982. *American Journal of Primatology* 3:345–47.

Chapter 8 Animal harm scales in public policy

American Psychological Association, 1985. *Guidelines for ethical conduct in the care and use of animals*. Washington, D.C. Page 6.

American Veterinary Medical Association, 1987. Panel report on the colloquium on the recognition and alleviation of animal pain and distress. *JAVMA* 191:1186–91.

Anderson, W., 1990. Australian Code of Practice for the Care and Use of Animals for Scientific Purposes. *ACCART News* 3(2):1–5. Canberra.

Animal Procedures Committee Report, 1988 and 1990. Home Office, London, UK.

Bateson, P., 1986. When to Experiment on Animals. *New Scientist* 109:30–32, February 20.

Balls, M., 1988. The weighing of benefit and suffering. *FRAME News*, 20:1–2. Nottingham, U.K.

Brenchley, J. E., Halvorson, H. O., and Wodzinski, R. J., 1987. Letter from the president and officers of the American Society for Microbiology on behalf of the Society dated June 30 addressed to Dr. R. L. Crawford, Animal and Plant Health Inspection Service, USDA Re: Docket No. 84-027, Animal Welfare, Definition of Terms (9 C.F.R. Part 1) and Docket No. 84-010 Animal Welfare Regulations (9 C.F.R. Part 2).

Canadian Council on Animal Care, 1989a. *Categories of invasiveness in animal experiments*. First adopted 1987, revised October, 1989. Ottawa, Canada.

————, 1989b. *Ethics of Animal Investigation*. Revised October. Ottawa, Canada. Similar wording to that quoted dates back to other CCAC material of 1980.

————, 1990. *CCAC Guidelines on Acceptable Immunological Procedures*. Revised February 19. Ottawa, Canada.

Dresser, R., 1989. Developing standards in animal research review. *JAVMA* 194(9):1181–91.

————, 1990. Review standards for animal research: a closer look. *ILAR News* 32(4):2–7.

Federal Register, 1987. Department of Agriculture, Animal and Plant Health Inspection Service. 9 CFR Parts 1 and 2, Animal Welfare: Proposed Rules, March 31, pages 10292–322. (pages 10313–14 for pain scale part).

Loesser, J. D., 1987. Letter from the president of the American Pain Society on behalf of the Society dated May 28 addressed to Dr. R. L. Crawford, Animal and Plant Health Inspection Service, USDA Re: Docket No. 84-027, Animal Welfare, Definition of Terms (9 C.F.R. Part 1) and Docket No. 84-010 Animal Welfare Regulations (9 C.F.R. Part 2).

National Health and Medical Research Council, 1991. Categories of experiments designated by NHMRC. *Animal Experimentation Ethics Committee Newsletter* No. 5. November, page 13. Medical Research Committee, GPO Box 9848, Canberra ACT 2601, Australia.

New York Academy of Sciences, 1988. Ad Hoc Committee on Animal Research. *Interdisciplinary principles and guidelines for the use of animals in research, testing, and education*. New York, NY.

New Zealand, 1988. *Guidelines for institutional animal ethics committees*. National Animal Ethics Advisory Committee, September. Pages 31–35.

Öbrink, K. J., 1982. Swedish law on laboratory animals. In: *Scientific Perspectives on Animal Welfare*, W. J. Dodds and F. B. Orlans, eds. Pages 55–58. New York, NY: Academic Press.

Orlans, F. B., 1980. Animal welfare. *Bioscience* 39(3):144–5.

————, 1987. Research protocol review for animal welfare. *Investigative Radiology* 22:253–8.

Porter, D., 1992. Ethical Scores for Animal Procedures. *Nature* 356:101–102. March 12.

Public Health Service Policy on Humane Care and Use of Laboratory Animals. Revised September 1986. Principle V, page 82. National Institutes of Health, Bethesda, MD.

Shapiro, K. J., 1987. A new scale of invasiveness in animal experimentation. *PsyETA Bulletin* 7(1):5–8. Published by Psychologists for the Ethical Treatment of Animals, New Gloucester, ME.

Smith, J. A., and Boyd, K., 1991. *Lives in the Balance: The Ethics of Using Animals in Biomedical Research*. Oxford University Press: Oxford. Pages 138–47.

Smyth, D. H., 1978. *Alternatives to Animal Experiments*. London: Scolar Press. Pages 144–5.

Spinelli, J. S., 1983. Testimony pertaining to the revision of the Guide for the Care and Use of Laboratory Animals, National Research Council, Institute of Laboratory Animal Resources, July 11.

Statistics of Scientific Procedures on Living Animals, Great Britain. Produced annually from 1974 to present by the Government Statistical Service, Her Majesty's Stationery Office, London, UK.

Chapter 9 Pain, suffering, and death

Alumets, J., Kåkanson, R., Sundler, F., and Thorell, J., 1979. Neuronal localization of immunoreactive enkephalin and β-endorphin in the earthworm. *Nature* 279:805.

American Veterinary Medical Association, 1987. Panel report on the colloquium on the recognition and alleviation of animal pain and distress. *JAVMA* 191:1186–91.

Anand, K.J.S., and Hickey, P. R., 1987. Pain and its effects in the human neonate and fetus. *NEJM* 317(21):1321–9.

Anderson, W., 1990. Australian Code of Practice for the Care and Use of Animals for Scientific Purposes. *ACCART News*, 3(2):1–5. Winter. Australian Council for the Care of Animals in Research and Teaching. Canberra, Australia.

Anonymous, 1987. Pain, anaesthesia, and babies. *The Lancet* 8558:543–4.

Arena, P. C., and Richardson, K. C., 1990. The relief of pain in cold-blooded vertebrates. *ACCART News*. 3(1):1–4. Australian Council for the Care of Animals in Research and Teaching.

Australian code of practice for the care and use of animals for scientific purposes, 1985, revised 1990. Australian Goverment Publishing Service, GPO Box 84, Canberra ACT 2601.

Barclay, R. J., Herbert, W. J., and Poole, T. B., 1988. *The disturbance index: a behavioural method of assessing the severity of common laboratory procedures on rodents.* Universities Federation for Animal Welfare: Potters Bar, Herts., England.

Beecher, H., 1959. *Measurement of subjective responses.* Oxford University Press: New York.

Berry, F. A., and Gregory, G. A., 1987. Do premature infants require anesthesia for surgery? *Anesthesiology* 67:291–3.

Beynen, A. C., Baumans, V., Bertens, A.P.M.G., Havenaar, R., Hesp, A.P.M., and Van Zutphen, L.F.M., 1987. Assessment of discomfort in gallstone-bearing mice. *Laboratory Animals* 21:35–42.

Broom, D. M., 1986. Indicators of poor welfare. *British Veterinary Journal* 142(6):524–6.

Bustad, L. K., 1987. Investigators' interrelationship with laboratory animals. In: Effective Animal Care and Use Committees. F. B. Orlans, R. C. Simmonds, and W. J. Dodds, eds. *Laboratory Animal Science.* Special Issue January 36:167–70.

Canadian Council on Animal Care, 1972. *Guiding Principles for Animal Experimentation at the Pre-University Level.* Ottawa, Ontario.

———, 1975. *Regulations for Animal Experimentation in Science Fairs.* Accepted by Regional Representatives, Canada-Wide Science Fair, May 23. Ottawa, Ontario.

Carter, L., 1979. NEI votes to protect cold-blooded animals. *Science* 206:1383.

Committee Report on Pain and Distress in Laboratory Animals, 1991. *ILAR News* 33(4):71–74. Committee convened by the National Research Council, National Academy of Sciences, Washington, D.C.

Cooper, J. E., Ewbank, R., Platt, C., and Warwick, C.. 1986. Euthanasia of reptiles and amphibians. *Vet. Rec.* 119:484.

Dawkins, M. S., 1980a. *Animal Suffering: The Science of Animal Welfare.* Chapman and Hall in association with Methuen: New York.

———, 1980b. The many faces of animal suffering. *New Scientist,* 20 November, 502–3.

Dennis, S. G., and Melzack, R., 1983. Perspectives on phylogenetic evolution of pain expression. In: *Animal Pain: Perception and Alleviation.* R. L. Kitchell and H. H. Erickson, eds. American Physiological Society: Bethesda, MD. Pages 151–60.

Dworkin, S. F., and Chen, A.C.N., 1983. As reported in *The NIH Record,* October 25, page 11.

Eisenmann, C. H., Jorgensen, W. K., Merritt, D. J., Rice, M. J., Cribb, B. W., Webb, P. D., and Zalucki, M. P., 1984. Do insects feel pain?—a biological view. *Experientia* 40:164–7.

European Council Directive of 24 November, 1986, on the approximation of laws, regulations and administrative provisions of the Member States regarding the protection of animals used for experimental and other scientific purposes. 86/609/EEC. *Official Journal of the European Communities* L358. 18 December, 1986.

Euthanasia of Amphibians and Reptiles, 1989. Report of a joint working party of the Universities Federation for Animal Welfare and the World Society for the Protection of Animals. Available from WSPCA, Western Hemisphere Office, 29 Perkins St., P.O. Box 190, Boston, MA 02130.

Field Research Guidelines, 1987 and 1988. (1) American Ornithologists' Union. Report of Committee on Use of Wild Birds in Research. *Auk* 105(1, Supplement):1A–41A:1988. (2) Acceptable Field Methods in Mammalogy: Preliminary Guidelines Approved by the American Society of Mammalogists. *Journal of Mammalogy,* Supplement to Volume 68(4):November 1987, 1–18. (3) Guidelines for Use of Fishes in Field Research. American Society of Ichthyologists and Herpetologists, American Fisheries Society, and the American Institute of Fisheries Research Biologists. *Copeia* Supplement, 1–27:1987. (4) Guidelines for Use of Live Amphibians and Reptiles in Field Research. American Society of Ichthyologists and Herpetologists, The Herpetologists' League, and the Society for the Study of Amphibians and Reptiles. *Journal of Herpetology,* Supplement 4:1–14:1987. For a discussion of these policies, see Orlans, F. B., 1988, ed. *Field research guidelines: impact on animal care and use committees.* Scientists Center for Animal Welfare: Bethesda, MD.

Fiorito, G., 1986. Is there pain in invertebrates? *Behavioural Processes* 12:383–8.

Flecknell, P. A., 1985–86. Recognition and Alleviation of Pain in Animals. In: M. W. Fox and L. D. Mickey eds. *Advances in Animal Welfare Science.* The Humane Society of the United States, Washington, D.C. Pages 61–77.

Fletcher, A. B., 1987. Pain in the neonate. Editorial. *NEJM* 317(21):1347–8.

Gilly, W. F., 1991. Review of book, *Squid as Experimental Animals,* D. L. Gilbert, W. J. Adelman, Jr., and J. M. Arnold, eds. Plenum: New York, 1990. *Science* 251:98.

Goodall, J., 1987. A plea for the chimps. *New York Times Magazine,* May 17. Pages 108, 109, 110, 118, 120.

Gray, J. A., 1982. *The neuropsychology of anxiety.* Oxford University Press: New York. Page 17.

Griffin, D. R., 1976. *The Question of Animal Awareness.* The Rockefeller University Press: New York.

———, 1978. Prospects for a cognitive ethology. *The Behavioral and Brain Sciences* 1:289.

Guide for the Care and Use of Agricultural Animals in Agricultural Research and Teaching, 1988, 1st edition. Consortium Executive Committee, Agricultural Animal Care Guide, Division of Agriculture, National Association of State Universities and Land-Grant Colleges, Washington, D.C. 74 pages.

Harlow, H. F., and Novack, M. H., 1973. Psychopathological perspective. *Persp. Biol. Med.* 16:461–178.

Home Office, 1986. Animals (Scientific Procedures) Act. London, UK.

Hughes, J., 1975. Isolation of an endogenous compound from the brain with pharmacological properties similar to morphine. *Brain Res.* 88:295–308.

Institute of Laboratory Animal Resources, 1989. *Principles and guidelines for the use of animals in precollege education.* National Academy of Sciences: Washington, D.C.

Jones, L. M., 1965. AVMA statement on proposed laboratory legislation. Testimony filed 'with the Subcommittee on Health and Safety, Committee on Interstate and Foreign Commerce, House of Representatives, 89th Congress, October 1.

Kavaliers, M., Hirst, M., and Teskey, G. C., 1983. A functional role for an opiate system in snail thermal behavior. *Science* 220:99–101.

Koehler, O., 1951. The ability of birds to "count." *Bulletin on Animal Behaviour* 9:41.

Laboratory Animal Science Association, 1990. Report of the Working Party on the assessment and control of the severity of scientific procedures on laboratory animals. *Laboratory Animals* 24:97–130.

Levine, J. D., and Gordon, N. C., 1982. Pain in prelingual children and its evaluation by pain-induced vocalization. Review article. *Pain* 14:85–93.

Lockwood, J. A., 1987. The moral standing of insects and the ethics of extinction. *Florida Entomologist* 70(1):70–89.

————, 1988. Not to harm a fly: our ethical obligations to insects. *Between the Species,* Summer issue, 204–11. P.O. Box 254, Berkeley, CA 94701.

Manser, C. E., 1992. *The Assessment of Stress in Laboratory Animals.* Royal Society for the Protection from Cruelty to Animals, Causeway, Horsham, West Sussex RH12 1HG, England.

Morton, D. B., and Griffiths, P.H.M., 1985. Guidelines on the recognition of pain, distress and discomfort in experimental animals and an hypothesis for assessment. *Veterinary Record* 116:431–6.

Morton, D. B., 1990. Adverse effects in animals and their relevance to refining scientific procedures. *ATLA* 18:29–39.

National Advisory Eye Council Policy Statement. *Procedures to Assure Freedom from Pain in Experiments upon Cold-Blooded Vertebrates,* December 1979. 3 pages. National Eye Institute, National Institutes of Health, Bethesda, MD.

Nielsen, M., Braestrup, C., and Squires, R. F., 1978. Evidence for a late evolutionary appearance of brain-specific benzodiazepine receptors: an investigation of 18 vertebrate and 5 invertebrate species. *Brain Res.* 141:342–6.

Orlans, F. B., 1977. *Animal care from protozoa to small mammals.* Addison-Wesley: Menlo Park, CA.

Public Health Service Policy on Humane Care and Use of Laboratory Animals. Revised September 1986. Principle IV, page 82. National Institutes of Health, Bethesda, MD.

Public Health Service Responds to Commonly Asked Questions, 1991. Report prepared by the staff of the Division of Animal Welfare, Office for Protection from Research Risks, NIH. *ILAR News* 33(4):68–70. Published by the National Academy of Sciences.

Rollin, B. E., 1981. *Animal Rights and Human Morality.* Prometheus Books: Buffalo, NY. Page 33.

Rose, M., and Adams, D., 1989. Evidence for pain and suffering in other animals. In: *Animal experimentation; the consensus changes.* G. Langley, ed. Macmillan Press: London, UK. Pages 42–71.

Rowan, A. N., 1984. *Of Mice, Models, and Men: A Critical Evaluation of Animal Research.* SUNY Press: Albany, NY. Page 83.

Royal Society for the Prevention of Cruelty to Animals, 1980. Report of the panel of enquiry into shooting and angling. Pages 7–10. RSPCA, Horsham, UK.

Schmidt, R. H., and Bruner, J. G., 1981. A professional attitude toward humaneness. *Wildl. Soc. Bull.* 9:289–91.

Spencer-Booth, Y., and Hinde, R. A., 1971. Effects of six-days separation from mother on 18–32 week old rhesus monkeys. *Anim. Behav.* 19:174–91.

Stephens, M. L., 1986. *Maternal deprivation experiments in psychology: a critique of animal models.* The American Anti-Vivisection Society: Jenkintown, PA.

Universities Federation for Animal Welfare and World Society for Protection of Animals, 1989. *Euthanasia of Amphibians and Reptiles.* Report of joint UFAW/WSPA working party. UFAW, Potters Bar, Herts., UK.

Verheijen, F. J., and Buwalda, R.J.A., 1988. *Doen pijn en angst een gehaakte en gedrilde karper lijden? (Do pain and fear make a hooked carp in play suffer?)* Publication of the University of Utrecht. English summary, pages 35–37. Obtainable from Dutch SPCA, P.O. Box 85980, 2508 CR, The Hague, The Netherlands.

Wallace, J., Sanford, J., Smith, M. W., and Spencer, K. V., 1990. The assessment and control of the severity of scientific procedures on laboratory animals. *Laboratory Animals* 24(2):97–130.

Watkins, V., 1990. *Frogs' legs Trade—India.* A report of the World Society for the Protection of Animals, Boston, MA.

Wigglesworth, V. B., 1980. Do insects feel pain? *Antenna* 4:8–9.

Zimmermann, M., 1980. International Association for the Study of Pain ethical standards for investigation of experimental pain in animals. Guest editorial by the IASP Committee for Research and Ethical Issues. *Pain* 9:141–43.

Chapter 10 Testing

Boxer, B., 1991. A "Dear Colleague" letter distributed from Congresswoman Boxer's office, dated November 26, about the Consumer Products Safe Testing Act of 1991, H.R. 3918, which she introduced in the 101st Congress.

Foundation for Biomedical Research, 1988. *The use of animals in product safety testing.* August. Washington, D.C.

Gettings, S. D., and McEwen, G. N., 1990. Development of potential alternatives to the Draize eye test: the CTFA evaluation of alternatives program. ATLA 17:317–24.

Griffith, J. F., Nixon, G. A., Bruce, R. D., Reer, P. J., and Bannan, E. A., 1980. Dose-response studies with chemical irritants in the albino rabbit eye as a basis for selecting optimum testing conditions for predicting hazard to the human eye. *Toxicology and Applied Pharmacology* 55(3):501–13.

Holden, C., 1988. Much work but slow going on alternatives to Draize test. *Science* 242:185–86.

Hunter, W. J., Lingk, W., Recht P. (undated). An intercomparison study conducted by the Commission of the European Communities on the determination of the single administration toxicity in rats. Communicated by the Health and Safety Directorate. Commission of the European Communities (unpublished data).

Kessler, D. A., 1991. Letter to The Honorable Bill Lockyer, Chair, Senate Judiciary Committee, California State Capital. April 18.

Lydenberg, S., 1987. *Rating America's corporate conscience.* Council on Economic Priorities, 30 Irving Place, New York, NY 10003.

Rowan, A. N., 1984. *Of Mice, Models, and Men: A Critical Evaluation of Animal Research.* SUNY Press. Albany, NY. Page 223.

Rowan, A. N. ed., 1991. *The Alternatives Report: Replacement, Reduction and Refine-*

ment in *Animal Research, Teaching, and Testing* 3(5–6):1–11. R. Scala's remarks on page 11.

Smyth, D. H., 1978. *Alternatives to Animal Experiments.* Scolar Press: London.

van den Heuvel, M. J., D. G. Clark, R. J. Fielder, P. P. Koundakjian, G. J. Oliver, D. Pelling, N. J. Tomlinson and A. P. Walker, 1990. The International Validation of a Fixed-Dose Procedure as an Alternative to the Classical LD50 Test. *Food Chem. Toxicol.* 28(7):469–82.

Welsh, H. J., 1990. *Animal testing and consumer products.* Investor Responsibility Research Center Inc., 1755 Massachusetts Ave., NW, Washington, D.C. 20036.

Zbinden, G., 1973. *Progress in toxicology: special topics.* New York: Springer-Verlag, page 23.

Zbinden, G., and Flury-Roversi, M., 1981. Significance of the LD50 test for the toxicological evaluation of chemical substances. *Arch. Toxicol.* 47:77–99.

Chapter 11 From sunshine laws and civil disobedience to raids

Animal Rights Direct Action Group, undated. *"Nonviolent Agreement for this action . . ."* Animal Rights Action Group, San Francisco, California.

Anonymous, 1984. Washington Report. *AALAS Bulletin* 24(1):8–9, 12.

———, 1985. Baboons Win Reprieve: Protests Pay Off. *The Animals' Agenda,* September, pages 1, 8–11.

———, 1990. Misguided Fanatics. *International Animal Action,* number 25, page 4, Autumn. Bulletin of the International Association Against Painful Experiments on Animals. St. Albans, England.

Brebner, S., and Baer, D., undated. "Becoming an Activist," PETA's Guide to Animal Rights Organizing. Published by People for the Ethical Treatment of Animals, Washington, D.C.

Fox, J. L., 1984. Lab Break-In Stirs Animal Welfare Debate. *Science* 224:1319–20.

Gennarelli, T. A., and Langfitt, T. W., 1985. Response of Drs. Gennarelli and Langfitt. *Almanac,* page 3. September 24. Published by University of Pennsylvania.

Hardin, P., 1988. Remarks to Faculty Council. University of North Carolina, Chapel Hill. November 18.

Henshaw, D., 1989. *Animal Warfare: The Story of the Animal Liberation Front.* Fontana/Collins: London, UK. Page 91.

Holden, C., 1990. Damage to Animal Research Mounts. *Science* 248:1308. June 15.

Hoyt, J. A., and Stephens, M. L., 1990. Animal Rights and Violence. *Science* 249:1358.

Jackson, C. M., 1989. The Fiery Fight for Animal Rights. *Hastings Center Report* 19(6):37–39.

Katz, E., 1992. "Waste, Mismanagement and Animal Abuse in Department of Defense Research Programs." Testimony given by the president of In Defense of Animals presented to the Research and Development Subcommittee of the U.S. House of Representatives Armed Services Committee, April 7.

Kilpatrick, J. J., 1985. Brutality and Laughter in the Lab. *Washington Post* July 23 Editorial Section, page A15.

Mangan, K. S., 1990. Universities Beef up Security at Laboratories to Protect Researchers Threatened by Animal-Rights Activists. *The Chronicle of Higher Education,* A16–A19. September 19.

Melville, M. A., 1992. Lab Break-in Pros and Cons. Letter to the Editor. *The Animals' Agenda.* June, page 3.

Miller, V., 1986. Animal Rights—Looking Ahead. *The Animals' Agenda,* January/February, page 8.

Molbegott, E., 1987. From transcript of her plenary address "Public Concerns about Animal Experiments" at an October 8–9 conference "Animal Research and Testing: Humane Frontiers" co-sponsored by the Scientists Center for Animal Welfare and The Rockefeller University and held at The Rockefeller University, New York City, New York.

Powledge, T. M., 1989. Locking up the Lab. *AAAS Observer, #*3. January 6.

Regan, T., 1987. *The Struggle for Animal Rights.* International Society for Animal Rights: Clarks Summit, PA. Pages 174–83.

Siegel, S., 1989. Grassroots Opposition to Animal Exploitation. *Hastings Center Report* 19(6):39–41.

Smith, J. A., and Boyd, K. M., 1991. *Lives in the Balance: The Ethics of Using Animals in Biomedical Research.* Oxford University Press: Oxford. Pages 148–82.

Society for Neuroscience, 1984. Report of the Ad Hoc Investigating Committee on Animals in Research. The Philadelphia Raid—The "Next Taub Case?" *Neuroscience Newsletter* 15(5):8–10.

Trankina, M., 1992. How Many Researchers are Really Happy in Their Work? *The Scientist* 6(4):11.

Wade, N., 1987. Animal Rights: NIH Cat Sex Study Brings Grief to New York Museum. *Science* 194:162–7.

Chapter 12 The use of animals in education

Barinaga, M., 1990. Where Have All the Froggies Gone? *Science* 247:1033–34.

Bentley, B., 1991. Animal Use in the Classroom. *The Quarterly Review of Biology.* 66:475–477. December.

Boddy, J., 1989. Animal Use: A Moral and Practical Dilemma. *Veterinary Practice Management* Summer/Fall, page 62. Whittle Communications, Knoxville, TN.

California Students' Rights Law, 1988, Education Code Sections 32255–32255.6, known prior to passage as Assembly Bill 2507. Copy and analysis of law available from Animal Legal Defense Fund, 1363 Lincoln Avenue, San Rafael, CA 94901.

Dunayer, E., 1990. *Alternatives to the harmful use of nonhuman animals.* Pamphlet issued by Association of Veterinarians for Animal Rights: Vacaville, CA.

Federal Register, 1989. Part IV Department of Agriculture. Animal and Plant Health Inspection Service, 9 CFR parts 1, 2, and 3. Animal Welfare; Final Rules, August 31, pages 36113–163.

Florida State Law, effective July 1, 1984. Known prior to passage as CS/HB 135, introduced by Representative Michael Friedman of Miami, and known as "The Treatment of Animals in Elementary and Secondary School Biological Experimentation."

German Law on Animal Protection, 1986. Federal Minister of Food, Agriculture and Forestry. Bundesgesetzblatt, Part 1, Bonn, 22 August. English translation by the Services of the Commission of the European Communities. Page 38.

Gibbs, E. L., Nace, G. W., and Emmons, M. B., 1971. The Live Frog is Almost Dead. *Bioscience* 21(20):1027–34.

Hairston, R. V., 1990. *The Responsible Use of Animals in Biology Classrooms Including Alternatives to Dissection.* Monograph IV. National Association of Biology Teachers, Reston, VA.

276   REFERENCES

Harbster, D. A., 1992. Use of Animals in the Classroom. Letter to Editor. *NSTA Reports*
April, pages 42 and 43. National Science Teachers Association, Washington, D.C.

Kramer, D. C., 1989. *Animals in the Classroom: Selection, Care, and Observations.*
Addison-Wesley: Menlo Park, CA.

Leib, M. J., 1985. *Dissection: A Valuable Motivational Tool or a Trauma to the High
School Student.* Master of Education dissertation thesis, a) pages 464–7, b) page
32.

Maine, 1990. Memorandum from Eve M. Bither, Commissioner of Education, Department of Educational and Cultural Services, to the Superintendents of Schools,
"Advisory Allowing Students to Refuse to do Dissection and Provisions for Alternatives to Dissection," January 30.

Massachusetts State Law, 1979. Chapter 439. "An act regulating the use of live vertebrate
for experimental or exhibitional purposes in certain schools."

Mayer, V. J., and Hinton, N. K., 1990. Animals in the Classroom. *The Science Teacher*
57(3):27–30.

Mayer, W. V., 1973. Biology: Study of the Living or the Dead? *The American Biology
Teacher* 35(1):27–30. Official publication of the National Association of Biology
Teachers.

Najarian, J. S., 1989. Presidential Address: the skill, science, and soul of the surgeon.
Annals of Surgery 210(3):257–67.

National Association of Biology Teachers, 1980. Guidelines for the Use of Live Animals
at the Pre-University Level. *The American Biology Teacher* 42(7):426.

National Association of Biology Teachers Policy Statements, 1989. Two policy statements
on animal use were issued: (a) "NABT Policy on Dissection and Vivisection."
News and Views, March/April; (b) "The Responsible Use of Animals in Biology
Classroom, Including Alternatives to Dissection—A NABT Policy Statement"
approved by NABT Board of Directors October 25. Available from NABT, 11250
Roger Bacon Blvd #19, Reston, VA 22090.

National Association of Biology Teachers, 1990. Two policy statements on animal use
were issued: (a) "NABT Guidelines for the Use of Live Animals." Revised January; (b) "The Responsible Use of Animals in the Biology Classroom: A Clarification." Approved by NABT Board November 7, 1990, *The American Biology
Teacher,* 1991:53(1):71.

National Science Teachers Association, 1980. The policy has two parts, (1) Study Living
Things (written at ninth-grade reading level), and (2) Code of Practice on Animals
in Schools (the same policy written at adult-reading level); both appear in *The
Science Teacher* 1980:47(6):58. This policy was revised in 1986 to be Code of
Practice on Use of Animals in Schools, *The Science Teacher* 53(1):172. Washing-
ton, D.C.

National Science Teachers Association, 1991. Guidelines for Responsible Use of Animals
in the Classroom. Adopted by the Board of Directors, July 1. *NSTA Reports*
December 1991/January 1992, page 6.

New South Wales, 1991. *Animals in Schools: Animal Welfare Guidelines for Teachers.*
Produced on behalf of the Schools Animals Care and Ethics Committee by the
NSW Department of School Education. Available from Sales Section, Curriculum
Resources and Marketing, Private Bag 3, Ryde, NSW 2112, Australia.

Orlans, F. B., 1977. *Animal Care from Protozoa to Small Mammals.* Addison-Wesley:
Menlo Park, CA.

————, 1985. Science Fairs—A Sampling of Misguided Experiments. *The Animal Welfare Institute Quarterly* 34(3):8–11. Fall. Washington, D.C.

————, 1988. Debating Dissection: Pros, Cons, and Alternatives. *The Science Teacher* 55(8):36–40. Official publication of the NSTA, Washington, D.C.

Pennsylvania Student Rights Option Measure, Public Law 30, number 14, 1992. Signed into law July 9 by Governor Robert P. Casey.

Physicians Committee for Responsible Medicine, undated. *Alternatives in medical education: non-animal methods.* PCRM, Washington, D.C.

Physicians Committee for Responsible Medicine, 1992. More Medical Schools Drop Animal Labs from Curriculum. *PCRM Update,* Spring. Page 2. Washington, D.C.

Public Health Service Guide for the Care and Use of Laboratory Animals, NIH Publication No. 86-23, Revised 1985. Pages 81–83.

Rowan, A. N., 1984. *Of Mice, Models, and Men: A Critical Evaluation of Animal Research.* SUNY Press. Albany, NY. Page 100.

Smith, J. A., and Boyd, K, M., eds., 1991. *Lives in the Balance: The Ethics of Using Animals in Biomedical Research.* Oxford University Press: Oxford. Page 234.

Snyder, M. D., Hinton, N. K., Cornhill, J. F., and Elfner, L. E., 1992. Animal Care Use Committees. *The Science Teacher* 59(2):28–35.

Strauss, R. T., and Kinzie, M. B., 1991. Hi-Tech Alternatives to Dissection, *The American Biology Teacher* 53(3):154–57.

Texley, J., 1987. Editor's Corner. *The Science Teacher.* December. Page 9.

United States Department of Agriculture, Animal Welfare Information Center. December 1989. *Animal-related computer simulation programs for use in education and research.* AWIC Series #1. National Agricultural Library, Beltsville, MD.

Chapter 13 The source of laboratory dogs and cats

American Humane Association, 1988, *Shoptalk,* 6(3), April/May, 1–2.

Anonymous, 1985. Some Preliminary Results. *Advocate* 3(4):14–15. The American Humane Association, Denver, CO.

Burke, R. E., 1985. The Role of Scientific Organizations in Humane Animal Research. In: *National Symposium on Imperatives in Research Animal Use: Scientific Needs and Animal Welfare.* US Department Health and Human Services, PHS, NIH. NIH Publication No. 85-2746:317–23.

DeBakey, M. E., 1987a. Are Animals More Important than People? *Buffalo News.* June 14. Reprinted from the *Washington Post.*

————, 1987b. So Where Will Researchers Get Their Dogs? *Washington Post,* July 25, A13.

Eckstein, R. A., 1987. *Use of Mongrel Dogs in Biomedical Research: An Assessment of Experimental Procedures.* Physicians Committee for Responsible Medicine: Washington, D.C. July.

Festing, M., 1977. Bad Animals Mean Bad Science. *New Scientist* 73(1035):130–31.

Foundation for Biomedical Research, 1990. *The Use of Pound/Shelter Animals in Biomedical Research and Education.* Washington, D.C. October, 9 pages.

Giannelli, M. A., 1985. Dogs and Cats by the Pound. *The Humane Society News.* Summer, 22-23.

Lederer, S. E., 1992. Political Animals: The Shaping of Biomedical Research Literature in Twentieth-Century America. *ISIS* 83:61–79.

McArdle, J., 1985. People You Should Know—John McArdle. *The Physiologist* 28(2):69–72.

Mrazek, R. J., 1987. The Least We Owe to Animals that are Sent to Shelters. *Washington Post,* June 25, A17. Mrazek herein quotes the authoritative source from NIH, Thomas L. Wolfle, the executive director of the NIH Interagency Research Animal Committee.

National Association for Biomedical Research, 1987. *Facts to Counter Assertions Made by Supporters of the Pet Protection Act of 1985 (S. 1457 and H.R. 778).* July 8, 2 pages.

Palmer, A. E., 1973. Diseases Encountered During the Conditioning of Random Source Dogs and Cats. In: *Research Animals in Medicine* ed. Lowell T. Harrison. The Proceedings of the National Conference on Research Animals in Medicine, National Heart and Lung Institute, NIH. DHEW Publication No. (NIH) 72-333. Pages 981–89.

Potkay, S., and Bacher, J. D., 1973. The Research Dog: Random Source or Colony Reared? In: *Research Animals in Medicine* ed. Lowell T. Harrison. The Proceedings of the National Conference on Research Animals in Medicine, National Heart and Lung Institute, NIH. DHEW Publication No. (NIH) 72-333. Pages 1061–65.

Potkay, S., 1989. Chief, Veterinary Resources, NIH. Personal communication, July 14. NIH intramural costs for routine maintenance of a small dog is $3.22 and for a large dog $3.86 per day. The amounts to $1095 and $1460 per year, according to size.

Rowan, A. N., 1991. *Tufts Center for Animals and Public Policy Newsletter.* 6(2), October.

Smith, S. J., and Hendee, W. R., 1988. Animals in Research. *JAMA* 259(13):2007–8.

Stevens, C., 1988. Individual Statement. In: *Use of Laboratory Animals in Biomedical and Behavioral Research.* National Research Council, National Academy Press. Washington, D.C.

White, R. J., 1988. The Facts About Animal Research. *Readers Digest* March, pages 127–32.

Wolfle, T., 1989. Director, Institute of Laboratory Animal Resources, National Academy of Sciences. Personal communication, July 11.

Zinn, R. O., 1968. The Research Dog. *Journal American Veterinary Medical Association* 153(12):1883–86.

Chapter 14 Editorial responsibilities and issues

American Medical Association *Animal Research Action Plan,* 1989, June. 15 pages. Also see article by William R. Hendee, vice president for Science and Technology at the AMA, and Jerod M. Loeb, Director of Biological Science at the AMA, in *The Chronicle of Higher Education,* May 30, 1990.

Anonymous, 1959. The care and use of animals. *Physiologist* 2(4):47.

Anonymous, 1980. Guidelines for authors. *American Journal of Veterinary Research.* Policy adopted by the American Veterinary Medical Association Council on Research in November.

———, 1986. Guidelines for the use of animals in research. *Animal Behaviour* 34:315–8.

Anonymous, 1990. Instructions to Authors. *Journal of Neuroscience* 10(1):no page number.

Barnard, N. D., and Hou, S., 1988. Inherent stress: the tough life in lab routine. *Lab Animal,* September, pages 21–27.

Barnard, N. D., 1990. Use of animals in research on panic disorder. Letter to editor. *Amer. J. Psychiatry* 147:5.

Beecher, H. K., 1966. Ethics and Clinical Research. *NEJM* 274:1354–60.

Broad, W., and Wade, N., 1982. *Betrayers of the truth: fraud and deceit in the halls of science.* Simon and Schuster, New York. Page 28.

Brobeck, J. R., Reynolds, O. E., and Appel, T. A., eds., 1987. *History of the American Physiological Society: the First Century, 1857–1987.* The American Physiological Society, Bethesda, MD. Page 392.

Bustad, L. K., 1987. Investigators' interrelationship with laboratory animals. *Laboratory Animal Science.* Special Issue January 37:167–70.

Cannon, W. B., 1914a. Report of Committee on the Protection of Medical Research. *JAMA* 63:94.

———, 1914b. Protecting medical research. *Chicago Medical Recorder* 36:359–60.

Council of Biology Editors Style Manual Committee, 1983. Writing the article. In: *CBE style manual,* 5th edition. Council of Biology Editors: Bethesda, MD. Page 22.

Dixon, B., undated. Manual for Authors. *Medical Science Research.* 8 pages.

Dodds, W. J., 1986. Animal welfare. Letter to editor. *Am. J. Vet. Res.* 47(10):2320.

———, 1987. Animal welfare considerations. Letter to editor. *Am. J. Vet. Res.* 48(6):1021.

Elston, M. A., 1992. Caught in the Crossfire of the Animal Wars. *New Scientist* 134(1822):32–35.

Goodall, J., 1990. *Through a window: my thirty years with the chimpanzees of Gombe.* Houghton Mifflin: Boston, MA. Page 15.

Hollands, C., 1989. Animal Experiments. *Nature* 339:248.

International Committee of Medical Journal Editors, 1988. Uniform requirements for manuscripts submitted to biomedical journals. *Annals of Internal Medicine* 108:258–65.

King, F. A., Yarbrough, C. J., Anderson, D. C., Gordon, T. P., and Gould, K. G., 1988. Primates. *Science* 240:1475–82.

Lederer, S. E., 1992. Political Animals: The Shaping of Biomedical Research Literature in Twentieth-Century America. *ISIS* 83:61–79.

Maddox, J., 1989. Can journals influence science? *Nature* 339:657.

Morton, D. 1992. A Fair Press for Animals. *New Scientist* 134(1816):28–30.

Nature, 1989. The original article that set off the debate is Dehay, C., Horsburgh, G., Berland, M., Killackey, H., and Kennedy, H., 1989. Maturation and connectivity of the visual cortex in monkey is altered by prenatal removal of retinal input. 337:265–7: January 19. Comments related to this article appeared in the following issues: 339:248:May 25; 339:324:June 1; 339:407:June 8; 339:414:June 8; 339:491:June 15; 340:10:July 6; 340:424:August 10; 340:672:August 31; 341:10:September 6; 341:341:September 14; 342:220:November 16.

New Scientist, 1992. A series of eighteen wide-ranging articles on the ethical issues of animal experimentation were published over a two-month period. The series was remarkable in that many articles had a definite slant toward welcoming reforms that enhance animal welfare; the authors included several persons well known for their espousal of animal welfare or animal rights positions. All are volume 134. Editorial (1815):15. Birke, L., and Mike, M., The Researchers' Dilemma (1815):25–28. Birke, L., and Mike, M., Views from Behind the Barricade

(1815):29–32. Arluke, A., Trapped in a Guilt Cage (1815):33–35. Hampson, J., The Secret World of Animal Experiments (1816):24–27. Morton, D., A Fair Press for Animals (1816):28–30. Silcock, S., Is Your Experiment Really Necessary? (1817):32–34. Wall, P., Neglected Benefits of Animal Research (1817):30–31. Bateson, P., Do Animals Feel Pain? (1818):30–33. Manser, C., Telltale Signs of a Stressful Life (1818):34–36. Balls, M., Time to Reform Toxic Tests (1819):31–33. Botham, P., and Purchase, I., Why Laboratory Rats are Here to Stay (1819):29– 30. Ward, L., Time for Talk Across the Trenches (1820):28–30. Smith, J., Dissecting Values in the Classroom (1820):31–35. MacKenzie, D., The Laboratory Rat's Guide to Europe (1821):29–31. Gavaghan, H., Animal Experiments the American Way (1821):32–36. Rogers, L. J., and Trémont, R., Australian Researchers Take on Animal Rights (1821):37. Elston, M. A., Victorian Values and Animal Rights (1822):28–31. Elston, M. A., Caught in the Crossfire of the Animal Wars (1822):32–35.

Phillips, M. I., 1986. Review Responsibilities of Scientists to Protect Animals from Pain. Transcript of presentation given at a conference "The Welfare of Laboratory Animals: Current Issues" organized by the Scientists Center for Animal Welfare and the University of Texas Houston, and held in Houston, October 16–17.

Porter, D. G., 1989. Letter to Editor. *Nature* 340:180, July 20.

Report of Editors-in-Chief, 1985. Publication of experimental animal research: ethical aspects. *The Veterinary Quarterly* 7(2):81–83.

Royal Society for the Prevention of Cruelty to Animals, 1988. *Animal Experimentation News,* November, #6, pages 2–6. Horsham, England.

Sternbach, R. A., 1976. The need for an animal model of chronic pain. *Pain* 2:2–4.

Wall, P. D., 1975. Editorial. *Pain* 1:1–2.

Wolff, S. P., and Hunt, J. V., 1990. Doing it wrong. *Nature* 348:104.

Young, J. D., Hurst, W. J., White, W. J., and Lang, C. M., 1987. An evaluation of Ampicillin pharmacokinetics and toxicity in guinea pigs. *Laboratory Animal Science* 37(5):652–56.

Zimmermann, M., 1980. International Association for the Study of Pain ethical standards for investigation of experimental pain in animals. Guest editorial by the IASP Committee for Research and Ethical Issues. *Pain* 9:141–43.

Chapter 15 Looking ahead

Baird, R. M., and Rosenbaum, S. E., eds., 1991. *Animal Experimentation: The Moral Issues.* Prometheus Books: Buffalo, NY.

Levine, C., ed., 1989. *Taking Sides: Clashing Views on Controversial Bioethical Issues,* 3d edition. The Dushkin Publishing Group: Guilford, CT.

Regan, T., and Singer, P., eds., 1976. *Animal Rights and Human Obligations,* 2d ed., 1989. Prentice-Hall: Englewood Cliffs, NJ.

Additional Readings

Dawkins, Marian Stamp, 1980. *Animal Suffering: the Science of Animal Welfare.* Chapman and Hall, New York.

This highly readable book examines how to recognize animal suffering. There are chapters on behavior, physiology, comparisons with wild animals, choice tests and analogies with ourselves, as methods for assessing suffering.

Frey, Raymond G., 1980. *Interests and Rights: The Case Against Animals.* Clarendon Press, Oxford, UK.

Frey attacks the claim that animals possess rights and that vegetarianism has a moral basis. He reaches conclusions that support animal experimentation.

Griffin, Donald R., 1984. *Animal Thinking.* Harvard University Press, Cambridge, MA.

This eminent scientist presents the evidence that animals have consciousness. This book provides a balanced view of both old and new evidence of animal thought, drawn from fields as diverse as behavioral ecology, neuroanatomy, and philosophy of mind.

Midgley, Mary, 1983. *Animals and Why they Matter.* University of Georgia Press, Athens, GA.

Midgley examines the barriers that our traditions have erected between human beings and animals. The book brings together two intellectual currents: an increased scientific understanding and public appreciation of animals, and an increasing tendency by philosophers to extend moral questions beyond the barrier of our own species.

Rachels, James, 1990. *Created from Animals: the Moral Implications of Darwinism.* Oxford University Press, New York.

Darwin's views on human origins, religion, and morality are treated here as one unified theory that requires a radical restructuring of our moral outlook. Rachels argues that Darwinism does indeed undermine the traditional idea of human dignity, but this is not a reason for rejecting Darwin's outlook. Instead, it is a reason for rejecting human dignity and replacing it with a better moral view. The book's detailed presentation of this new ethic includes its specific consequences for such matters as animal rights.

Regan, Tom, 1983. *The Case for Animal Rights.* University of California Press, Berkeley, CA.

Regan presents a scholarly, philosophical analysis of animal rights questions, examining the inherent worth of living organisms, and the criteria for assessing moral standing. Regan refutes the still current view that the animals we eat, hunt, and experiment on are, in the words of the seventeenth-century philosopher René Descartes, "thoughtless brutes."

Regan, Tom, and Singer, Peter, 1989. *Animal Rights and Human Obligations.* Second Edition. Prentice Hall, Englewood Cliffs, NJ.

This extremely useful book, edited by two leading philosophers in the animal rights movement, is essential reading for anyone interested in the ethical issues of animal experimentation. It provides a comprehensive overview of historical and contemporary writings, addressing both the nature of nunhuman animals and our duties to them. All viewpoints are represented.

Rollin, B. E., 1989. *The Unheeded Cry: Animal Consciousness, Animal Pain and Science.* Oxford University Press, New York.

Rollin believes that scientists have been cavalier about animal use, animal pain, and the moral questions they raise. He explores the damage done by this position, both morally and scientifically, arguing that the failure to take animal suffering into account distorts experimental results.

Rowan, Andrew N., 1984. *Of Mice, Models, and Men.* State University of New York Press, Albany.

Rowan's book is a readable, comprehensive treatment of all areas—empirical and conceptual—relevant to the use of animals in research. It combines a regard for the welfare of laboratory animals with a knowledgeable acceptance of the continuing need for research involving animals.

Singer, Peter, 1990. *Animal Liberation.* Second edition. New York Review of Books, New York.

Singer says, "This book is about the tyranny of human over nonhuman animals." This easily read book is the bible of the animal rights movement and is essential reading for anyone interested in these issues. The second edition has been revised to acknowledge the animal rights movement, which was nonexistent at the publication of the first edition.

Smith, J. A., and Boyd, K. M., 1991. *Lives in the Balance: The Ethics of Using Animals in Biomedical Research.* The Report of a Working Party of the Institute of Medical Ethics. Oxford University Press, Oxford.

This book, written in clear, nontechnical language, is in my view the best recent discussion of the ethical issues of animal experimentation. It sets out the facts and makes practical recommendations while leaving the readers to make up their own minds. The Working Party included scientists, officers of animal welfare organizations, physicians, veterinary surgeons, philosophers, theologians, and a lawyer.

Glossary

AAALAC	American Association for Accreditation of Laboratory Animal Care
AALAS	American Association for Laboratory Animal Science
AFAAR	American Fund for Alternatives to Animal Research
AHA	American Humane Association
ALDF	Animal Legal Defense Fund
AMA	American Medical Association
APA	American Psychological Association
APHIS	Animal Plant and Health Inspection Service
APS	The American Physiological Society
ASPCA	American Society for the Prevention of Cruelty to Animals
AVMA	American Veterinary Medical Association
AWA	Animal Welfare Act
AWI	Animal Welfare Institute
CAAT	Center for Alternatives to Animal Testing, The Johns Hopkins University
CCAC	Canadian Council on Animal Care
CTFA	The Cosmetic, Toiletry, and Fragrance Association
FASEB	Federation of American Societies for Experimental Biology
FBR	Foundation for Biomedical Research
FDA	Food and Drug Administration
FRAME	Fund for the Replacement of Animals in Medical Experiments
HSUS	The Humane Society of the United States
IACUC	Institutional Animal Care and Use Committee
IRB	Institutional Review Board
NABR	National Association for Biomedical Research
NABT	National Association of Biology Teachers
NIH	National Institutes of Health

OPRR	Office for Protection from Research Risks
PETA	People for the Ethical Treatment of Animals
PHS	Public Health Service
USDA	United States Department of Agriculture

Index